Smoke Signals

SYDNEY UNIVERSITY PRESS

Also by Simon Chapman

Over our dead bodies: Port Arthur and Australia's fight for gun control

Let sleeping dogs lie? What men should know before getting tested for prostate cancer

Removing the emperor's clothes: Australia and tobacco plain packaging

Coming in 2017: *Wind turbine syndrome: a communicated disease*

purl.library.usyd.edu.au/sup/chapman

Smoke Signals

Selected Writing

Simon Chapman

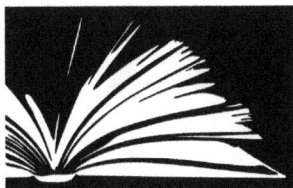

DARLINGTON PRESS

First published by Darlington Press
Darlington Press is an imprint of Sydney University Press
© Simon Chapman 2016
© Darlington Press 2016

Sydney University Press
Fisher Library F03
The University of Sydney NSW 2006
AUSTRALIA
sup.info@sydney.edu.au
sydney.edu.au/sup

National Library of Australian Cataloguing-in-Publication data

Creator:	Chapman, Simon, 1951– author.
Title:	Smoke signals : selected writing / Simon Chapman.
ISBNs:	9781921364594 (paperback) 9781921364617 (ebook: kindle)
	9781921364600 (ebook: epub) 9781921364624 (ebook: PDF)
Notes:	Includes bibliographical references.
Subjects:	Social problems.
	Public health—Moral and ethical aspects.
	Tobacco industry.
	Gun control
	Technological innovations—Health aspects.
	Essays.
Dewey number:	361.1

Cover image by Trish Kirby
Cover design by Miguel Yamin

*To Tricia, to Joe, Ali and Patrick, and my
curious grandchildren Florence and Jasper.
This is what I was doing in my study.*

Contents

Contents

Introduction

In April 2016, I was working in Christchurch for a few days. Christchurch is my idea of a very dull town so I spent hours in my hotel room, drawn to the pleasures of two essay collections I'd brought with me: Ben Goldacre's *I think you'll find it's a bit more complicated than that* (London: Fourth Estate, 2014) and Helen Garner's *Everywhere I look* (Melbourne: Text, 2016).

As I moved through these two favourite writers' selections of their very different work I wondered how my own earlier writing would read today. So I started browsing through it. I found many pieces I'd long forgotten and hoped others would have too. But there were a good few that I was pleased to have written. I began shortlisting those for what has now turned into this selection, thanks to Darlington Press.

I wrote my first academic research paper in 1976 for the *Medical Journal of Australia* (on psychotropic drug use in the elderly)[1] and in 1983, my first opinion piece for a newspaper (on tobacco advertising, published in the *Sydney Morning Herald*).[2] From the very start of my academic career, I was bewildered by the realisation that the vast majority of published research is totally inaccessible to anyone other

---

1   Chapman 1976.
2   Chapman 1983.

than other researchers and students in institutions with subscriptions to the often hugely expensive journals in which it appears. The idea of writing almost exclusively for other researchers instantly struck me as bizarre. In Australia, researchers spend sometimes months drafting and manicuring research grant applications. They then wait another eight months to hear if they were successful in getting the money (in 2015 only 17.6 percent of National Health and Medical Research Council research funding applicants were successful). They then spend three to five years doing the research, and finally waiting more months for their findings to be published in a journal that is highly likely to be pay-walled and therefore accessible only to other researchers. How crazy is it that all this effort would see only a vanishingly small number of fellow researchers ever read it, let alone that its messages and implications so seldom enter into public and political awareness?

This picture would be somewhat rational and understandable in highly technical or arcane research areas where very few outside such fields would have any hope of understanding or interest in them. But health is about all of us. It's about matters which we think about, act on, avoid, fear, enjoy and above all live with every day of our lives. As we headed toward the 2016 national election, a poll reported that health was the number one issue that voters were concerned about, with 75 percent of voters ranking it "very important", above "the economy" on 68 percent.[3]

In universities, there also remain large remnants of the attitude that scientists and researchers should refrain, in the words of one of the four foundational professors at Baltimore's Johns Hopkins Hospital, Sir William Osler (1849–1919), from "dallying with the Delilah of the press".[4] News media are frequently disdained by academics as trivialising and superficial, something from which those with ambitions of gravitas should keep well away.[5]

This results in a situation where publicly funded researchers can spend years of their lives developing specialist knowledge about health

---

3 Hudson 2016.
4 Osler 1905.
5 Chapman, Haynes, Derrick, Sturk, Hall and St George 2014.

issues but rarely bring the benefits of that knowledge to forums where individuals and policy makers might pay attention to it and use it to support change.

There is a Niagara of research demonstrating that people get a huge amount of their information and understanding of health issues from the news media. Equally, politicians and their advisors rarely if ever read scholarly papers in research journals. They form their understandings of the issues in their portfolios in a variety of ways. But like us all, they are exposed daily to information and discussion about health and medicine through the news media they consume. Work I did with colleagues in the last few years provided many insights into this.[6]

I had an instinct about the importance of all this right from the beginning of my research career and so quickly took to trying to get my research covered in the news media and giving high priority to making room in my day to provide media commentary about the areas in which I worked. And here I quickly learned that the constraints on time and space meant that something often richly nuanced and complex needed to be condensed into just two or three sentences in print media reports, or 7.2 seconds in television news.[7]

When I started making and taking opportunities to write opinion page and occasional feature articles, the access to my work and commentary on controversies in public health rapidly accelerated.

The visibility that this brought opened many doors to senior policy advisors and politicians. I also frequently had the experience of dozens of people at work telling me that they had read and enjoyed a piece I'd written in a newspaper that morning, or a prime-time breakfast radio interview as they got ready for work. Most of these colleagues worked in adjacent specialised areas of public health and would never have read my research work in journals. My own GP and other clinicians I knew often told me that patients had brought in articles of mine they'd cut out of a newspaper to ask about them. This was especially true about

---

6 Haynes, Derrick, Sally, Hall, Gillespie, Chapman and Sturk 2012; Haynes, Derrick, Chapman, Gillespie, Redman, Hall and Sturk 2011a; Haynes, Derrick, Chapman, Redman, Hall, Gillespie and Sturk 2011b.
7 Chapman, Holding, Ellerm, Heenan, Fogarty, Imison, McKenzie and McGeechan 2009.

pieces I wrote on the risks and benefits of prostate cancer screening (see Chapters 4 and 5). This feedback inspired a book on that issue in 2010.[8] We published it as a free ebook and to date it has been downloaded over 34,000 times.

Writers are often starved of information about how widely their work has been read. Journals are increasingly adding readership data to their pages. *The Conversation*, where I write a column with the same title as this book, is wonderful in that respect, automatically updating readership data ten to 12 times every hour. As of 8 September 2016, my 64 articles for *The Conversation* have been read 2,493,644 times. Just two of these (reproduced here as Chapters 62 and 63) have been read an astonishing 1,782,660 times, thanks largely to being republished in the massively read *I Fucking Love Science* blog.[9] The other 62 articles have been read 1,039 to 58,283 times (median 4,752).

By contrast, my most read research paper (by far) in my 40-year career has so far had over 147,000 readers (a paper in *Injury Prevention*, looking at the incidence of gun deaths ten years after the law reforms that followed the 1996 Port Arthur massacre).[10] Many have had just a few hundred.

Since that first piece in 1983, I've written over 310 opinion-page articles, commentaries and blogs, nearly 70 editorials for journals and 190 letters and news commentaries in research journals on top of my 260 peer-reviewed papers in journals. I wrote a column ("Focus") for the *British Medical Journal* for four years (1994–97), and one briefly for the *Weekend Australian* in 1999 ("Body Parts") until I was replaced by a writer about sex.

I've always loved writing. Early in high school I had the most English of English teachers, Bill "Spring" Lowe. He was firmly old school and wore his chalk-encrusted academic gown in the classroom. He would enter the room, go silently via his highly sprung purposeful walk (hence his nickname) straight to the blackboard, write a sentence and then command that we all parse it in silence in our exercise books. I loved parsing but I loved what he set us for homework even more.

---

8   Barratt, Stockler and Chapman 2010.
9   *I Fucking Love Science*: http://www.iflscience.com/
10   Chapman, Alpers, Agho and Jones 2006.

We had to write short essays twice a week. I imagine these were exercises in training us to write grammatically while turning our minds to the joys of creative writing. I never found these a chore, and always looked forward to settling down at the kitchen table that night to write. It's been pretty much like that ever since.

In 40 years as an academic, I took only eight months of study leave, on both occasions to finish books. I had seven months in Lyon in France in 2006 living 200 metres from the old town near the Saône River and then a perfect month at the Rockefeller Foundation's Villa Serbelloni in Bellagio on Lake Como in Italy in April 2014, where I had a writer's fellowship. During both of these I would begin writing after an early breakfast and didn't stop till about 4 pm. I had no phone to interrupt me and looked at email only once a day. Two books were finished during these retreats (*Public health advocacy and tobacco control: making smoking history,* published by Blackwell in 2007; and *Removing the emperor's clothes: tobacco plain packaging in Australia,* Sydney University Press, 2014).

The experience of these luxurious opportunities to write all day for weeks and months at a time ate away at me when I returned to the University of Sydney, where I had worked for most of my career. I loved academic work, but began to feel increasingly that the many administrative routines, teaching, and research supervision were quietly and obstinately destroying the years of writing pleasure that still remained for me.

So in October 2014, I retired from my position at the university, insofar as academics can ever "retire" (see Chapter 71) and started to write for pleasure nearly every day. In the 20 months since, I've published 56 articles and am half way through writing a book on wind-farm health anxieties as a "communicated" disease. I'm also writing a memoir of life in a country town (Bathurst) in the 1950s and 1960s – that one being just for family and close friends.

I write each day overlooking a tranquil Japanese pond we dug in our backyard 20 years ago, watching about 15 mature koi gliding among each other and getting drunk on oxygen under a rock waterfall.

In selecting the 71 pieces for this book, I passed over many that now seem uninteresting, being years away from the news on which they were commenting. These were often commissioned pieces where an editor asked for a quick commentary on a turn in events breaking that day.

I've chosen pieces which I hope best illustrate a range of issues that have been important to me across my career. Across the 40 years since my first publication I've researched and written in several main areas: tobacco control, gun control, studies of how the news media report on health matters, the practice of public health advocacy, the characteristics of influential public health research and researchers, and the fascinating field of low-risk but high-anxiety modern health panics like mobile phones, wi-fi and particularly wind turbines.

In public health, many challenges focus on trying to animate public and political concern about agents, policies and behaviours that are true threats to health and safety. But there are also a good many examples of the inverse situation as well: where we see people worried and anxious about "threats" that are of low or negligible risk. Here the task is one of trying to reduce that anxiety among the public and to derail it should it gain momentum and start adversely affecting evidence-based policies and people's lives.

I've always been deeply sceptical, and being named Australian Skeptic of the Year in 2013 was one of the most cherished awards I have received. One of my earliest sceptical awakenings was when I began questioning religion, having spent my early youth as both a chorister and an altar boy at the high-Anglican All Saints Cathedral in Bathurst. Years later I wrote about my rapid disillusionment with religion when invited by the *British Medical Journal* to describe a book that had influenced me (see Chapter 65). Bertrand Russell's *Why I am not a Christian* just leapt out when I got the invitation.

Other classics of scepticism I devoured around the same time were Arthur Koestler's *The roots of coincidence* (New York: Random House, 1972), Joachim Kahl's *The misery of Christianity* (Harmondsworth: Pelican, 1971) and George Orwell's collected essays and letters – all four volumes of them.

Public health issues provide many opportunities for a sceptical torch to uncover poorly examined assumptions, fragile but entrenched factoids, and the corrupting spell of conflicted interests all coalescing as disciplinary orthodoxy or the dominant ways that issues are talked about.

There are two large slabs of writing in the book about two topics
I've spent most of my work on: smoking (see Chapters 30–63), and
more recently, exposing the bizarre world of opposition to wind farms
(Chapters 22–26). There is a paen to the often maligned nanny state,
including 150 ways nanny is good for us all (Chapter 17) and an attempt
to imagine the dystopia that would unfold if the extremist libertarian
senator David Leyonhjelm was taken off the leash (Chapter 18) in his
selective contempt for government regulation.

My early career in tobacco control at the end of the 1970s exposed
me to daily oceans of tobacco-industry lies and duplicity as they sought
to publicly deny the health effects of tobacco, that nicotine was
addictive, and that they daily salivated over the prospects of making
smoking look as interesting and appealing as possible to children.
Privately, they of course knew very differently. I took great delight in
publicly pointing out the many contradictions and inconsistencies in
what they said in forums when they were speaking to each other. A
four-year grant from the United States National Cancer Institute to look
through (literally) millions of pages of previously internal, private and
sometimes secret tobacco industry documents was probably the most
productive phase of my academic career.

While I am often introduced as an anti-smoking "crusader", I am
considered a heretic by some in tobacco control, having spent years
challenging certain orthodoxies that some of my colleagues embrace.
Each of these is covered by essays in the book. I quickly came to
understand that the large majority of people you meet who used to
smoke quit by themselves. They didn't need any drug to help them quit
when they smoked their last cigarette. They didn't go along to a special
clinic or therapist and be walked through whatever psychological
fashion dominated at the time. In the ten years that electronic cigarettes
have been around, far more have quit without vaping (or any aid) than
quit with these methods. But you seldom hear about this.

I dropped an early, very pungent stink bomb on this issue in *The
Lancet* in 1985 (Chapter 34) and several more around 20 years later (for
example, Chapter 35) when I became fascinated by the resilience of the
dogma that it was foolish to try and quit alone when it was clear that
that was exactly how most former smokers had done it.

While I don't like tobacco smoke, what I dislike far more is the abandonment of evidence and ethical principles in the service of a goal. In tobacco control, we see that in the readiness that some have to ban smoking in wide-open outdoor spaces like parks and beaches, where there are near to zero health risks posed to others from drifting smoke (see Chapters 46–48), and the untroubled ease with which some have embraced North Korean-style censorship of films, arguing that movies should have smoking scenes removed or classified as suitable only for adult eyes (Chapters 55 and 56).

Most of the pieces in this selection were originally published as opinion-page articles in newspapers, particularly in the *Sydney Morning Herald* or, in more recent years, on websites like *The Conversation*, *Crikey* and ABC's recently axed *The Drum*.

However, I've included some that I published as short or sometimes long essays in research journals, most of which are not open access and therefore generally only available to subscribers or those who have access to them through institutional subscriptions, such as university libraries. Some of these papers are long-form essays in which I challenged prevailing dogma in public health, set out the case for a new policy (see Chapter 59) or tried to summarise emerging issues, like e-cigarettes (Chapters 60 and 61).

The selection starts with a reminder that we are all going to die: that death itself cannot be prevented and what considerations ought to follow from that in how we see the main tasks of public health. I end the book with two essays about my parents' deaths. Early pieces in the book include six on the prostate cancer screening debate, "fashionable" cancers and celebrity involvement in health causes.

When you write pieces that are sceptical or frankly critical of issues which attract impassioned supporters, there is inevitably spirited pushback from those who disagree with you. I've been a heavy Twitter user since 2009 and always promote my writing via Twitter. This frequently sees trolling by often anonymous brave souls who believe that anyone with a Twitter account should be obliged to engage with them. Like most sensible people who attract trolling, I have long instantly blocked and muted anyone who, experience tells me, has few if any interests in life other than their obsession. These include gun enthusiasts, anti-vaccination nut-jobs, electrosensitives who are convinced that they are being made ill by electro-magnetic radiation from wi-fi and wireless telephony, wind farm objectors and especially vapers, who make golf, wine and dope bores' preoccupations look utterly mild. In Chapter 67 I explain why I don't hesitate to block these (often anonymous) people.

I'm grateful to the publishers of all the pieces in the book for their permission to reprint them. In some cases, and particularly with the selections from *The Conversation*, permission was not needed as these were covered by Creative Commons agreements where authors very properly retain rights to use their own work as they see fit.

I have left each piece as it was when published, and so have not updated statistics or provided background information about facts, issues and events that may have slipped from some readers' memories. Where relevant, I have noted any important developments since original publication in the introductions to each piece.

Once again, I need to thank my editor, Agata Mrva-Montoya. This is my fourth book under her light-touch stewardship, and it's been a total delight. And thank you very much too, Stephanie Chan and Benjamin Fairclough, for your painstaking work in changing all the original hypertexted links to references.

Simon Chapman
Sydney, October 2016

1
Never say die?

For many years I gave a lecture on the first day of my school's Master of Public Health degree. I started by asking every student who was never going to die to raise their hand. We can't prevent death but we can do much to prevent early death and to make the years in which we live as disability-free as possible. We can add years to life, and life to years. I wrote this piece after receiving a phone call which inspired me to set down some thoughts about some of the core goals of public health.

An articulate 52-year-old woman recently telephoned me.

"Give the 'smoking kills' line a rest," she urged. "I've smoked for 30 years. I have emphysema. I am virtually housebound. I get exhausted walking more than a few metres. I have urinary incontinence, and because I can't move quickly to the toilet, I wet myself and smell. I can't bear the embarrassment, so I stay isolated at home. Smoking has ruined my life. You should start telling people about the living hell smoking causes while you're still alive, not just that it kills you."

Originally published as Chapman, Simon (2005). Never say die? *Medical Journal of Australia* 193: 622–3.

The call crystallised for me some diffuse unease I have long felt about some under-examined fundamentals in the entire public health enterprise. Here is how I see it.

We are all going to die. Advanced age is easily the strongest predictor of death. Nearly half of all deaths in Australia occur in a hospital.[1] These three truisms have acquired profane, almost unutterable status in contemporary healthcare debate. Each is banal in isolation, and they remain banished from polite discussion as indecent reminders of the pathos of the human dust-to-dust destiny, occasionally insisting to be heard amid the unbridled optimism of the scientific legacy. Huge energy is invested in avoiding their mention. Perhaps the most unabashed manifestation of this denial is the spamming American Academy of Anti-Aging Medicine, which boasts 11,500 members in 65 nations[2] and unblinkingly speculates about the virtues of people living to the age of 120 and possibly as long as 170.[3]

The decadence of such a first-world cosseted vision, in times when more than a billion people live on less than $1 a day and another 1–1.5 billion live on $1–$2 a day,[4] 37.8 million mostly young people are infected with HIV,[5] and 1 million people still die of malaria each year, would be remarkable were it not for the values it shares with mainstream health politics and the media-fuelled public expectations that sustain it. Today, anyone bold enough to suggest pausing to question the unrequited battle and conquest metaphors that dominate the politics of health risks being branded a medical heretic or even an apologist for involuntary euthanasia of the aged.

The dominant medical motto for our age might well be "Never say die". Recently, following on from Richard Nixon's declaration of war on cancer in 1971, the current head of the United States National Cancer Institute, Andrew von Eschenbach, caught the spirit of George Bush Junior's all-conquering zeitgeist, and challenged America to "eliminate suffering and death from cancer" by 2015.[6] In Sweden, it is government

---

1 Australian Institute of Health and Welfare 2004.
2 American Academy of Anti-Aging Medicine nd.
3 American Academy of Anti-Aging Medicine 2002.
4 United Nations Development Program 2005.
5 UNAIDS 2004.

policy to strive for a road toll of zero, not merely to have it fall.[7] If you scratch the surface of the human genome project, unstated assumptions about eternal life are not hard to find in the pitch to the often elderly biotech investors.

Single-issue health organisations often talk of research that might one day eliminate their diseases. The recent announcement of an imminent vaccine for cervical cancer[8] is self-evidently a wonderful thing. Here is a near-to-fully translated research advance that promises to end the collected misery, pain and indignity that millions of women would otherwise suffer over the years. The eradication of smallpox and the predicted departure of wild polio from the planet are astonishing achievements. So why not conquer everything else? In wealthy nations today, there are few causes of death that cannot boast a non-government agency and a research focus dedicated to eradicating the offending disease. Health agencies' mission statements are purged of anything that even hints that a point might be reached when an organisation might be content with a certain incidence of deaths from their cause. Defeat is anathema to medical progress when it comes to death.

Plainly, there is much to admire in all this. If the go-for-gold death eradication scenarios played out for each preventable cause, a huge number of young and middle-aged lives would be saved. But if no one died from cancer, was ever killed on the roads, or died from any given cause now subject to ever-onward mortality reduction targets, what would take their place? If the death toll from late-age cancer plummeted, if heart disease became something permanently able to be postponed, would this be progress? Which causes of death would increase when others declined? What would we die from?

Isolated from the wider "If not death from X, then what?" question, advances against deaths from particular diseases may be pyrrhic victories if all it means is that cause-of-death deckchairs are being shuffled on life's *Titanic*, only to sink around the same time.

---

6   Manley 2014.
7   Elvik 1999.
8   Khamsi 2005.

In at least six of the cases investigated in which patients died after being admitted to Sydney's Camden and Campbelltown hospitals in 2001, the patients were aged over 80. Several others had serious diseases likely to cause their deaths, sooner rather than later.[9] Yet an unexamined assumption in much of the outcry was that something was inherently wrong in very old or very sick people dying in hospital this month rather than in the next six.[10]

The discourses of shameful government neglect, of un-Australian inequitable health service provision in low socio-economic areas, have steamrollered the now endangered discourse of the innate decency of the "good innings". The "rule of rescue"[11] – the imperative people feel to rescue identifiable individuals facing avoidable death – similarly permeates health policy and resource allocation. Tucked deep away in the Productivity Commission's 2005 report on the economic implications of an ageing Australia[12] are examples of a very different kind from today's never-say-die epic, hinting at a lament among experienced doctors for times when if:

> pneumonia, the old man's friend, came to visit, that was regarded as quite a good outcome. That is not acceptable to the community anymore. There is a great tendency to do significant interventions in the very old . . . older people are able to undergo operations and procedures that previously were denied to them. For example, 10 years ago, 75-year-old people often were not dialysised if they had chronic renal failure, but this would be a common occurrence now.[13]

While there are ideological imperatives stoking apocalyptic visions of unsustainable ageing populations,[14] it is true that the elderly consume hugely disproportionate healthcare resources, particularly in the last years of life, when up to 40 percent of health care expenditure can

---

9   Health Care Complaints Commission (NSW) 2003, Table 5.1, 47–54.
10   Bradley 2004.
11   McKie and Richardson 2003.
12   Productivity Commission 2005.
13   Productivity Commission 2005.
14   Coory 2004.

occur.[15] If the healthcare costs for 25- to 29-year-olds are indexed at 100, those expended on 65- to 69-year-olds are 387.6, and those on 85- to 89-year-olds 614.2. Moreover, hospital separations in those aged 65 and over grew from 26 percent to 33 percent between 1991 and 2001, with the growth being only minimally explained by the growing number of aged people in the population.[16]

The director of the US Hastings Center, Daniel Callahan, has written of the deeply ingrained "pathology of hope" and its beneficiaries in the pharmaceutical, diagnostic and medical industries.[17] Together, these fuel exponential healthcare expenditure in ageing populations. Callahan's heretical proposal is that civil society should supplant medicine's present open-ended goal of prolonging life at all costs with a radical refocusing on quality of life and the compression of morbidity during a decent life span. He writes:

> The average person in good health in the developed countries of the world . . . already lives long enough to accomplish most reasonable human ends. A medical policy that could assure those now being born that they could live as long . . . and healthy lives as their parents, should be perfectly acceptable . . . This ideal of steady-state life expectancy at its present level would establish, happily, a finite and attainable goal: Enough, already.

Average life expectancy in Australia has risen from 51 for men and 57 for women at the beginning of federation, to 78 and 83, respectively, today.[18]Australia's non-Indigenous population has the world's fourth highest life expectancy after Japan, France and Switzerland. As a nation, we are near to being the healthiest in the world, with the exception of the national shame of the poor health status of our Indigenous population. Increasing longevity in the last 30 years reflects success in many areas, but particularly in preventing and treating heart disease,

---

15   Van Weel and Michels 1997.
16   Productivity Commission 2005.
17   Callahan 1998.
18   Australian Institute of Health and Welfare 2016.

declining disease caused by reduced smoking in men, and big reductions in motor vehicle and child-injury deaths.

These and other major preventable causes of death kill Australians early, often well before their retirement, still causing tens of thousands of person-years of life lost (PYLL) before age 75. Indeed, the PYLL concept enshrines the idea that years of life lost after 75 do not "count", and do not enter into national calculations of the national state of health.

A hallmark of a civilised society is valuing life at all stages, and not simply when its citizens are in the peak of their economically productive powers. The revulsion that many expressed at news of the study sponsored by Philip Morris (which advised the Czech government that early deaths of smokers each saved the country $1,227 on healthcare, pensions and housing[19]) is an index of these values. However, the corollary is not to hold the door of life open unquestioningly and indefinitely, regardless of the quality of such life or the costs of doing so.

A recent systematic review of the rate of functional decline in older people in the US has shown a significant reduction in this decline in the past three decades, suggesting some success in compressing morbidity (i.e., delaying the onset of illness) through both disease prevention and medical care.[20] However, the demographic wave of people entering old age will mean that the number of people who are disabled, dependent and living with reduced functionality through multiple chronic conditions will grow to be larger than ever before.[21] With this trend compounded by the rapidly growing obesity epidemic,[22] we seem likely to see an unprecedented prevalence of disability in ways that may not have been anticipated in previous modelling. The number of people with Alzheimer's disease in Australia (presently around 200,000) is expected to reach 580,000 by 2050.[23]

---

19   Fairclough 2001b.
20   Mor 2005.
21   Rosen and Haglund 2005.
22   Thorburn A.W 2005.
23   Access Economics 2003.

Death, and particularly early death, is typically privileged above suffering in the formulae used by health planners to set priorities. Health ministers boast about disease survival rates all going in the right direction, but spare relatively little thought about how to reduce the burden of chronic disability in the living. A reorientation that saw improvements in quality-of-life indices like chronic pain, immobility, isolation, sensory impairment and depression as being just as, if not more, important than the slavish pursuit of prolonging lives, would see a major rechannelling of research and expenditure. National audits of the morbidity arising from such quality-of-life-eroding variables deserve more attention and public policy discussion.

The medical specialties that would benefit from such a reorientation would include pain management, public health efforts dedicated to keeping people physically and mentally active, and efforts to improve the much-discussed Bhutanese-inspired concept of "gross national happiness".[24] More importantly, considerations of such qualities of life would force the health and medical enterprise to engage more with other sectors, like financial and residential planning and ergonomic design, to facilitate greater independence for the aged, rather than focusing so much on simply keeping people alive in old age. And we need to embrace "Enough already".

---

24   Revkin 2005.

2

The paradox of prevention

My clinical colleagues tell me that they often get gifts and long letters of thanks from patients and their families. But how often do we think about the public health advances that save lives without us even noticing? We don't wake up each morning and thank some nameless road safety committee for helping us not to die or be injured yesterday. In this article, I considered the unlikely prospect of a TV reality program about the heroes of prevention.

Health and medicine make good TV news and drama. Charles Sturt University's Professor Deborah Lupton found that a third of all front pages of the *Sydney Morning Herald* ran a health story and that doctors were centre stage in many of these. When not starring in fall-from-grace news sagas as radiological-scan scammers or drug-company perk dippers, doctors could fill a casting-agency catalogue with archetypes, each of whom speaks to us about fundamental issues like trust, dedication, the taming of nature and the power to heal. From the dedicated and tireless family practitioner Dr Finlay of *Dr Finlay's Casebook* (BBC TV, 1962–1971), to his sagacious and avuncular partner

Originally published as Chapman, Simon (2001). The paradox of prevention. *Good Weekend*, 12 May.

Dr Cameron. From the nightly news diet of pointy-head medical researchers announcing breakthroughs, to oracle-like pronouncements about avoiding the latest infectious disease, doctors, their healthcare citadels and technological accoutrements are ubiquitous in our lives. The death of Victor Chang in 1991 drew headlines like "A brilliant giver of life", "A man in a million", and "Patients mourn a friend and saviour", suggesting a Christ-like popular meaning for this doctor who could do all but raise the dead by transplanting that most sacred of organs, the heart. In television dramas, doctors are often portrayed as successful, benevolent and authoritative, with almost mystical power to dominate and control the lives of others and restore order and justice from chaos.

RPA, the eponymous *cinéma vérité* series set in Sydney's Royal Prince Alfred Hospital, has rated the house down since it commenced seven years ago. Last year more than 2.5 million people couldn't get enough of it every week, making it the 12th most watched program on Australian television. From the comfort of our homes we follow patients and their families as they put themselves in the healing and comforting hands of hospital staff, enduring heart- and often gut-wrenching operations. These are real people, not the buffed and scripted patients and staff of *ER*, another hospital drama that rates its socks off. They're like our parents or workmates. Like us.

The seamless blending of the ordinary with the heroic in infotainment like *RPA* reinforces notions of medicine as an almost sacrosanct activity: healing the sick and saving lives. The idea that such services could ever be cut, or that every glimmer of hope should not be pursued relentlessly, have become popular profanities. Hospital waiting lists can be used at will by a political opposition to bludgeon governments. But when it comes to saving lives and improving quality of life through health improvement on a massive scale, the contributions of hospital clinicians need to be considered against the relatively unsung contributions of prevention and public health.

Prevention can come in the form of drugs, like blood pressure controlling medication and asthma inhalers, and through screening for disease in cases like cervical, breast, bowel and skin cancers where early detection is known to make a difference to survival or to quality of life if the Big Clock has already started speeding up. It can also come in more obtuse forms, like laws to deter high-risk behaviours and public awareness and advocacy campaigns designed to alter – sometimes over timeframes lasting years – the ways we perceive health-related issues, like affirming self-worth in children, or the idea that it's irresponsible to drink and drive.

So imagine if the producers of *RPA* decided to develop a parallel series on saving lives through prevention. Immediately problems would arise about how to make it work as television. "Tune in next week to see if Betty's blood pressure is still down!" Swallowing pills or generational cultural shifts about smoking just don't have the same televisual appeal as a patient like your mum navigating a life-or-death operation. The paradox of prevention is that it succeeds when nothing happens. Few people sit up in bed at 3 am astonished at the thought they have not yet been badly injured or were born without a birth defect. It's hard to make riveting TV out of a change across 20 years on the slope of a graph showing disease incidence. While every grateful patient knows their doctor's name and hangs on every bedside word, who has any idea of those behind the epidemiological detective work that first leads to understanding of what causes disease? Or of the years of unglamorous expert committee work and community trials of ways to have people change health-related behaviours?

The first segment on the new program would be called *Trojan horses*, in which things invented for other purposes and later found to have other tricks up their sleeves get applauded. The first guest wheeled onto the set could well be not a doctor or health advocate, but the humble refrigerator. The invention and proliferation of refrigeration has had profound effects on world health. The ability to preserve food through cooling saw a rapid decline in the consumption of smoked, pickled and salted food, which was followed by huge falls in the incidence of stomach cancer in nations affluent enough to afford widespread use of domestic refrigeration. Add to this the benefits of reduced salt in a population's diet for the incidence of hypertension and stroke, and we start to see a superhero in action.

Aspirin, first synthesised from willow bark by Felix Hoffmann in Germany in 1897, was first used for pain relief and remains the leading painkiller used worldwide, with hundreds of billions swallowed year round. But in the last 30 years, its value in preventing death from heart disease has added to its extraordinary reputation. It has been repeatedly shown that aspirin substantially reduces the risk of death and non-fatal heart attacks in people who've had a previous myocardial infarct or unstable angina pectoris, which often precedes a heart attack. Moreover, a randomised controlled trial in the USA studied over 22,000 male physicians between 40 and 84 with no prior history of heart disease to see if aspirin could prevent cardiovascular deaths in healthy people. The study was stopped early and the findings shouted from the rooftops when investigators found that the group taking aspirin had a substantial reduction in the rate of fatal and non-fatal heart attacks compared with the placebo group after four and a half years.

The next regular segment would be called *Grandma was right*, where folk wisdoms eventually anointed by epidemiology get invited up on stage. First up in this segment might be Professor Cres Eastman from Westmead Hospital and South Australia's Professor Basil Hetzel, for over 20 years leading figures in a worldwide effort to reduce the incidence of iodine deficiency disorders (IDD). Onto the desk they would place a small pile of iodised salt to symbolise what 1.5 billion people who live in iodine-deficient areas can't get without help from the outside world. Iodine deficiency is by far the world's leading cause of mental retardation. Endemic mental retardation in turn causes untold other health problems downstream associated with the inability to learn, retarding entire regional health profiles. In 1990, UNICEF estimated that 750 million people were affected by goitre, 43 million had IDD brain damage and 100,000 children were born each year with iodine-deficiency cretinism. Since the launch of the 1990 program to end iodine deficiency, each year 85 million newborns have been protected from IDD. The achievements of this program have been nothing less than revolutionary.

Tasmania, for years the butt of national jokes about family sleeping patterns, is home to Professor Terry Dwyer of the Menzies Centre for Population Health Research. But for parents of newborns, Dwyer and his team have changed forever the way we think about sleep. They were among the first to show through research that babies who slept on their stomachs were at higher risk of cot death (SIDS). Along with warnings about not smoking in homes with babies, advice to parents about sleeping babies on their backs has halved the national incidence of SIDS in a decade. Their photos deserve to be on the cover of every good-parenting magazine.

Perth's Professor Fiona Stanley would then come on down for her research and advocacy in reducing neural tube defects. Each year about 80 babies in Australia are born with the birth defect spina bifida. At least 80 percent of those with spina bifida have an Arnold-Chiari malformation (where two parts of the brain, the brainstem and the cerebellum, are longer than normal and protrude down into the spinal canal) and associated hydrocephalus or fluid on the brain requiring a mechanical shunt to relieve the fluidic pressure. Other chronic problems include impaired mobility, bladder and bowel dysfunction, and curvature of the spine.

Neural tube defects can be prevented by reducing the incidence in all pregnancies, or by terminating affected pregnancies. Folate can be acquired naturally through fruits, dark-green leafy vegetables, and dried beans and peas, through folic acid fortified cereals or via folic acid vitamins. It is now well established that supplementation with folic acid plays a role in reducing by more than 70 percent the risk of neural tube defects in babies. In Australia the rate of spina bifida in live births more than halved between 1987 and 1996, from 7.1 to 3 per 10,000 births, reflecting both widespread advocacy about the importance of folate and increased in-utero investigation and terminations.

The next segment in our program, *Nanny for a day*, allows viewers into the world of those who never tire of trying to get us to stop doing dangerous things. The undisputed Australian champions here are in road safety and smoking control. Despite the ritual post-holiday weekend calls for all cars capable of travelling more than 120 kilometres per hour to be banned (and that's all of them, right?), Australia's road toll has fallen faster than that of any other nation. In 1981, 3,321 Australians were killed on the roads. Despite population growth, 18 years later this had fallen 47 percent to 1,759.

When intergalactic archaeologists one day rake over Australian soils they will find the ashtray started disappearing from public life around now, joining in antique shops the spittoon, which left restaurant tables for oblivion early last century thanks to efforts by hygienists to prevent the spread of tuberculosis. In the early 1960s, nearly 70 percent of men smoked. Today, it's down to 22 percent. Women's smoking has fallen from a high of 33 percent in the mid-1970s to be today around that of men. Adult per capita tobacco consumption fell 61 percent between 1961 and 1998. Reflecting this, male lung cancer, the leading cause of cancer death, has fallen 17 percent in the ten years from 1987 to 1997, but in the same period has risen 24 percent in women, reflecting changing smoking patterns that commenced 20 to 30 years ago.

Everyone likes to see a prodigal son return home, so a routine segment in the new series would be *Jekyll and Hyde*. Here much-maligned public health villains would be publicly rehabilitated. The motor car, vilified for decades for killing, maiming and polluting, would be demonstrated to have also saved an incalculably large number of lives and immeasurably improved the standards of living of billions. Next to be released from the public stocks would be the mobile phone. Smeared in recent years as a cancer-causing suspect, interviews with ambulance drivers, firemen and police would reveal how one in four mobile users have used them to call up 000, truncating the critical golden hour in emergency cases of profuse bleeding, head injury and heart attack. Mobile phones almost certainly save far more lives than they might claim through their as yet unproven contribution to rises in relatively uncommon cancers like brain cancer.

Finally, alcohol – and not just red wine – would be brought in from its health Siberia. The Australian Institute of Health and Welfare's latest attempt to quantify national death and hospital usage from drugs showed that the net health effect of alcohol consumption in the community is now positive in the over-65 age group: more older people have heart disease prevented by their alcohol use than their livers pickled or their bodies mangled by drunk drivers. While most attention has been on wine's health-enhancing properties, population evidence on other forms of alcohol shows that they have similar protective effects too.

3

The commodification of prevention

In 1996, government health promotion campaigns were being cut amid austerity rhetoric (so what's changed?), but "health" has long been a selling point for foods. A dubious news-media pitch for fish in asthma control made me reflect on what often gets lost when "health" becomes commodified in advertising.

In the 1980s Australian television viewers were stuffed with a diet of big-budget, government-sponsored health-promotion campaigns. Most of these have now been pared to the bone, partly because of government austerity but also because of a growing recognition that huge media coverage can be obtained without cost via "infotainment" programs, help with soap-opera scripting, and the media's appetite for health as news.

A recent study of a full year of the *Sydney Morning Herald*'s front page found that 38 percent of editions contained at least one health story. After politics, health and medical topics consistently rank highest of all news categories, and for virtually any health issue the public will nominate the news media as their main source of information.

Originally published as Chapman, Simon (1996). The commodification of prevention. *British Medical Journal* 312: 730.

So for health promoters the media present enormous opportunities. But, as one Australian group found out recently, the road to health promotion is also paved with banana skins. A recent study in the *Medical Journal of Australia* reported a significantly reduced risk of asthma among 8- to 11-year-old children who regularly ate fresh, oily fish. After controlling for most of the relevant confounders and discussing the biological plausibility of their findings, the authors concluded that consumption of oily fish "may protect against asthma in childhood".

An accompanying editorial was less sanguine, cautioning that the estimated mean intake of eicosapentaenoic acid in the subjects' diets was much less than that which would plausibly predict anti-inflammatory effects on leucocyte mediator and cytokine generation. It suggested that the oily fish was likely a proxy for some undiscovered wider dietary or social factor in fish-eating families.

About 20 percent of Australian children experience wheezing, so the story leapt to the top of every news bulletin, featuring interviews at Sydney's fish market with the first author. A "miracle food", "Grandma was right" subtext swept the critical "*may* protect" caveat from all but one bulletin. Whatever cautious note the author may have uttered wound up on cutting-room floors.

The next week *Media Watch*, ABC TV's scathing weekly review of journalistic standards, denounced the reportage as irresponsible in ignoring the editorial caveat while trumpeting the "discovery". While the study acknowledged the financial support of the fishing industry, only one bulletin mentioned this. The incident exemplified the problems central to the popular communication of research and to the question of when health promoters should be able to translate epidemiology into take-home messages about more of this, less of that. Other studies contradict the results of this one, so aficionados of evidence-based medicine would probably judge that this fish story should go back into the water for now.

But is it reasonable to expect journalists to adopt the same standards of evidence and to take a meta-analytic perspective on every report published in journals? As governments privatise more and more of their responsibilities, we may well see much of health promotion being "commodified" into messages about goods and services that have health as their main selling point. The private sector has many health-promotion selling angles – for foods and drinks, drugs, sunscreens, safety innovations for cars and houses, and exercise equipment – that leave those of government campaigns in the shade. But the price of these advantages seems bound to lie in the abandonment of the cautious language of benefit and risk. Try as they might to avoid this, scientists taking research money from industry will find themselves regularly exposed to such dilemmas thanks to the media's lack of interest in what it would probably regard as scientific onanism.

4
A testing time for prostate

In 1995 I was 44 and increasingly aware of the nascent prostate cancer screening movement having men of my age and even younger in its sights. This was the first of several pieces I was to write drawing a deep breath of caution. I would eventually write a book on the subject with two colleagues (*Let sleeping dogs lie*, Chapman, Barratt and Stockler 2010).

The Australian Institute of Health and Welfare's latest data on deaths from prostate cancer in Australia show that in 2013, the median age of death from the disease was 82 years. However, the median age of death in men from all causes combined was 78, four years younger than the median for prostate cancer. Prostate cancer is a disease that kills most men very late in life, and, as I discussed in Chapter 1, we must all die from some cause.

In an adult population of about 12 million, some 3.58 million people have had voluntary tests for HIV since 1988. Fifty-three percent of the adult population has had a cholesterol test.

Originally published as Chapman, Simon (1995). A testing time for prostate. *Sydney Morning Herald*, 6 January.

Much in the same way that astrology and other forms of fortune telling beckon the curious and those starved of ordinary feedback about their personalities, a medical test offers unique information that may bring relief from anxiety with the probability of good news about one's most precious yet mysterious possession: one's body. Occasionally bad news from a fortune teller can result in actions that ruin lives. Mostly, though, it causes momentary disquiet, soon rationalised away. The same benign scenarios cannot be drawn for many medical tests, which is why serious ethical issues need debating before screening procedures are promoted by groups, some of which stand to gain from their use.

Three drug companies (Merck Sharp & Dohme, Schering, and Abbott), the RSL, the Australian Kidney Foundation, the Combined Pensioners & Superannuation Association of New South Wales, and sections of the emerging men's health movement are currently leading the charge for the Next Big Thing in screening – prostate screening. Surfing the 1990s zeitgeist of men trying to redress the balance lost to affirmative programs for women, the men's health movement is brandishing a compelling rhetoric that can be summed up as "Women are getting all this stuff for breast cancer, what are we getting?" Bruce Ruxton is among their champions.

Aside from considerations of cost (to screen Australia's 1.5 million men aged 50-plus, $300 million, 20 times the total cancer research budget, is required), the decision to promote screening for asymptomatic disease ought to be based firmly on evidence that there will be benefit to those being screened.

This benefit can lie in increased lifespan and improved quality of life compared with the consequences of not screening. With breast cancer, considerable evidence shows that early detection can prolong survival. The main argument for HIV screening has always been that knowing one is HIV positive may well promote safer sexual practice, while a high cholesterol reading might motivate dietary change or cholesterol-lowering drug therapy.

It seems that the drift of these analogies, together with the fairness imperatives of the new male health movement, have ignited enthusiasm for men to be next in line for what to some is a screening gravy train. With their very own organ as candidate, some superficially appealing statistics (one in 23 men will develop prostate cancer in his lifetime, compared with one in 14 women who will develop breast cancer) and entrepreneurial sections of medicine and the drug industry beating the drum, this issue won't be hiding from minister for health Carmen Lawrence's office in 1995.

Any aggressive and well-promoted prostate-cancer screening campaign will detect many hitherto undiscovered cancers. But this is not the point. The aim of screening, except where it is solely designed to measure prevalence of a disease in a population, is not to find more cancers. It is to find candidates for treatments where there is a high probability of success (although what is "high" enough will always be subject to debate). And this is where the prostate screening exercise starts to go horribly wrong.

Aside from the general trauma of being labelled as having cancer and the traumas of surgery and radiotherapy, international research shows that urinary incontinence occurs in up to 8 percent of men given radical prostatectomy or radiation. Impotence is more frequent and about 1 percent of men die within 30 days of prostate removal. Of more fundamental importance is that while one in 23 men will be diagnosed with prostate cancer, one-third of deaths from the disease occur in men over 80 years. Two-thirds of men with diagnosed prostate cancer die from a cause other than their prostate cancer. Thus any large-scale prostate screening campaign is guaranteed to uncover a large number of men in good spirits and apparently in good health, who would have gone to their graves from something other than prostate cancer, many without any significant symptoms or decrement to their quality of life.

The Australian Cancer Society opposes the screening of asymptomatic men for prostate cancer, arguing that, as yet, there are no prospective studies which demonstrate reductions in death following any treatment currently available. It goes further, criticising "the identification of innocuous disease which would never have made itself clinically apparent is a serious, unethical and iatrogenic consequence of any screening activity, particularly if the complications of unnecessary treatment are substantial". "Street corner" screening facilities for prostate cancer, now common in the USA, seem certain to develop rapidly here, thanks to entrepreneurial medicine, a community poorly informed about the natural history of disease, and the prevalence of the view that it is negligent not to treat.

We all have to die from something and, as far as we know so far, old age is the best predictor of prostate cancer. A recent national poll showed that Australians' personal fear of cancer is way ahead of any other disease (77 percent naming it first, ahead of AIDS with 13 percent). Health policy on screening should not be influenced by ideological views about men's health.

5
Prostate screening not worth it

A decade after I wrote the last piece, the prostate cancer screening push was in full swing. I'd published research (Mackenzie, Chapman et al. 2007) documenting many of the worst excesses of these efforts and wrote this piece to point people to that research.

Most of us assume that finding cancer early rather than later is always sensible. Early detection finds cancer before it might spread, before one becomes "riddled" with inoperable cancer. Cancer-control agencies have worked hard at driving home the importance of early detection and are united in promoting screening for breast, cervical and colorectal cancer and promoting awareness of skin changes. But with screening for prostate cancer, things get complicated. No government anywhere recommends prostate screening. The International Union Against Cancer does not support it, nor has any major review of the evidence on whether screening saves lives.

This is not the message that Australian men are getting about prostate cancer screening, where the main messages overwhelmingly promote screening as a lifesaver, play down the common, serious side

Originally published as Chapman, Simon (2007). Prostate screening not worth it. *Sydney Morning Herald*, 5 November.

effects of treatment and, appropriating the rhetoric of gender equality, simplistically urge: "Hey guys, women have their screening tests. We have ours. Be a man!"

There are inaccuracies in news media reports about prostate cancer, as my colleagues and I report in this week's *Medical Journal of Australia*. We found many examples of blatantly incorrect statements. One said, "every single hour at least one man dies of prostate cancer". Channel Nine's *What's Good for You* told us that "prostate cancer is second only to heart disease in killing Australian men".

Both statements are wrong. If prostate cancer killed one man an hour there would be 8,760 deaths each year – 317 percent more than the 2,761 who died in 2003. Prostate cancer is the fifth leading cause of death in men, running well behind heart disease, which kills 16,442 a year, stroke (4,826), lung cancer (4,733) and chronic obstructive pulmonary disease (2,986).

Nowhere in the media coverage did we find any explanation that prostate cancer tends to kill late in life, when death *per se* increases – and we all have to die of something. Instead, there were many examples of survivors pleading with men to be screened from as early as 40. A large proportion of those who die from prostate cancer are around or have exceeded normal life expectancy – 85.2 percent of prostate cancer deaths occur in men aged over 70, with 47 percent occurring in men over 80.

The counterintuitive, unpopular conclusion today is that there is no reliable evidence that prostate cancer screening saves lives. If you test millions for cancer you find lots of cancer. But the idea of screening is not just to find cancer, but to find disease that has a high probability of turning ugly and needs to be treated early. A lot of the cancers found by screening are "indolent", meaning that many men would achieve normal life expectancy without them being found. Autopsy studies of men who have died from other causes show that significant percentages live with prostate cancer without knowing it, let alone it causing their deaths.

The consequences of treating cancers that never needed to be treated can be serious: permanent incontinence, impotence and a not insignificant rate of serious infection like septicaemia arising from biopsies. A review in the *Lancet* put it plainly: if one million men over 50 years of age were screened, "about 110,000 . . . will face anxiety of possible cancer, about 90,000 will undergo biopsy, and 20,000 will be diagnosed with cancer. If 10,000 of these men underwent surgery, about ten would die of the operation, 300 will develop severe urinary incontinence and even in the best hands 4000 will become impotent".

It is important that men talk to their doctors about prostate screening, asking specifically for accurate information about downsides. If your doctor is a man, ask whether he has had the test, and how he weighed up the pros and cons. The former head of Cancer Council Australia, Professor Alan Coates, declared in 2003 that he had not been tested and was not planning to be. He was by no means Robinson Crusoe in that regard. The vilification he received was deplorable.

The key aim of medicine is not to prolong life indefinitely, but to give priority to preventing and treating those diseases that reduce what decent societies call "a good innings". It is early deaths and those preceded by significantly eroded quality of life that deserve our greatest attention. Unnecessary medical intervention can significantly reduce quality of life. What is urgently needed is a diagnostic test that will accurately predict those prostate cancers which will turn nasty. The tests we have now have poor reliability in that regard. Research funding into the development of such tests is vitally important.

6

Why do doctors keep silent about their own prostate cancer decisions?

Sometimes I come across data about doctors' own preventive health practices. When I saw a report that 55 percent of male middle-aged Victorian GPs had not had a prostate-specific antigen test, I thought this needed some sunlight and wrote this.

Across 38 years in tobacco control, I have been asked countless times in media interviews if I ever smoked. It's often an early question. I always unhesitatingly explain that I did: I stopped in my mid-20s. The tone of the interview immediately relaxes because the subtext of the question is about authenticity. If this person has never smoked, what would he really know about quitting? If I chose to stammer something about it being private or "not the point here", most would become preoccupied with my evasiveness. Fudging and equivocal replies tend to suggest disingenuousness or lack of personal conviction about the information being given.

Clinicians tell me they're frequently asked by patients, "What would you do, doctor?" The question might mean, "What would you do if you were *me*?" But it might also be an invitation to a doctor to explain their own personal health decisions. The question can refer to anything

Chapman, Simon (2015). Why do doctors keep silent about their own prostate cancer decisions? *The Conversation*, 19 January.

from diet, dietary supplement use, organ donation, beating jetlag, travel medicine or exercise. It's normal to ask friends and family what they do in health matters, so when you come face to face with someone who's supposed to know a lot about health, wanting to know if they personally practise some behaviour is an obvious question.

Many health-related practices are openly observable. So if you know or associate with health workers, you can see if they are wear a hat in the sun, walk or cycle to work, take the elevator when stairs are available, or hit the drink at social events. But many health practices are not obvious and require disclosure if we are to know what someone does.

Few would ask their doctor about his or her alcohol intake, and even fewer would ask about their doctor's sexual behaviour (for example condom use or contraception), because these questions cross obvious privacy boundaries. A corpulent doctor is unlikely to be asked about their diet or the extent of their exercise regimen but a lean doctor might well be because of differences in the social meaning of body size. But it's not obvious that screening tests, check-ups, dietary practices and supplementation cross privacy boundaries, particularly when patients are likely to have read conflicting information and material inviting them to discuss testing with their doctors.

But when it comes to prostate cancer screening, men in the medical profession – with rare exceptions[1] – keep their heads well down from public disclosure. In 2003, the then head of the Cancer Council Australia, Professor Alan Coates (then aged 59), told Jill Margo, health reporter at the *Australian Financial Review*, that he had not personally been tested for prostate cancer and did not plan to be. Despite there being no government position on prostate-specific antigen (PSA) testing and considerable professional criticism of the practice, Coates was subjected to astonishing vilification, including a vicious spray on national television from senior Labor politician Wayne Swan, who had personal experience of the disease.[2]

I know that many people privately thanked Coates for his frankness, which did much to open up much-needed public discussion of prostate screening in Australia.

---

1 Haines 2014.
2 Scott 2003.

With two other colleagues, I wrote a book in 2010, *Let sleeping dogs lie: what men should know before getting tested for prostate cancer.*[3] The free-to-download book has had a remarkable 26,500 downloads. Knowing it was likely that I would be asked if I had been tested, I decided to be open about it and explain why I had not when the book was published.

Discussion about the book with colleagues in my own faculty quickly revealed that many men past their 50s had also chosen not to have a PSA test. Several had not consented to be tested, but were given their PSA result after their GP had taken the decision for them and added PSA testing to a blood sample drawn for other reasons. I suggested to some that they might do men's health a service by explaining publicly why they have chosen not to be tested.

About five years ago, the Clinical Oncology Society of Australia allowed me to survey its members about their personal cancer prevention and screening practices. Confidentiality was assured, but the response rate was so low that the data were unusable. The most recent information I know about Australian doctors' own prostate screening practices is now 18 years out of date (1997). Then, 55 percent of a sample of Victorian male GPs aged over 49 had chosen to not have a PSA test themselves.[4]

With widespread publicity being given to problems of unnecessary over-diagnosis and the very serious problems that can follow from this (anxiety or depression in living with a cancer diagnosis, permanent impotence and incontinence), it is possible and even likely that an even higher proportion of Australian doctors today will have elected not to be tested. But we don't know.

The recent draft report from the Prostate Cancer Foundation and Cancer Council Australia recommends men and their doctors fully explore the risks and benefits of prostate testing.[5] In that spirit, if the subject comes up when you are next seeing your (male) doctor, ask him whether and why he has chosen to be tested or not. What you hear (or don't hear) might be very revealing.

---

3   Barratt, Stockler, and Chapman 2010.
4   Livingston, Cohen, Frydenberg, Borland, Reading, Clarke and Hill 2002.
5   Cancer Council Australia 2015.

7
How famous faces muddle the message on cancer

Celebrities endorsing health issues can give them huge oxygen.
But sometimes it can be rather complicated . . .

What is it about breast cancer that attracts prominent glitterati into
fundraising but sees most of them comfortable with ignoring – or
sometimes even helping promote – lung cancer?

The leading couturier Peter Morrissey is featuring in full-page ads
for the National Breast Cancer Foundation. Yet Morrissey assisted
Philip Morris with a fashion parade at an illegal "Wavesnet"
promotional event successfully prosecuted by the Health Department
in November last year. These events were built around Alpine cigarette
promotions targeting young women.

The model Sarah O'Hare is another whose views on cancer
prevention are hard to read. A new book just out by Kathy Buchanan,
Quit for chicks, has a foreword by O'Hare in which she spoons it on
about how she'll never smoke again. So what then should we all make
of a full-page photo showing her miming a deep, unmistakably ecstatic
pull on a lung buster in *Who* magazine's 20 October issue, "100 years

Originally published as Chapman, Simon (2003). How famous faces muddle the
message on cancer. *Sydney Morning Herald*, 3 November.

of glamour"? Only doing her job? I guess she needs the cash. O'Hare is patron of the National Breast Cancer Foundation.

Nicole Kidman has also thrown her stick-figure weight behind fighting breast cancer. Meanwhile millions of young women note her unabashed public smoking. Breast cancer bad. Lung cancer OK. Mixed messages indeed.

There are a bewildering number of breast cancer charities, foundations and support groups, often fronted by high-profile women. While men occasionally get breast cancer, it is overwhelmingly a women's disease. In New South Wales in 2001 there were 4,067 new cases and 871 deaths. Screening and better treatment have reduced the death rate by 22 percent in the past decade, and 85 percent of newly diagnosed women will still be alive in five years. Fund-raising is helping to save and extend lives.

But compare this with lung cancer, where in the same year there were 2,326 deaths – nearly three times more than breast cancer. Only 15 percent of people diagnosed with lung cancer will be alive five years later, giving it one of the worst prognosis profiles of all cancers. When we add all the heart disease, other smoking-caused cancers and emphysema, smoking-caused diseases leave breast cancer well in the shade.

Unlike breast cancer, lung cancer is almost entirely preventable. In 1919 the famous surgeon Alton Ochsner was summoned as a young intern to see a lung cancer operation, something he was told he may never see again. He didn't see another case for 19 years. Today lung cancer is the leading cause of cancer death in Australia, with 85 percent occurring in smokers.

If we knew what caused breast cancer, the thought of celebrities promoting it would be unimaginable. However, music stars like Craig David, Alanis Morissette, Savage Garden and Jewel have all appeared in tobacco-sponsored concerts in developing countries. The Deveaux promotions agency in Sydney is supplying young hunks and babes to act as Marlboro salespeople in nightclubs and World Cup events. So where are the celebrities lining up to criticise all this and demand the government fund the pathetically emaciated Quit campaign?

Breast cancer authorities have no evidence-based advice on preventing the disease, so the mission becomes one of promoting early detection and treatment. For all the apple pie of prevention being better than cure, the promise of curing disease beats prevention every time as a wallet opener and headline grabber. Resurrecting the dying provides endless life dramas of despair, hope and redemption. This is why there are no medical soaps about prevention, despite it saving more lives than cures ever dreamt of.

This is where lung cancer loses out. By contrast, lung cancer offers little hope for cure or survival and its victims labour under the spectre of self-blame. It's argued that smokers choose to smoke. But with 85 percent of smokers starting when children, and tobacco company chemists working into the night to fine-tune nicotine addiction, shrugging off lung cancer with indifference is victim-blaming. Thanks to prevention, male lung cancer rates have been falling by an average of nearly 2 percent a year since 1984, with rates for females remaining steady. These trends mirror the avalanche of men who've quit, and hold the line in preventing women's smoking rates from rising.

Today it is fashionable to work to help breast cancer, and many are reaping the benefits. Yet an article in this month's *Journal of the National Cancer Institute* on lessons for cancer control states: "Tobacco is the big gorilla in all of cancer control. Just a few percentage points' shift in tobacco use makes a huge difference [in total cancer death rates] compared to, for instance, mammography." The new NSW Cancer Institute will add important weight to the fight against all cancers and the early death they can bring. Let us hope it remembers the gorilla.

8

Patient consent in spectator surgery not the only consideration

One evening my rock band played at a fundraiser to raise money to support research into rare cancers. Among the standard fundraising items like dinners at restaurants, wines, and stays in holiday cottages was the opportunity to observe high-profile Sydney neurosurgeon Charlie Teo operating on someone's brain. In the band at the time were three people who worked in health and medicine. We all immediately looked at one another, aghast. I went home and wrote an essay (Chapman 2011) for the *British Medical Journal* (*BMJ*) on the ethical issues that this incident raised for me. The piece below was a follow-up for Australian readers who wouldn't have read the *BMJ*.

The debate occurring over Dr Charlie Teo's "spectator surgery" was precipitated by a report of an article I wrote for the *British Medical Journal*. In the article I never used his name, being concerned to discuss the principles involved rather than the individual. Its title, "Should the spectacle of surgery be sold to the highest bidder?", invited debate that is now occurring both inside and outside medicine.

Originally published as Chapman, Simon (2011). Patient consent in spectator surgery not the only consideration. *Sydney Morning Herald*, 31 January.

There are important reasons why other surgeons don't offer the same opportunity to the paying public. Many, I am certain, are equally concerned to donate to good causes, support cancer research, demystify surgery and urge people to get treatment. Remarks by the Royal Australian College of Surgeons, the Australian Medical Association and a leading bioethicist suggest that I am not Robinson Crusoe.

So is Teo the only surgeon marching in step here? The ethical argument he advances is that the patients involved consent to being observed by paying strangers. They are approached by his staff, not him. Some refuse, so he believes there could be no coercion. But judgements about the adequacy of the cardinal ethical principle of informed consent in medicine and research are never left to individual practitioners or researchers. They are referred to human research ethics and professional standards committees who set rules designed to preserve patient interests. As Teo's own hospital has reported that it does not endorse paying spectators, is it therefore sensible to defer to his judgement here?

There are many examples where societies deem there to be wider considerations involved than simply consent, and that a person's agreement is not all that matters. Here, Teo's patients are under the care of a man whose skills they may sometimes believe represent their last hope. This is likely to produce a highly loaded decision-making context. Patients would instantly understand that this was something that Teo wanted. Few would want to incur the slightest risk of displeasing him. A large body of research on the process of consent makes it clear that patients have feelings of obligation towards doctors: "He's asking for my co-operation. If I refuse, he may be disappointed. I'd better agree."

Teo says no one criticises medical reality TV programs like *RPA*, in which millions of viewers follow the treatment of real patients. In fact there are many parallel problems and some differences. It would be unimaginable if RPA patients being filmed were unable to withdraw their consent at any time before broadcast. Patients or families may decide they no longer wished to share developments: to have millions witness their grief and anxiety, for example. But the "live" viewing of an operation by strangers cannot be erased. There is no cooling-off period between the operation and the "viewing": it has already happened.

Equally, it would be unimaginable if the *RPA* film crew were not bound by journalistic ethics to respect the privacy of patients and families. All hospital staff encounter public figures, neighbours, colleagues, friends and acquaintances as patients. The same possibility arises for film crews and paying spectators. If hospital staff or medical students were to gossip about patients to others outside the hospital, major consequences would follow. No such sanctions are available for members of the public.

My good friend Andrew Penman, from the Cancer Council, defended his charity's acceptance of surgery-viewing auction money on the grounds that patient participation was not "materially different" from things like inviting patients to join a research trial. I disagree. Research trials involve health professionals being bound by enforceable ethical protocols. Researchers are frequently removed from the provision of healthcare to the patient to minimise confounding of effects caused by patients wanting to please their doctors. I know of people who have lost their jobs by breaching the ethical requirements.

Important questions remain about Teo's spectator surgery. Does he impose restrictions on who can bid to watch him? Does he run security or character checks on those who win? Most importantly, if his hospital does not endorse the practice, how has it been allowed to happen?

In the early days of surgery, operating "theatres" were packed with spectators. A historian of medicine records that "Patients put up with the audience to their distress because they received medical treatment from some of the best surgeons in the land." When I grew up in Bathurst in the 1950s, freak-show tents appeared at the local show each year, and people with malformations were displayed for paying customers. Those displayed presumably "consented" to appearing. Thankfully, society has moved on by recognising that consent alone is sometimes not in a person's or society's best interests.

9
Does celebrity involvement in public health campaigns deliver long-term benefit? Yes

Bucketing celebrity involvement in public health campaigning is a common snooty reaction we see from professionals, usually on the sidelines of these efforts. The *British Medical Journal* invited me to put the case for the "yes" case for such involvement (you can find the "no" case in Rayner 2012. Sorry, but it's paywalled).

Celebrities appear often in news reports about health and medicine. Since 2005, my research group has recorded all health-related content on all five free-to-air Sydney TV channels. As of 21 August 2011, 1,657 of 29,322 (6 percent) news items have featured celebrities, a rate substantially below those experiencing disease or injury (60 percent), experts and health workers (50 percent) and politicians (49 percent).[1] They often get involved because of personal experience with a disease or because they share the concerns of other citizens about an issue and

---

1   Chapman, Holding, Ellerm, Heenan, Fogarty, Imison, McKenzie and McGeechan 2009.

Originally published as Chapman, Simon (2012). Does celebrity involvement in public health campaigns deliver long-term benefit? Yes. *British Medical Journal* 345: 6364.

want to help by offering the publicity magnet intrinsic to their celebrity. And like experts, some probably calculate that a public profile on good causes might also be good for their careers.

Celebrities are by definition newsworthy before they embrace any subject. When they do, again just like experts, they turn in a range of performances. Those concerned about celebrities in health campaigns invariably point to examples that have gone badly wrong or that fail to change the world forever. They hone in on celebrity endorsement of flaky complementary medicine or quack diets, or ridicule feet-in-mouth incidents where celebrities have wandered off message or blundered, or point out cases where celebrity "effects" are not sustained,[2] a problem of course not confined to campaigns using celebrities. But they are silent about the many examples of celebrity engagement that have massively amplified becalmed news coverage about important, neglected issues or celebrity involvement in advocacy campaigns to promote evidence-based health policy reform.

Is there anyone concerned about action to mitigate anthropogenic climate change who is not delighted when celebrities stand side-by-side with climate scientists and thereby attract attention that a phalanx of impeccably credentialed researchers could only dream of? And on the flipside, is there anyone in public health who is not appalled when celebrities speak up for smoking (David Hockney, Joe Jackson); promote prostate cancer screening for men even younger than 40 (Australian hard rocker Angry Anderson); or blather about the odious nanny state (Formula 1 driver Mark Webber after having his car impounded for driving dangerously on suburban streets)? What does it say that we can be disgusted when celebrities try to set back public health agendas but get all bothered about celebrity efforts in campaigns that could influence millions positively?

There are some uncomfortable subtexts just beneath the disdain for celebrity engagement in health. The main one seems to be an arrogant "What would they know?" reaction. Celebrities are not experts: they can use embarrassingly naive language and may have no idea about levels of evidence or all the work that has gone before in advocating for an issue. But just as the media have an appetite for those experiencing

---

2   MacArthur, Wright, Beer and Paranjothy 2011.

health problems, celebrities often speak personally and bring compelling authenticity to public discourse. A leading Sydney health and medicine reporter told me once that "Experts are fine, but they are not a living thing."[3] She went on to explain a litany of problems that journalists routinely encountered in using experts, like a common inability to imagine an audience outside their own often middle- to high-brow cliques. *Nature*'s online editor, Ananyo Bhattacharya, has just reminded us of all the ways that scientists can be hopeless news participants.[4]

Why do we expect perfect outcomes following celebrity engagement, yet are realistic about the need to sustain public campaigns beyond their first burst? In 1999, cricketer Shane Warne accepted a six-figure sum to use nicotine replacement therapy to quit smoking.[5] The challenge rapidly became a paparazzi sport: who would be first to photograph him smoking again? It didn't take long. Warne was a world-class cricketer, but a very ordinary, relapsing smoker. This was an important message that many experts failed to exploit, instead climbing on a cynical populist bandwagon about his alleged motives.

Publicity about the then 36-year-old Kylie Minogue's breast cancer, meanwhile, led to an increase in unscreened women in the target age-range having mammograms,[6] but also to an increase in young women at very low risk seeking mammograms and thus being exposed to unnecessary radiation and false positive investigations.[7] But what if such a celebrity had instead had precancerous cervical lesions detected by a pap smear and her story went viral, generating increased awareness of the importance of pap smears? The ambivalence about "the Kylie effect" reflects enduring debate about the wisdom of breast screening, but it should not blind us to the potential value of celebrity engagement in important causes.

---

3   Chapman, McCarthy and Lupton 1995.
4   Bhattacharya 2012.
5   Chapman and Leask 2001.
6   Chapman, McLeod, Wakefield and Holding 2005.
7   Kelaher, Cawson, Miller, Kavanagh, Dunt and Studdert 2008.

10

A nation of flashers should show some modesty

When people flash their car lights at us, it's often a warning
that there is a police car with a camera up ahead. We check our
speed and if we are over the limit, feel very thankful for these
little acts by strangers that might save us lots of money. But
should we do it as well?

As with drivers who flash their lights at you, most of us think that
radio announcements about the locations of police speed cameras are
godsends. Flashing at your fellow motorists and phoning up special
radio hotlines to breathlessly join in foiling those hapless coppers
sitting there is becoming part of what it means to be an Australian.
Traffic reports are tagged with coy little asides about a "photo
opportunity on Boundary Road". Radio stations gain loyalty points
from their listeners, thousands of whom each week would personally
ease off as they were about to hit a just-announced surveillance section.
Wow, thanks guys! I'll stay tuned to my radio friends who just saved me
my licence or $600.

The police actually encourage these announcements. Over the
recent Queen's Birthday weekend, New South Wales police publicised

---

Originally published by Chapman, Simon (1999). A nation of flashers should show
some modesty. *Weekend Australian*, 10–11 July.

camera locations. The idea is that publicity will cause a general increase in awareness that the cameras are "out there". Little by little, the theory goes, motorists given these daily reminders will have the message sink in and we'll all slow down. We'll all be safer and in joining in the camera-spotting will have gained some fuzzy communal capital too. Nice idea: shame though about the lack of *any* evidence to support it.

If they really believe all this, why, then, don't radio stations and the police use the same rationalisations and blow the cover on random breath testing units? The New South Wales police say they would take a totally different attitude to what the PR plod I spoke to described as "a criminal and highly dangerous offence that only relatively few people do". But it's the randomness of random breath testing that gives the process its deterrent potency. If you know there's a booze bus in the direction you're travelling, you can take a different route home from the pub. But if it's random and unannounced, you think about the wisdom of driving every time you're out and drinking. If you know there's a speed camera up ahead, you can take your foot off until you've passed it and flash the lights at other motorists. Tricked the bastards, didn't we!

The talkback take on speeding is that it's all a grubby money-grab, clinging to the shirt tails of a worthy cause. The police are just errand boys for the Treasury. So why don't we hear the same argument run about drink driving, where the fines are even larger? It's because we make the assumption that drink driving is so much more dangerous than speeding. Professor Jack McLean and Craig Kloeden from the University of Adelaide's Road Accident Research Unit investigated 151 Adelaide crashes requiring ambulances in 60 km/h zones on non-rainy days where drivers were not drunk and not undertaking illegal manoeuvres like U-turns. Using computer-aided crash reconstruction techniques, and matching each crash vehicle with four other randomly selected comparison vehicles – all speed-timed, and all drivers breath tested – they found that each 5 km/h increase in speed above 60 km/h in urban areas increased the risk of a casualty crash by roughly the same amount as each increase in blood alcohol concentration of 0.05 g/100 mL. In other words, speed and drink are about equal as predictors of serious crashes.[1]

---

1   See Kloeden, McLean, Moore, and Ponte 1997.

In 1979, 3,573 people were killed on Australia's public roads. More than half of them were aged 15–34, the main audience group for the stations that broadcast the speed camera locations. By 1997, despite population growth, this carnage had fallen to 1,800 – an amazing 99 percent reduction in 18 years. But the relentless pursuit of an ever-falling road toll always comes at a price. For example, if all drivers were obliged, like motor cyclists, to wear crash helmets, then deaths from head injury would fall way further. But would the community be prepared to trade such inconvenience for further reductions?

Historically, the debate on the road toll has seen the hotel industry opposing random breath testing, arguing po-faced that it would cost jobs. Undertakers and the wheelchair trade apparently decided to cut their losses. Civil liberties groups once opposed compulsory seat belts and helmets. Some car manufacturers resisted the introduction of compulsory high-mounted brake lights, and barriers in station wagons designed to restrain luggage rocketing through the car and snapping the necks of passengers. Speed enthusiasts have long strenuously objected to speed laws. Like the gun lobby, they argue that there are safe drivers and unsafe drivers and the answer is more driver education. The apparent enthusiasm of radio stations and their young audiences for the sport of speed camera dobbing may well be a sign that the community values the right to speed more highly than shaving more lives and quadriplegics off the annual road toll. There are probably few who would feel comfortable in saying upfront, "Look, I think I do enough already to play my part in reducing the road toll. I don't want to be restricted anymore – too bad if this means there are going to be a few hundred or so lives ruined. It's not my responsibility."

We prefer to surreptitiously cast our vote in this continuing opinion poll by flashing our lights. Next time you're tempted to flash or phone up and ruin the police camera party, ask yourself what's more important: the petty satisfaction of fleeting solidarity with other anonymous drivers at having thwarted the police, or the thought that someone, ego-bruised by having their licence cancelled for a cooling-off period, might hit the road next time a little calmer.

11
A long, winding road to end the carnage

We often hear people say, "If it saved just one life, it would be worth it!" And advocates for the reduction of health problems generally seem to agree that efforts should not abate until all cases of a preventable problem have disappeared. Below, I looked at this reasoning when it comes to road injury.

The concern about the holiday road toll invites a good many questions. Before any are addressed, the community needs to discuss the fundamental matter of what level of road toll should be considered too high, and its indelicate corollary of what annual road carnage the community would be willing to accept.

The idea that the road toll will inexorably inch closer to zero seems implicit in most of the outrage over the toll for this holiday season and the annual tally, as is the notion that anything worse than the year before is self-evidently a national disgrace, regardless of population growth.

A zero road toll is a concept for science-fiction writers with visions of collision-proof cars tracked onto an electromagnetic national grid.

Originally published as Chapman, Simon (2001). A long, winding road to end the carnage. *Sydney Morning Herald*, 8 January.

Even Luddites like the Amish who eschew cars are occasionally killed by bolting horses and drays.

International comparisons give some idea of what lower road death rates are possible. Among the 25 OECD countries, between 1987 and 1997, Australia's rate of road deaths ranked tenth, at 9.5 per 100,000 of the population. That is behind Iceland (5.5), Britain (6.3), Sweden (6.1), Finland (8.5) and Japan (8.9). At the other end lie Portugal (28.9), Greece (20.9), and the United States (15.7).

We could strive to reach Iceland's level, although with a total population of only 280,000, mostly in the capital, there is hardly basis for comparison. Several of the low-toll nations such as Britain and Japan also have among the world's highest rates of public transport use, promoted by far-sighted infrastructure development and cultures that demand and are willing to pay for its development. Western European rates of public transport use in cities of more than 250,000 people are more than double those in Australia and nearly six times those of the USA, which has a road toll among the highest in the developed world. Even Italy, with its reputation for road anarchy, has lower pedestrian and motorcycle death rates than Australia. But Rome's urban rail, for example, carries 9.1 million annual passengers per line mile, compared with Sydney's much-lamented low usage. (The Department of Transport was unable to supply me with the comparable figure for New South Wales.)

If more people use public transport, fewer will use private cars. Unless dangerous drivers somehow disproportionately self-select out of using trains and buses, this means that we might expect a corresponding reduction in their ventures onto roads. But would the Australian community be willing to support, through tax, the major expenditure that would be necessary to significantly improve access to public transport? If not, then the recipe for further improvements to the road toll must be drawn from added doses of driver education, threats and disincentives, and harm reduction through car and road engineering.

These have clearly worked to some extent up to now: Australia leads the OECD in reducing its road toll (38 percent between 1988 and 1997). Theoretically, of course, we can imagine the annual road toll being zero, and anyone who has ever lost family or friends would probably agree that almost anything that could have saved those lives should have been done. No price seems too high when it's your child or partner who has been killed or maimed. But when such an implied vision is addressed at the policy level, the community has a right to debate its acceptance of liberty-restricting and punitive preventive measures like speed fines, traffic calming and car safety modifications. While such debates are always generated by reference to the road toll, they are often resolved by the ascendancy of other values that reveal plainly that for all the public anguish about road carnage, the community has higher priorities.

Consider head injury, among the leading causes of death and lifelong brain damage in vehicle crashes. The logic of extending the argument for compulsory motor cycle helmets to car occupants is obvious. Just as injury-conscious motor racing has long required drivers to wear helmets, why not cars on roads, too? Acting from wholly paternalistic precepts, we inconvenience motorcyclists, arguing that the decision to risk one's head being slammed against a road obstacle at 60 km/h cannot be a rational and informed decision. The state therefore makes the decision for motorcyclists by making helmets mandatory. So why not car occupants, given the imagery of heads as bursting watermelons that we have all been exposed to in motivational advertising? The resounding unpopularity of such a proposal and the ridicule it would bring to any proponent would reflect the overwhelming rejection of a major increment in car-user safety over the importance of keeping one's coiffure intact.

Equally, Bob Carr's rejection last week of the Pedestrian Council's bullbar-ban proposal may owe as much to electoral sensitivity as to his reading of the estimated, relatively small number of lives that could be saved by such a move. Opponents of a ban on bullbars in the city engage a mental calculus that puts their concerns about damaging their cars ahead of the perceived unlikelihood of cutting pedestrians in two. Perceptions of risk are all about perceptions of control: bullbar owners feel that, being impeccable drivers, the risk of them hitting a pedestrian is infinitesimal, whereas the risk of a roo jumping out of the bush in Killara is presumably perceived as higher.

Just as seat belts, random breath testing and suburban traffic calming were all vigorously opposed by the public and many politicians, so is it likely that bullbars in urban areas will one day be popularly reviled as viciously anti-social. The years ahead are likely to see refinements of this debate, with city-registered vehicles opting for bullbars being hit with huge registration fees as a disincentive. The Pedestrian Council's Harold Scruby may have his historical status upgraded from public nanny to public health visionary. There is a vast science of road injury prevention, resplendent with controlled experimental trials of different strategies, international comparisons and instructive longitudinal data. While the conclusions of this continue to be debated at the margins, the road toll will not fall further without further impositions on all of us.

As gun control did for those who like to own lethal weapons, the road toll debate draws heavily on the insult and resentment felt by those who like to drive fast but have impeccable safety records. "We've never hurt anyone . . . restrictive laws are unjust . . . it's somebody else's problem." This has all the moral force of a law-abiding passenger being insulted at having to walk through an airport metal detector. The real questions that remain all come back to the balance that must always be struck between the cost of saving further lives and the price we are willing to pay to do so.

12
Drink and drive? Not the publican's problem

A High Court judgement that a hotelier had no duty of care to act to prevent a very intoxicated patron from driving a motor vehicle highlighted where the legal rubber met the road when it came to testing libertarian philosopher John Stuart Mill's (1806–1873) famous dictum on liberty: "The only purpose for which power can be rightfully exercised over any member of a civilized community, against his will, is to prevent harm to others. His own good, either physical or moral, is not sufficient warrant." But perhaps the judges missed something Mill also wrote? "A person may cause evil to others not only by his action but by his inaction, and in either case he is justly accountable to them for the injury." (Mill 1998)

A unanimous decision handed down this week by the High Court will cause jubilation in the hotel industry in its ongoing efforts to shift all responsibility for the harms caused by drinking onto drinkers. In the judgement, a duty-of-care negligence claim against a Tasmanian hotel owner was dismissed. He had handed back motorcycle keys, which had been lodged with staff for safe-keeping, to an insistent, belligerent

Originally published as Chapman, Simon (2009). Drink and drive? Not the publican's problem. *Sydney Morning Herald*, 11 November.

patron, who on leaving the pub was killed in a crash while showing a blood alcohol level of 0.253. A reading of 0.05 doubles the risk of a crash. At 0.08, the risk increases seven times. At 0.15, it is 25 times higher. Data are too scant to reliably calculate the stratospheric increase in risk at the level shown by the dead man.

The man had drunk seven or eight cans of bourbon and cola between 5.15 pm and 8.30 pm. According to the judgement, the licensee told him he had had enough, that it was time to go home, and asked for his wife's phone number so that she could fetch him. The patron became agitated and said, "If I want you to ring my f'ing' wife, I'd f'ing ask ya." The licensee responded, "Whoo hang on, whoo, whoo, whoo, this is not, you know, don't go crook at me, this is not the arrangement that was made." Not having the wife's phone number, and not wanting to push the issue into further confrontation, the licensee then gave the keys to the patron, after asking him three times if he was OK to drive.

While the verdict in no way removes all duty of care from hoteliers, it will surely set a benchmark that will be enthusiastically incorporated into bar staff training sessions for years to come. Bar staff will be told that there's no apparent problem in continuing to serve patrons till their blood is almost pickled with alcohol and that they have no duty of care to take steps to prevent a drink patron getting behind a wheel.

The High Court's judgement, steeped in precedent, contains some startling reasoning. It first enshrines the right of people to get as intoxicated as they please, noting that a hotelier has no business in "impairing the autonomy" of a patron wanting to do this. While the court agreed that the licensee had a statutory duty to refuse an intoxicated person service if he or she appeared to be drunk and to require that they leave the hotel, it ruled that no one other than the police had a right to restrain a person from driving when intoxicated, and that if the hotelier had refused to return the keys to the intoxicated patron or somehow restrained him, he would have been guilty of "false imprisonment".

The legal defence of necessity allows citizens to break laws if they judge that some higher responsibility or good will be served by their actions. If I were to forcibly enter a house on fire on a reasonable expectation that I might save the lives of occupants, any charge of

wilful damage or trespass would be dismissed. Here, if a bar worker
– hopefully having attended a mandatory course on the responsible
service of alcohol, at which they would have learned about the
increased risks of motor vehicle crashes caused by drinking – were to
try and prevent a plainly drunk person from driving a motor vehicle,
the law as it stands appears to say they have no right to do so.

In this incident, the apparently inviolable exercise of the dead man's
autonomy resulted in his own death. But every year drink drivers kill
and permanently injure hundreds of Australians. One-third of all road
deaths involve alcohol.

The alcohol industry profits hugely from heavy-duty alcohol
consumption. The National Drug and Alcohol Research Centre has
calculated that 39 percent of alcohol is consumed in Australia at levels
posing long-term health risks. For all its posturing about the
responsible service of alcohol, it knows there is a low probability that
courts will see cases involving serving those who are drunk.

In 2006, a magistrate dismissed charges against two bar staff who
had served a West Australian woman who then fell 15 stories to her
death with a blood alcohol reading of 0.342. The woman had been
unable to walk unaided, and the bar staff had to help her to the toilet. At
the time, an Australian Hotels Association spokesman said cryptically,
"The industry sat up and took notice of what had happened here". Bar
staff are told that the law says they cannot serve intoxicated persons, but
they know they will rarely be charged if they do so. There have been just
17 such prosecutions a year in Queensland in the past five years.

This judgement should unleash momentum for the mandatory
fitting of ignition interlocking devices on all vehicles. These devices
require the driver to blow into a tube to detect alcohol consumption.
The lock will not deactivate if alcohol is detected. Evidence from many
trials show the success of this measure. For example, a New Mexico
study of 437 drink-driving offenders ordered to have interlocks
installed found a reduction in recidivism of 65 percent after installation,
compared with a comparison drink-driving group that did not have the
devices installed.

13
The AIDS myth that will not die

In the early years following the advent of HIV/AIDS, there were apocalyptic forecasts of the disease running rampant throughout the population. I had several friends and colleagues in infectious disease epidemiology who were highly sceptical of these claims, but worried about challenging the zeitgeist. I drew a deep breath and published the piece below and two years later followed it up with another one (Chapman 1992b). I was subjected to some hostility from sections of the HIV/AIDS activist community, but looking back 26 years later, I didn't get much wrong.

One of the more striking AIDS advertisements in the renewed campaign to heighten public awareness of the menace is headed "Most parents suffer from AIDS" and goes on to urge parents to "talk, plead, shout, cry" but not to "suffer in silence" about their teenage children's chances of contracting the disease. It makes the claim that if a teenager's latest girlfriend or boyfriend has shared needles, "They would [sic] pass the virus on through unprotected sex".

Chapman, Simon (1990). The AIDS myth that will not die. *Sydney Morning Herald*, 18 June.

This is a highly tendentious claim which, accompanied by the suggestion that parents should encourage their children to "simply not have sex at all at this stage", suggests the public health agenda has been hijacked, to a degree, by neo-puritan ideology.

It also raises many important questions about how decisions are made about priorities in AIDS prevention and control. It asks, in particular, why authorities are persisting with expensive strategies aimed at the low-risk population when, for example, only four people are now employed as Outreach counsellors to cover the hundreds of public toilet beats in the state where thousands of men, many bisexual, meet every day to have anonymous, often unprotected sex.

How infectious, then, is the HIV virus? Studies of the sero-conversion rates of the regular heterosexual partners of HIV-infected bisexual men, intravenous drug users (IVDUs) and haemophiliacs have come up with answers that may surprise many people. A study of 93 women published in *JAMA*, the *Journal of the American Medical Association*, estimated that a woman having 100 or more episodes of unprotected intercourse in a year with an infected partner has about a 31 percent chance of acquiring the virus, a much lower infectivity rate than occurs with hepatitis B, herpes and other STDs. Others have estimated from this and other partner studies that any single act of intercourse without condoms with an infected person has about a one in 500 chance of passing on HIV.

But what about the odds with "one-night-stand" sex with someone with no high-risk history? Estimates based on data from the USA, where the incidence of HIV is higher than in Australia, suggest that the chances of a heterosexual acquiring the virus during one sexual encounter with someone undiagnosed as having HIV is one in 5 billion. When fatalities from bee stings run at one in 5 million, such odds are hardly suggestive of a major health crisis requiring multi-million-dollar scare campaigns.

What, then, about the argument that the pool of infected heterosexuals is slowly building, but hasn't yet reached a critical mass that will cause it to explode and rapidly spread the virus? A later review of heterosexual infection published this year in the journal *AIDS* states that "new infections in heterosexuals, acquired either through intra-venous drug use or heterosexual contact, are not increasing at the rates observed among cohorts of homosexual men and IVDUs during the early 1980s".

The review states that of 8,810 heterosexual AIDS cases reported in the USA to September 1989, 83 percent occurred among intravenous drug users and 7 percent among the heterosexual contacts of people at risk, primarily female sexual partners of male IVDUs. This leaves 10 percent – some 880 individuals in the USA – who may be true members of the so-called third wave of transmission: those who have caught the virus from a sexual partner twice removed from a primary infection.

Even in this case, there is much doubt about the authenticity of people's reports of their not being in a high-risk group. The report states: "Although some of these cases may represent secondary or even tertiary heterosexual transmission, most are found to be IVDUs or sexual partners of men at risk" when they are more intensively interviewed and investigated. The review concludes that among identified cases, the proportion that may represent unrecognised heterosexual transmission has remained relatively constant for men and women since 1986.

In Australia, despite regular prophecy that the incidence of HIV will skyrocket and that recorded cases are only the tip of the iceberg, all available indicators suggest that the incidence in the overall population is low. For example, from May 1985 to 30 June 1988, 2,662,593 separate blood donations were made in Australia. Twenty HIV-positive cases were found in this group, representing eight cases per million donors. The Australian rate decreased from 0.004 percent in 1985 to 0.00004 percent in 1987, probably reflecting the voluntary withdrawal of infected donors from the donor population. All military recruits have been screened in Australia since late March 1988. Between March and June of that year, 5,000 people were screened; none was found to be seropositive.

Experts themselves are largely guessing about the extent of HIV in the population. By the end of March this year, the cumulative total of notified cases stood at 12,552. Yet in 1988, 35 Australian epidemiologists were asked to estimate the likely prevalence of HIV in the Australian population. Estimates appearing in press reports had ranged up to nearly 100,000. The figures I have cited are easily accessible to anyone acquainted with the voluminous scientific literature on AIDS and are yet to be coherently disputed by anyone other than those carrying alarmist or sexually conservative baggage.

The tone and wording of the current AIDS campaign thus raises important questions about why official policy on AIDS education appears willing to condone rampant exaggeration and unfounded scare tactics. Whenever this criticism has been raised in the past, the response from people like the former federal minister of community services and health, Dr Neal Blewett, has been to argue that it is better to be accused of scaring people needlessly than not taking the epidemic seriously enough. Certainly, there is plenty of anecdotal evidence that a significant section of the population is scared of contracting the virus.

The goal of AIDS education efforts should be to give the public a realistic sense of the seriousness of AIDS and what is involved in its prevention. But AIDS publicity also appears to have done a great deal more than inform the population about the fundamentals of the disease. It has aroused considerable unwarranted anxiety in a large section of the population and has either spawned or reinforced socially divisive and hostile attitudes about gay men, drug users and even children who have been infected.

Serious and coherent challenges are now being made to the wisdom of continuing to direct AIDS control messages to the whole population, a large proportion of which is at negligible risk, instead of more intensively targeting the high-risk groups to which the disease appears to be confined in Australia. Given the disturbing extent of hysterical and exaggerated perceptions of AIDS, and of potentially socially divisive attitudes, these challenges should prompt AIDS-control authorities to consider whether the means (scaring the population unnecessarily) can continue to justify such stigmatising and neurosis-producing ends. Not least among these ends may be the unforeseen legacy of the distortion of public perceptions about the size and nature of the AIDS problem on future efforts to have the public at large show concern for issues where they really are at distinct risk.

14

A shattering of glass in Tasmania

The outrage among some religious moralists about homosexual men who enjoy sodomy has been going on for millennia. But tellingly, you never hear the same outrage about heterosexuals who enjoy it occasionally or more often. In this piece, I "did the math" with Juliet Richters to show that on any night there's much more of it happening between men and women than between men and other men. Strangely, we never hear the moralists railing about this.

The caterwauling in Tasmania over sodomy raises at least one interesting question: why is the outrage always focused on gay men, when heterosexuals not uncommonly engage in the practice, too?

In fact, on any given night in Tasmania, it is almost certainly the case that more heterosexual couples engage in sodomy than do male couples. If, as the Liberal state attorney-general, Ronald Cornish, argues, "sodomy is an unnatural act and unhealthy", where is the chorus of commensurate outrage about what a large number of men and women do together?

Originally published as Chapman, Simon and Juliet Richters (1994). A shattering of glass in Tasmania. *Sydney Morning Herald*, 31 August.

Australia has not yet conducted a national random survey of sexual activity, as has been done in recent years in France and Britain. The British study of nearly 19,000 adults, the results of which were published this year, points to a situation that, in the absence of any evidence to the contrary, is likely to be very similar to that which applies in Australia. And if "No sex please, we're British" is a deserving description, the findings of the British study may well be a rather conservative guide to sexual conduct in this country.

The British study, the National Survey of Sexual Attitudes and Lifestyles, funded by the Wellcome Trust after Margaret Thatcher refused government money, was conducted in a way that allowed those surveyed to answer extremely detailed and intimate questions without jeopardising their anonymity.

It found that 6.5 percent of men and 5.9 percent of women aged 16–59 reported having anal intercourse with a person of the opposite sex in the past year, with 2.8 percent of men and 2.4 percent of women claiming to have engaged in the practice in the past month.

Note that these figures refer to all men and women aged 16–59 sampled in households throughout Britain – not just to people in relationships. The small discrepancies between men and women in the reported rates result from lower rates reported by older women compared with men. This suggests either that older women under-report anal intercourse, that men over-report it, or that the sample somehow uncovered a group of women who were multi-partnered in this activity. By comparison, only 1.1 percent of all men interviewed reported having any sexual contact with men in the past year, compared with a rate of lifetime ("ever") male-to-male sexual experience of 6.1 percent.

Contrary to what some Tasmanian supporters of the Liberal MP Chris Miles and the anti-gay TasAlert group might believe, not all gay and bisexual men routinely engage in anal intercourse. A long-running Macquarie University study reported that only 56 percent of the men interviewed who had sex with men in the past six months had had anal intercourse. This study was expressly designed to reach gay and bisexual men. Internationally, such studies invariably report higher rates of anal intercourse than studies which randomly sample the general population. The 56 percent estimate almost certainly overstates the true rate of male-to-male anal intercourse among gay and bisexual men in the general community.

So what might all this mean for Tasmania? There are about 136,000 men aged 16–59 in Tasmania. If 1.1 percent of them are actively homosexual or bisexual, and 56 percent of these engage regularly in anal intercourse, then there might be about 840 male-to-male sodomites (as Cornish might call them) on the island.

By contrast, there are about 270,000 people aged 16–59 in the state (135,800 men and 134,200 women). If we subtract the 1,500 gay and bisexual men from this number (although this would not be completely warranted, for a considerable proportion who are bisexual may also have anal intercourse with women) then going by the British percentages, about 8,730 men and 7,920 women in Tasmania could be expected to have had anal intercourse with a person of the opposite sex in the past year. This suggests there are nearly 20 times the number of people who have had recent experience of anal intercourse with a member of the opposite sex than men who have had anal intercourse with another man. While our calculations have been for Tasmania, there is no reason to expect that they would not apply across Australia.

We can almost hear the howls of protest from across Bass Strait. "We're not like those British!" We can also hear murmurings about the predilection of certain ethnic groups to use anal intercourse as a form of birth control – "Greek" has long been brothel slang for the practice. The British study found no evidence of any class differences in the practice, nor of any racial differences between white, black or Asian groups. (Intriguingly, only the racial group described in the report as "Other" had a higher rate.)

15
Gun lobby on shaky ground

In the 1990s, I was actively involved in gun control advocacy through the Coalition for Gun Control. On 9 July 1995, Senior Constables Robert Spears and Peter Addison were killed by a man with a semi-automatic gun while attending a domestic violence call-out at Crescent Head on the mid-north coast of New South Wales. Gun registration was one of the policies we were calling to be introduced. It was finally introduced after the Port Arthur massacre in April 1996.

Three weeks on from the Crescent Head police shootings, the calls for tighter gun controls have predictably moved off the news pages. The same headlines and the same for and against advocates will be back again at the next inevitable incident.

Gun registration is at the heart of gun control policy while being utter profanity to the gun lobby. Those urging registration advance a simple argument in its favour: that registration allows police to match shooters' licences and addresses with a gun register. As they drive to a domestic violence incident, police can check the address on a computer register to find out how many guns to expect.

Originally published as Chapman, Simon (1995). Gun lobby on shaky ground. *Sydney Morning Herald*, 30 July.

The best illustration of how this might have worked was in the case of the Terrigal gunman, Malcolm Baker. Baker was on an apprehended violence order and, as such, had had his shooter's licence revoked and his guns confiscated. The trouble was, with New South Wales having no gun registration, the police could only confiscate the guns they could find. Baker had hidden the gun he used to kill four people.

The anti-registration lobby advances three arguments: registration is useless because it will be ignored; it is iniquitous because it is a slur on the character of law-abiding citizens; and it is capricious because it is fixated on guns rather than (for example) knives as instruments of death. They say such schemes are useless because, as has been shown in other states, tens of thousands of shooters simply won't register their guns out of concern that registration is just a pretext for the guns eventually being confiscated in some Fabian plot to disarm the community.

If failure to register a gun were elevated to being a serious offence and backed by "dob in a gun hoarder" schemes like those used for drugs in Operation Noah, it is likely that those choosing to hide unregistered guns would diminish greatly. Truly law-abiding gun owners would have nothing to fear.

The gun lobby is offended by the insult that the ordinary, law-abiding gun owner is in any way a danger to the community. Here they contrast the number of guns in the community (estimated at well over 3 million) with the number of violent incidents (some 600 annual deaths), arguing that effort should be spent locating and controlling those known or predicted to be dangerous. This is the focus of a current NSW Cabinet inquiry. The trouble with this argument is that, like the Crescent Head incident, most gun violence is perpetrated by people who would never have come to the attention of police or psychiatrists.

It is curious indeed that those insulted by the implication of gun registration do not seem to feel the same way about registering their cars or boats. The fact that a small proportion of car owners deliberately drive unregistered or falsely registered cars is never used as an argument for abandoning the registration system at large. It is plainly recognised that vehicle registration will have many public and administrative benefits. As the gun lobby would put it, "No law or registration system is going to prevent the determined criminal or suicide getting hold of a gun." This ignores the fact that most domestic shootings and suicides involve people who were not premeditating violence when they were required to register their guns. In essence, the gun lobby's argument here follows the logic of "If you can't fix all of the problems, don't attempt to fix any of them."

There are also those who keep unregistered and often savage guard dogs, presumably seeking to avoid a visit from authorities should their dogs stray and maul people or even foul the footpath. Again, your average Chihuahua owner may see dog registration as insulting to the proclivities of their well-behaved little darlings but probably accepts that there are good reasons for wanting to trace the owners of anti-social dogs. Since no reliable predictive tests of savagery or footpath fouling exist, registration of all dogs seems only fair.

If we all must register our cars, boats and dogs for the sake of community, why should the argument be any different for guns? If this argument were anything other than an Alamo fantasy, why then does the gun lobby support hand-gun registration? What is it about pistol owners that allows them to co-operate with the pistol registration law in ways that long-arm (rifle) owners allegedly cannot? And, persuasively, pistols – with the tight controls that apply – are used in far fewer incidents of gun violence than are long-arms.

Finally, the gun lobby argues that with stabbings being more prevalent than gun attacks, it is just fashionable and convenient to pick on guns. If you are serious, why not register knives too? The rhetoric of this argument invites us to consider that guns should be considered as commonplace and as utilitarian as knives and treated accordingly. However, every house has dozens of knives and these are used for eating and food preparation and only occasionally misused in acts of violence. By contrast, other than for target shooting (which should be confined to secure gun clubs), a gun is designed and purchased with lethal or threatening intent.

A browse through gun lovers' magazines in any newsagent reveals the vehemence of the gun lobby's objections to gun registration. Repeatedly, letter writers and columnists in these magazines revealingly show their preoccupations with the potential for malicious false reporting of threats by disgruntled ex-wives and girlfriends, with *Dad's Army* fantasies about defending Australia from invading forces, and with conspiracies about socialist plots to disarm the population so that a totalitarian regime can be established.

These hysterical analyses never include a further concern close to the hearts of many in the gun lobby. Lack of national registration of guns allows a tax-avoidance cash market in guns to flourish through gun collectors' fairs, licensed dealers and word of mouth. Registration would severely inhibit this trade as well as reduce (not eliminate) gun violence in the community.

16

Now, about those guns . . .

I wrote this open letter to Australia's police ministers, who were meeting on the day it was published in the aftermath of the Port Arthur massacre, which had taken place 11 days earlier. The next day, the National Firearms Agreement was announced. It was the most sweeping template for uniform national and state gun control ever legislated. My book *Over our dead bodies: Port Arthur and the fight for gun law reform* (2013c [1998]) gives a detailed account of the advocacy we engaged in to encourage those reforms.

An open letter to Australia's police ministers:

Gentlemen, tomorrow each of you is a key player in what can be a proud national moment or a giant squib in Australian history. You stand at a fork in a road, where one path is paved with the pre–Port Arthur excuses to continue to embrace US-style policies that consider it reasonable for virtually anyone to own a gun – an instrument de-signed for one purpose: to kill. The USA in 1994, with 250 million people, had 39,250 deaths from firearms, a 64 percent increase from 1968. The other fork takes us down the path of Britain and Japan, where, in populations of 57 million and 124 million respectively, and

Originally published as Chapman, Simon (1996). Now, about those guns . . . *Sydney Morning Herald*, 8 May.

with tougher gun laws now being promised, they had 70 and 34 gun deaths each in a recent year.

John Howard speaks for all civilised Australians in understanding that we've been staring at a sign on the first road. It reads: "Go back. You're going the wrong way!" It has taken 35 gruesome deaths to finally drag bipartisan support to this issue. Thirteen other massacres in the past ten years in Australia and New Zealand, where between five and 13 victims died, were apparently not horrendous enough to motivate political courage. Neither were the 522 gun deaths in Australia in 1994, dominated by suicides and domestic killings.

Many Australians have found the pandering to the gun lobby to be the low-water mark of Australian politics. Many are also bracing for the excuses. Let's rehearse some of the main ones.

"Killers will always get guns." Britain's tough gun laws didn't stop Dunblane, they argue. But no laws will eliminate all gun violence. Just as our internationally acclaimed policies on road deaths have given us our lowest ever road toll, John Howard's proposals will almost certainly reduce gun violence in Australia.

"Restrict military-style guns, OK. But most models of semi-automatic rifle are not dangerous." Not true. Although two-thirds of the victims of local mass shootings were shot with military-style semi-automatic rifles using "high power" centrefire ammunition designed for the battlefield, a large proportion also died at the hands of men wielding the most common semi-automatic rifle of them all: the ubiquitous .22 calibre "bunny gun". Although these fire "low-power" rimfire rounds, .22 semi-automatic rifles have been used as the principal weapon in four mass shootings in Australia and New Zealand. The police killed at Crescent Head were shot by such a gun.

"Victoria has gun registration&nbps;.&nbps;.&nbps;.&nbps;tens of thousands of gun owners refuse to register their guns." Oh really? Without registration, no one knows how many guns are in the community. If the gun lobby claims to know the size of this group, and claims to represent law-abiding shooters, why doesn't it report them? The gun lobby likes to talk up the number of shooters and guns in the community. My files on John Tingle's utterances on unlicensed shooters in New South Wales include "half a million" (11 July 1995) "as high as 700,000" (13 July 1995), and "as many as 750,000" (8 August 1995) –

a 50 percent growth in less than a month! Ted Drane of the Sporting Shooters' Association said on Channel 7 this week that there were "2 to 3 million" shooters in Australia, which means nearly one in four is said to have guns. Yet the New South Wales Health Department's recent survey found that only 11.7 percent of those interviewed reported a gun in their house. This translates to some 250,000 houses in a state with 32 percent of the national population. And if many lied, having refused to be licensed, are we not entitled to ask why?

"Many won't register their guns." Some, often with criminal intent, don't register their cars, boats or vicious dogs either. So do we hear a call for the abandonment of car registration? Registration will only work if it is accompanied by a high-profile confidential hotline, like Operation Noah for drugs, where people can report those they know who are keeping illegal guns. Penalties for possession of unregistered guns after the amnesty period must also be spectacular and police directed to take all reports seriously. Anything less will be an abject failure.

"Let's have a prohibited persons register." The gun lobby argues that 99.9 percent of gun owners are totally law-abiding: leave us alone and crack down on criminals and the mentally ill, they argue. If there are a million gun owners in the country, by the gun lobby's own rhetoric this means there are 1,000 who are dangerous. The AMA's code of ethics already allows doctors to report those who endanger the community, whether it be the poorly sighted who refuse to stop driving or the shooter who exhibits violent intent. However, prior to Martin Bryant, Australia and New Zealand's 13 gun massacres in which five or more people died resulted in 92 deaths. Seventy-one (88 percent) of the victims in these incidents were killed by someone with no record of mental illness. Besides further stigmatising the mentally ill, a register of the mentally suspect would still allow the majority of potential killers to get guns.

"How can we possibly fund a buy-back?" Yacht owners pay mooring fees. Recreational pilots pay landing fees. Car drivers pay licence fees, hefty registration and parking fees. The users pay. It is likely that there will be many more legal guns remaining in the community than the semi-automatics that the prime minister wants recalled. These hundreds of thousands of legal guns that will remain will each need to be registered. Some would argue, "Why should their owners escape the sort of fees that are standard and accepted for other user groups?" If each gun cost, say, a one-off $300 to register, a pool of money would gather that would more than pay for the one-off buy-back of prohibited weapons. Such a fee for each gun will give many pause to wonder if they really want to keep a gun. However, being a voluntary "tax", it may motivate many shooters to ignore registration. A rise in sales tax on new guns and on all ammunition should therefore be considered.

The buy-back should also have extended to guns not proposed to be banned. There will be many with single shotguns who will be inspired by Port Arthur to hand them in. A buy-back incentive can only increase this response.

John Howard has shown remarkable leadership in setting an uncompromising minimum standard for reform. New South Wales premier Bob Carr, leader of the Opposition Peter Collins and leader of the National Party Ian Armstrong's belated common ground has neutralised the Shooters' Party. New South Wales Farmers, through Ian Dungess, has given its support to a total ban on semi-automatics. All that remains is for you to fulfil the will of over 90 percent of the community who want strong gun laws.

17
150 ways (and counting) that the nanny state is good for us

Those who use the epithet "nanny state" almost always do it pejoratively. But everyone in public health knows how important so many of our laws, regulations and product safety standards are in protecting us from a vast array of life-ending and life-ruining consequences that remain all too common in nations with rudimentary or non-existent consumer protections and public health regulatory systems. I wrote this piece after sending an email to all staff in my school, inviting them to give me examples of such measures. I stopped at 150 but could easily have gone on for much longer. I've had many, many people thank me for writing this one.

In February 1985, the *Age* reported that at least three Australian children had been disembowelled in the previous two years after sitting on swimming pool skimmer-box covers shaped like children's seats. Before the advent of mandatory shatterproof safety glass for showers, over the years many people suffered major lacerations and occasionally died after bathroom accidents. Before 2008, it was legal for fast-buck retailers to sell children's nightwear that could easily catch fire: many children were

Originally published as Chapman, Simon (2013). One hundred and fifty ways the nanny state is good for us. *The Conversation*, 2 July.

hideously burnt and scarred for life. Random breath testing was first introduced in 1976, to the chagrin of the Australian Hotels Association.[1] In New South Wales it was followed by "an immediate 90 percent decline in road deaths, which soon stabilized at a rate approximately 22 percent lower than the average for the previous six years".

These are just four of many examples of changes to laws, regulations, mandatory product standards and public awareness campaigns that were introduced following lobbying from health advocates. With these, as with nearly every campaign to clip the wings of those with the primitive ethics of a cash register, there was protracted resistance. I was a board member of *Choice* magazine for 20 years and lost count of the number of times manufacturers staunchly resisted voluntarily making changes to their dangerous, ineffective or substandard products.

These bans and brakes on personal and commercial freedoms are routinely ridiculed as the interventionist screechings of that reviled harridan, the nanny state. And the cathedral of the anti-nanny state in Australia is the Institute of Public Affairs (IPA). One of its high priests is Tim Wilson, who pumps out an incontinent flow of the doctrine regularly on ABC's *The Drum* and in numerous blogs and op-eds.

Similar attacks once rained down on Edwin Chadwick, the architect of the first Public Health Act in England in 1848. He proposed the first regulatory measures to control overcrowding, drinking-water quality, sewage disposal and building standards. After he was sacked for his trouble the *Times* gloated: "We prefer to take our chance with cholera and the rest than be bullied into health. There is nothing a man hates so much as being cleansed against his will, or having his floors swept, his walls whitewashed, his pet dung heaps cleared away." And yet on the 150th anniversary of the Public Health Act a *British Medical Journal* poll saw his invention of civic hygiene, and all of its regulations, voted as the most significant advance in public health of all time.

In May this year, Wilson, Australia's champion of contemporary pet-dung-heap rights, railed that "Nanny state critics understand that incremental attacks on our freedom to choose are single steps down a longer road to remove individual choice and responsibility."[2] He wrote

---

1   http://bit.ly/2cLclD6.

of the "rising groundswell of Australians who are sick of increasing local, state and federal government regulations of their choices"; denied that people like him want to "selfishly put their wants above the safety and happiness of others"; and argued that we should all "learn to manage risk through our choices" and that it is not "the job of government to coddle us from the world's evils, avoid risk and use taxes, laws and regulations to either steer or direct our behaviour".

The IPA has academic pretentions and calls its associates "fellows". But it has not the first idea about academic principles like funding transparency, and refuses to name its corporate sponsors (which include British American Tobacco[3]). It has an infamous list of 75 policies[4] and institutions it would like to see abolished. These include the Australian Consumer and Competition Commission, the Australian National Preventive Health Agency, renewable energy targets, plain cigarette packaging and the alcopops taxes, and mandatory food labelling.

Those, like Wilson, opposed to state intervention in markets subscribe to often-unarticulated social Darwinist values that imply that those with the misfortune to be killed, injured or made chronically ill by their participation in untrammelled marketplaces had it coming to them. The unregulated marketplace and community is a kind of noble jungle where the fittest survive thanks to their better education and judgement in their consumer choices, and to their better ability to pay for superior, less dodgy products, to keep up repairs on their cars and homes, and to get employment in work that is not dangerous or toxic. Children living in poorer housing near busy roads in the leaded-petrol era had only their parents to blame for their lead-lowered IQs: they didn't have to live there! When a toddler drowned in a backyard pool before mandatory pool fencing laws, it was the fault of the feckless parents for not being more vigilant, and nothing to do with the failure of government to mandate the cost of a fence as part of the cost of a pool. When kids ingested lead or other heavy metals from dodgy toys when these were legal, their parents should have just done their homework and not bought them.

---

2   Wilson 2013a.
3   http://bit.ly/2ciSu2h.
4   Roskam, Paterson and Berg 2012.

Those who can't keep up find their way into national health statistics, where, across almost every area of public health, the poor and less educated have higher rates of disease, injury, major disease risk factors and death.

Below is a big list of nanny state coddlings and protections that a profoundly ignorant Wilson would say are "rarely supported by credible research".[5] I stopped at 150 and could have doubled, tripled or even quadrupled the list. We don't hear much from the IPA and its ilk on any of these because they are all immensely popular, taken-for-granted safeguards on our health, safety and quality of life. Other countries are climbing over themselves to emulate many of these as best practice. Australia is one of the healthiest nations on earth. The precious freedoms that they "erode" are almost always trivial, and the industries that were regulated (with some exceptions, like asbestos and hopefully tobacco) reluctantly rolled over and still make money, now from safer products and procedures. No one could care less that their "choice" to buy leaded petrol has been removed, or that women are being "coddled" by the criminalisation of domestic violence. Only the most rapacious libertarians swoon at the unregulated, let-it-rip free market that would wind back the clock of civil society many decades if unleashed by their ideology.

So, a public invitation to the IPA: which of these 150 heinous intrusions on people's freedoms and the right to unbridled commerce does it wish to see abolished?[6]

Access to drugs	(1)	Drug scheduling
	(2)	Pharmaceutical Benefits Scheme
Access to healthcare	(3)	Compulsory third-party motor injury insurance
	(4)	Medicare
Alcohol control	(5)	Minimum legal drinking age
	(6)	Responsible serving of alcohol
Building standards	(7)	Balustrade and railing-height regulations

---

5   Wilson 2013b.
6   Links to more information about each of the 150 examples below can be found here in the original article: http://bit.ly/2cLcpCX.

	(8)	Elevator standards and inspection requirements
	(9)	Fire-safety building regulations
	(10)	Floor-space provision to prevent overcrowding
	(11)	Mandatory smoke alarms
	(12)	Mandatory swimming pool fences
	(13)	Maximum water-temperature regulation
	(14)	Safety-glass standards
	(15)	Swimming pool skimmer-box standards
	(16)	Mandatory residual current devices (electricity)
Cancer control	(17)	Sunsmart regulations for schools and daycare centres
Child protection	(18)	Background checks for staff working with children
	(19)	Child pornography laws
	(20)	Mandatory reporting of child protection incidents
Congenital malformation prevention	(21)	Folate fortification
Dental health	(22)	Fluoridation of water
Disability	(23)	Disability parking permits
Disease management	(24)	Mosquito control
	(25)	Cancer registries
Drug control	(26)	Pseudoephedrine pharmacy controls
	(27)	Regulation of illicit drugs
	(28)	Pharmaceutical drug regulation
Emergency services	(29)	24-hour emergency services phone lines
	(30)	24-hour poisons information service
Environmental health	(31)	Backyard burning controls
	(32)	Burial standards
	(33)	Air-quality standards controlling industrial emissions into the air
	(34)	Controls on industrial discharges into rivers
	(35)	Emission controls on cars

(36) Lead in paint banned

(37) Lead in petrol banned

(38) Legionella control standards for cooling towers

(39) Petrol and diesel fuel standards (for emission controls)

(40) Planning regulations around open spaces

(41) Recycled water standards for reuse applications

(42) Septic-tank standards

(43) Sewage discharge standards

(44) Storm-water drainage

Farm safety (45) Tractor rollover harm reduction

Food safety (46) Abattoir standards

(47) Food-additive labelling

(48) Food-allergy labelling

(49) Food-handling standards

(50) Food standards (many)

(51) Regulation of genetically modified organisms

(52) Pasteurisation of milk

(53) Publication of the names of filthy restaurants

(54) Regulation of food additives

(55) Regulation of food-store refrigerator temperatures

Health promotion (56) Mandatory physical education in schools

(57) Mandatory school canteen standards

(58) Rights to breastfeed in public places

Infection control (59) "Blood rules" in sport

(60) Autoclaving of dental equipment

(61) Bans on public spitting, urination and defecation

(62) Chlorinated water supplies

(63) Dog faeces disposal

(64) Drinking-water quality A124 standards

(65) Immunisation standards and infrastructure

(66) Infection-control standards and protocols

(67) Legalisation of brothels

	(68)	Mandatory immunisation for healthcare workers
	(69)	Mandatory sewerage and sanitation in urban areas
	(70)	Notifiable disease laws
	(71)	Sex-worker health checks
	(72)	Sharps disposal and blood-borne virus controls
	(73)	Skin penetration legislation for hairdressers, dentists, tattooists and body piercing
	(74)	Veterinary and animal-husbandry standards
	(75)	Water standards in public swimming pools
Information control	(76)	Advertising standards
Mental health	(77)	Mental-health scheduling
Occupational health	(78)	Workers' compensation
and safety	(79)	Asbestos building ban
	(80)	Dust standards
	(81)	Hard hats
	(82)	Harness standards
	(83)	Noise standards
	(84)	Personal protective equipment regulations
	(85)	Scaffolding standards
	(86)	Smoke-free workplaces
	(87)	Asbestos removal standards
Product safety	(88)	Condom standards
	(89)	Controls and bans on the use of lead and other heavy metals in toys
	(90)	Myriad of standards, bans, recalls, etc
Professional	(91)	Standards for childcare facilities
standards	(92)	Continuing medical education for medical professionals
	(93)	Licensing of healthcare facilities
	(94)	Medical and allied health-worker registration
	(95)	Nursing home regulation
Public amenity	(96)	Noise regulations

Public safety	(97) Agricultural and industrial chemicals regulation
	(98) Child-resistant cigarette lighters
	(99) Child-resistant medical packaging
	(100) Design rules for babies' cots to reduce the risk of asphyxiation
	(101) Dog licensing
	(102) Engineering standards for roads and bridges
	(103) Extraordinary powers under the *Public Health Act* to deal with emergencies
	(104) Gun laws
	(105) Hair-dryer standards to prevent bath electrocution
	(106) Hazard reduction in children's playgrounds
	(107) Mandatory standards for children's nightwear
	(108) Registration and control of pesticide use
	(109) Poisons Act
	(110) Poisons labelling
	(111) Quarantine Act
	(112) Reduced ignition-propensity cigarettes
	(113) Regulations around provision of footpaths
	(114) Safety standards for fitness and leisure equipment
	(115) Sunglasses standards
	(116) Total fire bans
	(117) Toy standards
Radiation control	(118) Regulation of the carriage and transport of radiated material
	(119) Dental X-ray equipment standards
	(120) Sun-bed bans
	(121) Uniformity in the control of radiation use
Road safety	(122) Air bags in cars
	(123) Mandatory bicycle helmets
	(124) Double demerit points
	(125) Drink-driving penalties

(126) Breath-alcohol ignition interlock devices for repeat drink-driving offenders

(127) Energy-absorbing steering columns

(128) Graduated driver licensing schemes

(129) Infant and child vehicle seat restraints

(130) Mandatory motorcycle helmets

(131) Motorcycle helmet standards

(132) Motor vehicle design standards

(133) Pedestrian crossings

(134) Provisional and learner drivers' licensing

(135) Random breath testing

(136) Seatbelts in cars and school buses

(137) Speed limits

(138) Speed limits near schools

(139) Standards for medical assessment of fitness to drive

(140) Third brake lights on cars

(141) Traffic regulation in general

(142) Vehicle roadworthiness inspections

(143) Dedicated bicycle lanes

Tobacco control　　(144) Health warnings on tobacco products

(145) Outlawing "light" and "mild" descriptors on tobacco

(146) Plain packaging of tobacco

(147) Smoke-free public transport

(148) Bans on tobacco sales to minors

(149) Tobacco tax

Violence control　　(150) Criminalising domestic violence

18

Tardis travelling into David Leyonhjelm's post-nanny state dystopia

David Leyonhjelm is a senator in the Australian parliament who by his own public admission owed his first tenure there, from 1 July 2014 until 1 July 2016, to having had the fortune to be drawn in the lottery for the coveted number-one position on the senate ballot paper and fronting a party with a name (the Liberal Democrats) that would have confused many political inattentives into thinking they were voting for the Liberal Party. Leyonhjelm is a "conviction libertarian" who, on principle, appeared to oppose anything that diminished even the most trivial of personal freedoms. During his first term he let all manner of lunacy off the leash. Perhaps my favourite was an item defending battery caging of chickens in which he argued: "Those pushing for much lower densities are motivated either by animal rights arguments (not the same as animal welfare) or visions of hens happily wandering in green pastures. There is a very strong anthropomorphic aspect to these; that is, they are based on the question: 'How would you like to live at that density?' What they overlook is that it only takes a visit to a sporting event to see that humans choose to congregate at high

Originally published as Chapman, Simon (2015). Tardis travelling into David Leyonhjelm's post-nanny state dystopia. *The Conversation*, 1 July.

densities. And when they do, not everyone goes outside for some peace and quiet" (*Farm Online*, 8 July 2015). I wrote this piece soon after he commenced a Senate witch-hunt into the nanny state.

Australian Liberal Democrat Senator David Leyonhjelm is a "conviction libertarian". He loathes excess government regulation, bureaucracy and taxes. He'd also like to see Australians able to carry concealed weapons[1] unrestricted, as is allowed in six US states. This, he argues with his compelling logic, would help prevent the sort of gun massacres[2] that occur so often in the USA, but have not occurred once in Australia in the 19 years since the 1996 law reforms that banned the semi-automatic firearms favoured by those intent on killing many people quickly.

He readily admits his place in the Senate is largely due to luck,[3] having drawn the coveted first "donkey vote" place on the ballot paper at the last election. This political equivalent of Steven Bradbury, the Australian speed skater who in 2002 won an Olympic gold medal after all of his opponents fell over,[4] is currently enjoying the fruits of heavy-duty courtship from the government, as it seeks to secure the cross-bench support essential for the passage of its legislation through the Senate.

Leyonhjelm has expressed great concern about the globally discredited health hazards of wind farms, but has grasped $35,000 for his party from the Philip Morris tobacco company,[5] the second largest contributor to a global death toll from tobacco predicted to cause a billion deaths this century.

His libertarian philosophical footwork allows him to wave away any apparent inconsistency here. He subscribes to John Stuart Mill's principle[6] that people should be allowed to do anything as long as

---

1 http://bit.ly/2cItrER.
2 Follman, Aronsen and Pan 2016.
3 Colebatch 2013.
4 http://bit.ly/1d5GgCW.
5 Bourke and Cox 2014.
6 http://stanford.io/2cLck1K.

they are not harming others in the exercise of their freedoms. What he counts as harm appears to change from issue to issue.

On 24 August, submissions will close on another Senate enquiry, which Leyonhjelm will head, into what he's promoting as an anti-nanny-state regulation pogrom.[7] Much of this is likely to be air cover for him to grease the political rails for his tobacco industry benefactors to break down barriers to market e-cigarettes in Australia, with one of his senior advisors, Helen Dale (formerly Demidenko[8]), having recently attended a small meeting of vaping activists in Poland. Some focus will be given to bicycle helmets, cannabis, tobacco and pornography, but the terms of reference don't hold back and include attention to "any other measures introduced to restrict personal choice 'for the individual's own good'".[9]

Car seatbelts and motorcycle helmets are the apotheosis of "for your own good" paternalistic health legislation, and so for consistency should be under threat too, as may be decades of hard-fought consumer protection legislation that keeps shonky and unsafe goods out of the charmed circle of free consumer choice.

Leyonhjelm's veneration of choice naturally extends to the freedom to do dangerous and very unhealthy things. But his antibodies to corporate regulation and even to public warning signs (on 29 June he told SBS TV that of nanny-state intrusions, "Probably one of the silliest ones is signs") together form a toxic mixture of corporate indifference to health consequences, and efforts to minimise the information environment for consumers to make informed choices. The social Darwinist philosophy here is that consumers who are stupid enough to make unwise choices, including those shaped by their economic disadvantage, deserve what's coming to them. The noble consumer is the intelligent one with the wherewithal to research health information unencumbered by annoying ingredient labelling, warning labels or imposed health and safety standards.

---

7   Stokes 2015.
8   http://bit.ly/2cAUO2J.
9   http://bit.ly/1HkKRA3.

So let us climb briefly aboard a time-travelling Tardis for a taste of what life in the future might be like in Leyonhjelm's utopia. A couple of examples might give us the flavour.

Arriving at Bondi Beach in the aftermath of a storm surge, we find that a massive surf is running, but we notice that there are no signs about the beach being closed. A tourist is being resuscitated, clinging to life, while two others lie dead beside her. All warning signs have gone in the Leyonhjelm utopia, including the age-old flagging of lifesaver-patrolled areas.

But there are no lifesavers, either. A Liberal Democrat spokesman explains: "We helped Australians come to see that lifesavers were the archetypal nannies: telling us where we had to swim and blowing their annoying whistles at people who were exercising their choice to swim where they pleased. We didn't mind them rescuing people when they got into trouble, but we drew the line at them trying to prevent people getting into dangerous rips, so they had to go."

We learn that the burns and emergency units in all hospitals (long since privatised) have tripled in size to cope with the increased demand. Laws regulating the maximum domestic water temperature were repealed after the party's spin-meisters began repeating an old but prescient tobacco industry line: "Pretty soon these people will want to adjust the water temperature of your shower because they know what's good for you". The repeal was soon followed by a spike in emergency admissions of bath- and shower-scalded children, many scarred for life. Cheap water heaters have flooded in and the victim-blaming rhetoric of slack parenting is given a megaphoned workout by fellow-travelling shock jocks.

The good old days of cheap non-safety-glass shower screens are also back. The wealthy and intelligent can get the safety glass but the poor and ill-informed take their chances. Many suffer major injuries when slipping in showers.

My list of 150 ways that nanny-state legislation is good for us has become the legislative hit-list. Much credit for the shredding of public health regulation went to Leyonhjelm's senior staff member Helen Dale, who got traction for her observation on Twitter that it made good economic sense for people to die early ("Evidence is unhealthy choices are cheaper for the state – the person dies instead of staying on life support").[10]

The party spokesman tells us: "Helen correctly pointed out that tobacco is a great commodity because it kills so many people toward the end of their working lives but before they start being an economic dead weight. But we soon thought, hang on, the very same reasoning can be applied to just about everything that kills people before they start to need serious healthcare. So we expanded our deregulatory vision and targeted anything that might help the state in this way. Someone unkindly pointed out that some nasty regimes in history took a pretty similar attitude to the aged, infirm and disabled. But we always need to be true to our principles."

*

Every person who has had their life saved or quality of life enhanced by the nanny-state laws, regulations and standards should flood Leyonhjelm's inquiry with personal accounts that will flavour those that will be submitted by agencies and experts, who will send him data on why Australia is today among the world's healthiest and safest nations, thanks to nanny.

---

10   http://bit.ly/2cIN8uE.

19
Torture by omission

When you are in severe pain, little else matters until you find
relief from that pain. So why is relief from pain not a basic
human right?

In 1809, 47-year-old Jane Crawford risked scalping and the tomahawk
to ride her horse 60 miles in four days to the practice of Dr Ephraim
McDowell in Danville, Kentucky. Mrs Crawford's ovarian tumour was
giving her unremitting, labour-like pain. While several men held
Crawford's arms and legs and she recited psalms, McDowell took 25
minutes to cut a 14-centimetre incision in her lower belly, remove a
1.2-kilogram tumour and then sew her up with interrupted sutures.
Outside the house, an angry and incredulous mob, not unlike those
who would today seek to close heroin injecting rooms that minister to
a different sort of pain, waited, ready to lynch McDowell should his
patient die. Five days later she was out of bed and lived for another 30
years. McDowell's pioneering operation and his patient's courage are
historical landmarks in the annals of surgery.

While opium and cocaine have been used since antiquity for pain
relief, it was not until 1846, when Thomas Morton first used ether to

Originally published as Chapman, Simon (1999). Torture by omission. *Sydney
Morning Herald*, 18 September.

anaesthetise a patient for a tooth extraction, that lengthy and detailed surgery more subtle than crude hacking could be performed under general anaesthesia. The next year, chloroform was used for the first time to relieve pain in childbirth and went on to become the anaesthetic of choice for more than a century. Today, pain management specialists estimate that more than 90 percent of postsurgical, post-trauma and cancer pain can be fully relieved, and 75 percent of chronic, non-cancer pain such as arthritis. Thirty years ago, these figures hovered around 10 percent. Worldwide, though, only half of those suffering from these conditions have access to services and drugs that can provide this relief.

Proust wrote that "Illness is the doctor to whom we pay most heed; to kindness, to knowledge, we make promises only; pain we obey." People in pain are preoccupied by the experience. Pain bulldozes all emotions aside, including hope. Yet pain produces a bewildering range of ambivalence. While aspirin and paracetamol are the most commonly used drugs, and around one in five people experience pain that has lasted longer than three months, so often we conspire to deny the reality of pain. We feel obliged to cheer the injured footballer who returns to the fray after losing teeth or being knocked unconscious. Many couples make a virtue out of refusing pain relief in childbirth. While a woman begs for an epidural, her husband gently counsels, "Remember we agreed . . . no drugs". Many who have lived with pain tell of the scepticism of others ("You don't *look* like you're in pain") but also of the subtle imperatives to stop their misery infecting those around them. Anglo and Asian women tend to be stoic in childbirth, while southern European and Arabic women are uninhibited in their expression. Moralists, including many in medicine, have often denied the dying sufficient morphine, fretting that they might become addicted.

Recently, television allowed us to consider the abandoned Serbian torture chamber, where unspeakable degradations were wrought on its Kosovar captives. Torture is the active infliction of pain on its unwilling victims. Professor Michael Cousins, head of the Pain Management Research Centre at Sydney's Royal North Shore Hospital, describes unrelieved pain as "torture by omission". The United Nations Declaration of Human Rights codifies civilised society's most basic standards and aspirations for its citizens. Yet as Cousins points out, the

Declaration says nothing about the most elemental concern of all: the right to be relieved from pain.

This remarkable omission is a testimony to our ambivalence about pain. Its consequence is that pain management as a medical speciality lives a Cinderella existence, shining occasionally as an island of enlightenment in a sea of misery. The most recent and exciting developments involve discoveries about the way that damaged nerve endings sprout pain fibres, the growth of which can be inhibited; the pain can then be controlled through drugs administered through surgically implanted mini pumps. People who have lived for years in desperate pain are now being assisted to live largely pain-free lives again through such developments. Yet there are only seven pain management training centres in Australia, and for all the pious political talk of the need for palliative care after the overturning of the Northern Territory euthanasia legislation, cruelly token budgets have found their way into health expenditure in the period since.

As historically unprecedented falls in fecundity, better living standards and the successes of public health combine to cause the age distribution of the world's populations to balloon increasingly to the right of the graph, more people will live with the pain of chronic degenerative conditions and cancer. Despite this, the disabling and all-absorbing nature of pain often militates against its victims becoming potent advocates for pain relief to be declared a basic human right, and all that would flow from this. If Cousins' and his colleagues' mission were to succeed, what a gift to the world this would be.

20

It's the government's call over phone tower debate

In the 1990s, risk-o-phobics had a field day, hyperventilating their anxieties about the proliferation of mobile phone transmission towers. These were obviously going to cause . . . well, just name any disease of concern here. With Sonia Wutzke, I wrote about the predictability of this upsurge in health fears in Chapman and Wutzke 1997. Today this anxiety has all but disappeared, as it has done for each successive wave of technological panics that has arisen since electricity and the household phone excited concern in the late 19th century.

Local councils in Sydney have struggled to respond to growing resident action about the placement of mobile phone towers across their municipalities. Recently I received a letter from one informing me about decisions regarding minimum distances towers can be located from people.

Note here that it is "distances" not "distance". If you live in the council district, the council will not allow a tower within 300 metres of your house. But it you work in the area, the towers can come as close as specified in any deal struck between your employer or a landowner

Originally published as Chapman, Simon (1997). It's the government's call over phone tower debate. *Sydney Morning Herald*, 6 March.

and a phone company. They can plonk one right outside your office or factory window, in your car park, wherever. The council wrote that it had taken "potential health impact" into account in fashioning its resolutions. From this, we can draw one of two conclusions: that the council believes people at work are somehow more robust than people in houses in resisting the alleged health effects of radio frequency radiation (RFR) emitting from the towers; or that it finds this a preposterous idea and instead believes that workers are less uptight about exposure than residents and won't mind a cosier acquaintance with a tower or two. What the thousands who work and live in the area are supposed to make of this is anyone's guess.

But wait, there is more. If you are in a school, any sort of childcare facility, a hospital or, most intriguingly, an aged-care centre or "any recreational facility", you won't find a tower within 450 metres of you. Observe that yet further layers have now been added to this emerging hierarchical model of radiation susceptibility.

Someone playing golf, bowls or having a picnic apparently cannot resist RFR like a worker can. Along with infants, children, the sick and the elderly, those taking recreation get to enjoy an extra 150 metres buffer zone. Or at least while the kids are in daycare or school. When they go home in the afternoon, the council thinks it's OK to locate the towers up to 150 metres closer. Given that children spend more time at home than in school, the two different minimum distances cannot reflect any rational concern to minimum exposure.

If, and this is a very big if, there is any demonstrable health risk from phone tower RFR, this risk is almost certainly not acute, but medium to long term and small by any ordinary sense of the word "risky". If there is any group which would escape the health consequences of exposure it is the very old, who, to put it bluntly, won't be around to suffer any consequences. So lumping the elderly in nursing homes in the same category as infants in daycare suggests the intriguing possibility that there might be a hotbed of reincarnationism inside the council. Curiouser and curiouser.

During the 1995 debate about the towers near a kindergarten in Harbord, an angry parent jabbed his finger in the air at hapless Telstra officials and told them, "There's no way that even if there's [RFR at] even one hundred millionth of the Australian standard that I'm going to let my little girl go to that place and be exposed to that sort of risk. No way!" This vignette says a great deal about the debate on phone towers. It suggests that when it comes to anything industrial, imposed and close to populations perceived as vulnerable, many in the community demand zero risk – a notion that of course does not exist anywhere but in the minds of totally risk-averse people. These dimensions to the debate have nothing to do with the actual hazard but are in every way as "real" and measurable as the RFR itself. Just ask the nervous members of local councils struggling to accommodate them.

In all probability, this particular council's bizarre resolutions may go some way towards assuaging community concerns, in that it has incorporated distinctions between domestic and industrial exposure and between population groups generally considered "vulnerable" and the (residential) population at large. Many, on hearing that towers can be located nearer factories and homes than childcare centres, will assume this to be a sensible policy despite its rampant internal contradictions.

Instead, the misplaced precision of the guidelines reflects a confused interpretation of both what we know about the true level of risk over the long term (not much, but equally, not a cacophony of ominous warning bells either) and of risk communication principles. The starting point of any sane policy would place the towers equidistant from any residence, workplace or gathering place.

But the unsung side of the health debate about mobile phone towers has nothing to do with any possible effects from radiation. There are countless examples that can be given of mobile phones being used to call for help – breakdowns on freeways and isolated roads where danger was imminent; calling ambulances to attend the injured; people fearing assault and rape; families who give an elderly relative who is prone to wander a phone so he or she can be traced – not to mention the health-promoting aspects of allowing ordinary, often unexceptional contact between people. "I just called to say I love you". Any decisions by governments that reduce the reach of the mobile phone net which claim to be driven by public health concerns must factor in the loss of such health benefits, and balance these against the estimates of what even the doomsayers calculate as modest rises in dreaded diseases like cancer.

The prospect of the farce I have described being repeated in different versions throughout Australia cries out for leadership from Canberra and from the phone companies. With Australia having the highest rate of mobile phone ownership in the world and indecent levels of profit being made by suppliers, would a major public consultation and education campaign be too much to ask for?

21

No, we're not all being pickled in deadly radiation from smartphones and wi-fi

I've long been interested in low-risk threats to health that cause panic and outrage in some parts of the community. There's a fascinating branch of social medicine focused on the study of "modern health worries", and to the ways these spread and then die out. "Electrosensitives" are people who believe they are highly sensitive to electromagnetic radiation and believe they are adversely affected by ubiquitous sources of this such as radio and television signals, mobile phones and transmission towers, wi-fi, wireless microphones and smart electricity meters. In 2016, I published a paper with colleagues looking at the incidence of brain cancers (cancers that EMR-phobics argue are increasing because of this exposure) (Chapman, Azizi et al. 2016). We found no evidence of any increase across 29 years that could be plausibly attributed to mobile phones.

Tomorrow at TedX Sydney's Opera House event, high-profile neurosurgeon Charlie Teo will talk about brain cancer. Last Saturday Teo was on Channel 9's *Sunrise* program talking about the often

Originally published as Chapman, Simon (2015). No, we're not all being pickled in deadly radiation from smartphones and wi-fi. *The Conversation*, 20 May.

malignant cancer that in 2012 killed 1,241 Australians. During the program he said:

> Unfortunately the jury is still out on whether mobile phones can lead to brain cancer, but studies suggest it's so.

Teo's name appears on a submission[1] recently sent to the United Nations. If you Google "Charlie Teo and mobile phones", you will see that his public statements on this issue go back years.
The submission he signed commences:

> We are scientists engaged in the study of biological and health effects of non-ionizing electromagnetic fields (EMF). Based upon peer-reviewed, published research, we have serious concerns regarding the ubiquitous and increasing exposure to EMF generated by electric and wireless devices. These include – but are not limited to – radiofrequency radiation (RFR) emitting devices, such as cellular and cordless phones and their base stations, wi-fi, broadcast antennas, smart meters, and baby monitors as well as electric devices and infra-structures [sic] used in the delivery of electricity that generate extremely-low frequency electromagnetic field (ELF EMF).

That list just about covers off every facet of modern life: the internet, phones, radio, television and any smart technology. It's a list the Amish and reclusive communities of "wi-fi refugees"[2] know all about.
Other than those living in the remotest of remote locations, there are very few in Australia today who are not bathed in electromagnetic fields and radiofrequency radiation, 24 hours a day. My mobile phone shows me that my house is exposed to the wi-fi systems of six neighbours' houses as well as my own. Public wi-fi hotspots are rapidly increasing.[3]
The first mobile phone call in Australia was made over 28 years ago, on 23 February 1987. In December 2013, there were some 30.2 million

1 http://bit.ly/2d4EeeA.
2 O'Brien and Danzico 2011.
3 The Research and Analysis section 2014.

mobile phones being used in a population of 22.7 million people.[4] Predictions are that there will be 5.9 billion smartphone users globally within four years.[5] There are now more than 100 nations which have more mobile phones than people.

So while Australia has become saturated in electromagnetic field radiation over the past quarter century, what has happened to cancer rates? Brain cancer is Teo's surgical speciality and the cancer site that attracts nearly all of the mobile phone panic attention. In 1987 the age-adjusted incidence rate of brain cancer in Australia per 100,000 people was 6.6. In 2011, the most recent year for which national data is available, the rate was 7.3.

The graph below shows brain cancer incidence has all but flat-lined across the 29 years for which data are available.[6] All cancer is notifiable in Australia.

Age-standardised incidence rate by year

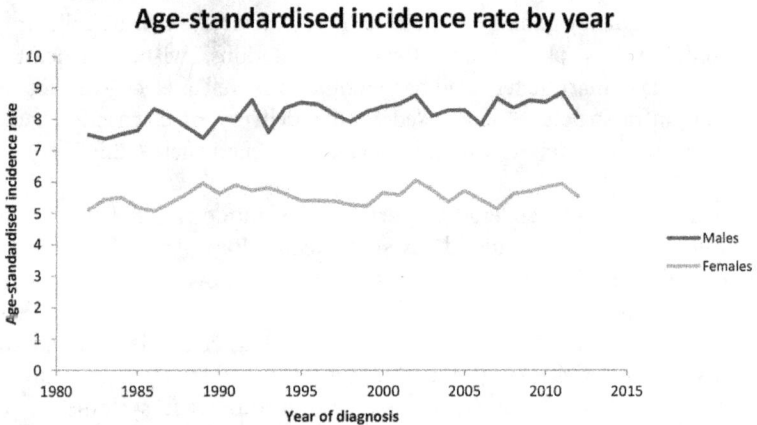

Figure 21.1 New cases of brain cancer in Australia, 1982 to 2011 (age-adjusted). Australian Institute of Health and Welfare, CC BY.

4 http://bit.ly/2cATCfM.
5 Worstall 2014.
6 http://bit.ly/2cURBuO.

Brain cancers are a relatively uncommon group of cancers: their 7.3 per 100,000 incidence compares with female breast (116), colorectal (61.5) and lung cancer (42.5). There is no epidemic of brain cancer, let alone brain cancer caused by mobile phones. The Cancer Council explicitly rejects the link.[7] A US National Cancer Institute fact sheet summarises current research, highlighting rather different conclusions than Charlie Teo.[8]

Another Australian signatory of the submission, Priyanka Bandara, describes herself as an "Independent Environmental Health Educator/ Researcher; Advisor, Environmental Health Trust and Doctors for Safer Schools". Last year, a former student of mine asked to meet with me to discuss wi-fi on our university campus. She arrived at my office with Bandara, who looked worried as she ran an EMF meter over my room. I was being pickled in it, apparently.

Her pitch to me was one I have encountered many times before. The key ingredients are that there are now lots of highly credentialed scientists who are deeply concerned about a particular problem, here wi-fi. These scientists have published [pick a very large number] of "peer-reviewed" research papers about the problem.

Peer review often turns out to mean having like-minded people from their networks, typically with words like "former", "leading", "senior" next to their names, write gushing appraisals of often unpublished reports.

The neo-Galilean narrative then moves to how this information is all being suppressed by the web of influence of vested industrial interests. These interests are arranging for scientists to be sacked, suppressing publication of alarming reports, and preventing many scientists from speaking out in fear.

Case reports of individuals claiming to be harmed and suffering Old Testament-length lists of symptoms as a result of exposure are then publicised. Here's one[9] for smart meters, strikingly similar to the 240+

---

7   "Mobile Phones Do Not Cause Brain Cancer – Cancer Council NSW." 2014.
8   "Cell Phones and Cancer Risk." 2016.
9   Powell 2015.

symptom list[10] for "wind turbine syndrome". Almost any symptom is attributed to exposure.

Historical parallels with the conduct of the tobacco and asbestos industries and Big Pharma are then made. The argument runs: "We understand the history of suppression and denial with these industries, and this new issue is now experiencing the same." There is no room for considering that the claims about the new issue might be claptrap, and that the industries affected by the circulation of false and dangerous nonsense might understandably want to stamp on it.

Bandara's modest blog offers schools the opportunity to hear her message:

> Wireless technologies are sweeping across schools exposing young children to microwave radiation. This is not in line with the Precautionary Principle. A typical classroom with 25 WiFi enabled tablets/laptops (each operating at 0.2 W) generates in five hours about the same microwave radiation output as a typical microwave oven (at 800 W) in two minutes. Would you like to microwave your child for two minutes (without causing heating as it is done very slowly using lower power) daily?[11]

There can be serious consequences of alarming people about infinitesimally small, effectively non-existent risks. This rural Victorian news story features a woman so convinced that transmission towers are harming her that she covers her head in a "protective" cloth cape.[12] This woman[13] was so alarmed about the electricity smart meter at her house that she had her electricity cut off, causing her teenage daughter to study by candlelight. Yet she is shown being interviewed with a wireless microphone.

Mobile phones have played important roles in rapid response to life-saving emergencies.[14] Reducing access to wireless technology

---

10 Chapman 2016a.
11 Bandara 2015.
12 http://bit.ly/2cWh2Pr.
13 http://bit.ly/2cLbVg2.
14 Chapman and Schofield 1998.

would have incalculable effects on billions of people's lives, many profoundly negative.

Exposing people to fearful messages about wi-fi has been experimentally demonstrated to increase symptom reportage when subjects were later exposed to sham wi-fi.[15] Such fears can precipitate contact with charlatans, readily found on the internet, who will come to your house, wave meters around and frighten the gullible into purchasing magic room paint, protective clothing, bed materials and other snake oil at exorbitant prices.

As exponential improvements in technology improve the lifestyles and wellbeing of the world's population, we seem destined to witness an inexorable parallel rise in fearmongering about these benefits.

---

15   Witthöft and Rubin 2013.

22
Wind turbine sickness prevented by the money drug

In 2010 I started noticing alarmist writing about the health hazards of being exposed to wind turbines. These accounts bore all sorts of tell-tale signs that here was the latest kid on the block of non-diseases, so I was instantly captivated. This set of problems even had its own portentous sounding medical name: "wind turbine syndrome". I took a look at its provenance.

Last week an American pediatrician, Nina Pierpont, gave video evidence to a Senate inquiry into the social and economic impacts of rural wind farms.[1] Pierpont is the global medical guru for a small movement virulently opposed to wind farms because of "wind turbine syndrome", Pierpont's very own entry into the long line of doomsday claims about diseases of modernity that are said to threaten us. She calls it "an industrial plague." Plagues throughout history have killed millions, while wind turbines have so far killed no one and seem likely instead to contribute to saving hundreds of millions of lives over future

---

1   Clarke 2011.

Originally published as Chapman, Simon (2011). Wind turbine sickness prevented by the money drug. *ABC Unleashed*, 29 March.

decades through reducing greenhouse gases. So Pierpont's language gives us an immediate sense of her objectivity.

Her reputation as an authority on "wind turbine syndrome" is a 2009 self-published book[2] containing descriptions of the health problems of just ten families (38 people, 21 of them adults) in five different countries who once lived near wind turbines and who are convinced the turbines made them ill. With approximately 100,000 turbines worldwide and uncounted thousands living around them, her sample borders on homeopathic-strength representativeness.

Her book says that her research has been peer reviewed. What this means is that she showed it to people she selected and then published some of their responses, including that by Oxford University's Lord Robert May, whose subsequent public silence on the issue may suggest a re-think. Predictably, they all said her study was important. But this is a peer review process that is frankly laughable. If only independent peer review was a matter of authors selecting their own reviewers and publishing the complimentary ones.

So what are some of the problems with her research that any independent reviewer would raise? First, she says nothing about how the ten families she interviewed were selected. She says, "I chose a cluster of the most severely affected and most articulate subjects I could find." Why choose "articulate" subjects and not randomly selected residents living near wind farms? More fundamentally, why did she not make any attempt to investigate controls (people living near turbines who do not report any illness or symptoms they attribute to turbines)?

Amazingly, she interviewed them all over the phone, and did not medically examine any of her subjects nor access their medical records. So her entire "study" is based on her aggravated informants' accounts. Even here, she does not describe who among the ten families she interviewed, nor consider for a moment questions of accuracy about people giving "proxy" reports about others in their family. This is beyond sloppy.

Pierpont provides pages of information on her informants' claims about their health while living near turbines. She also provides summaries of the prevalence of various health problems in these

---

2 http://www.windturbinesyndrome.com/.

families prior to the arrival of the turbines. These are revealing. A third of the adults had current or past mental illness and a quarter had pre-existing migraine and/or permanent hearing impairment. These rates are much higher than those in the general population. In other words, her subjects were a group who are unrepresentative of the general population.

Pierpont's Australian counterpart is Sarah Laurie, an unregistered doctor who describes herself as the "medical director" of the Waubra Foundation.[3] Laurie claims that in addition to a long list of health problems, poor school performance, juvenile mental-health disturbance and acute suicidal tendencies are associated with exposure to wind farms. Like Pierpont, she has not had her claims considered by independent peer review in any publications in research journals.

Money: a highly effective antidote?

Those most exposed to wind turbines include those who have them on their land. Yet miraculously, there are no known cases of such people making claims about being adversely affected by turbines. Strangely, it is always those who see the turbines on the land of their neighbours. Money, it seems, is an astonishingly effective preventive agent in warding off wind turbine syndrome.

Landowners with topography favourable to the installation of turbines who are approached by power companies can receive substantial annual payments, apparently around $10,000 per turbine each year. A landowner with the good fortune to have 15 turbines on topographically favourable land will thus be on a nice little earner for life. But close neighbours living on unsuitable land miss out. This may cause resentment and anxiety about the impact of not having wind turbines on relative land values within rural neighbourhoods. The turbines thus become a symbol of perceived "unfairness", and features of the turbines such as the "swoosh" sound that might otherwise be unremarkable when compared to natural wind sounds become anxiety-generating preoccupations.

---

3   Second Sight 2010.

One recent Dutch study found that "people who benefit economically from wind turbines have a significantly decreased risk of annoyance, despite exposure to similar sound levels", and that "High turbine visibility enhances negative response, and having wind turbines visible from the dwelling significantly increased the risk of annoyance. Annoyance was strongly correlated with a negative attitude toward the visual impact of wind turbines on the landscape."[4]

Pierpont's book repeatedly asserts that wind energy companies require those whose land they have bought to sign gag clauses, which include not talking about any illnesses. Energy companies have bought properties from neighbouring residents who have complained about the turbines. These people therefore have form in complaining and have succeeded in selling land that might otherwise have attracted little buyer attention in depressed rural markets. Complaining can turn a property with poor sales prospects into cash-in-hand. Energy companies weigh the costs and benefits of buying out such complainants and understandably want to shut down any further attempts by such people to cash in, particularly when the symptoms of wind turbine syndrome are highly subjective,[5] inviting protracted and expensive disputation.

But the companies can't require those with turbines on their land to waive their common law rights to claims of negligence should there be any health damage arising from exposure. So the apparent immunity to wind turbine syndrome caused by payment to those with turbines in their own backyard is a salient consideration.

Wind-farm opponents also complain that turbine blades kill bats and birds. But these newly aroused advocates for bird and bat protection have been strangely silent on decades of bird and bat strikes from aircraft, cars, plate glass and cats. A US National Academy of Sciences report calculated that it takes 30 turbines to reach a kill-rate of one bird a year, while national bird deaths from domestic cats are put at "hundreds of millions".[6]

---

4   Pedersen, van den Berg, Bakker and Bouma 2009.
5   National Health and Medical Research Council 2010.
6   Marris and Fairless 2007.

In the 21 September 1899 issue of the *British Medical Journal*, Britain's doctors were warned of the dangers of a new technological scourge: the telephone. The report noted that:

> not in women only, but in strong-minded and able-bodied men, symptoms of what we may call "aural overpressure" caused by the condition of almost constant strain of the auditory apparatus, in which persons who use the telephone much have to spend a considerable portion of each working day . . . The patients suffered from nervous excitability, with buzzing noises in the ear, giddiness, and neuralgic pains . . . The victims of "telephone tinnitus", if we may so baptise this latest addition to the ills that flesh is heir to, seem all to be of markedly nervous organisation, and the moral may be drawn that such persons should not use the telephone.

Ever since, there has been a long history of sometimes protracted episodes of community concern about health risks said to be caused by new technologies. Some examples include television sets, computer screens, microwave ovens, electric blankets and other household electrical appliances, mobile telephones, and base stations. Wind turbines seem likely to enter the annals of technophobic history.

23

Wind turbine syndrome: a classic "communicated" disease

As I read more about "wind turbine syndrome" it became rapidly clear that here was a "disease" that spread by it being talked about. Communicable diseases spread by organisms passing from person to person by direct contact or via aerosols like sneezing and coughing. I coined the term "communicated" diseases for those that could be spread by people just hearing or reading about them. In 2017 Sydney University Press will publish my book on this topic, *Wind turbine syndrome: a communicated disease*.

At the beginning of this year I started collecting examples of health problems some people were attributing to wind turbine exposure. I had noticed a growing number of such claims on the internet and was curious about how many I could find. Within an hour or two I had found nearly 50 and today the number has grown to an astonishing 155 (Chapman 2016a).

I have worked in public health on three continents since the mid 1970s. In all this time, I have never encountered anything in the history of disease that is said to cause even a fraction of the list of problems I

Originally published as Chapman, Simon (2012). Wind turbine syndrome: a classic "communicated" disease. *The Conversation*, 20 July.

have collected. The list of 155 problems includes "deaths, many deaths", none of which has ever been brought to the attention of a coroner. It includes several types of cancer, and both losing weight and gaining weight. You name it. Haemorrhoids have not yet been named, but nothing would surprise me.

Many of the problems are those that affect large proportions of any community: hypertension (high blood pressure); mental health problems; sleeping difficulties; sensory problems (eyes, hearing, balance); and learning and concentration difficulties. Every day in Australia many hundreds of Australians receive their first diagnosis with these problems, and most live nowhere near wind farms.

So is it reasonable to suggest that all these problems – or even a fraction of them – are caused by wind turbines? Wind farm opponents repeatedly argue that turbines cause both rapid and long-gestation health problems. It is common to read accounts of people having been adversely affected within hours or even minutes of being exposed. If this were true, there would be a big problem here.

Wind farms existed in Australia long before the first claims about health ever surfaced. The Ten Mile Lagoon wind farm near Esperance, Western Australia has been operational for 19 years. Victoria's first, the Codrington wind farm, just celebrated its 11th birthday and has 14 turbines, each capable of producing 1.3 megawatts. And yet health complaints are relatively recent, with the few in Codrington post-dating a visit to the area by a vocal opponent, spreading anxiety.

In this sense, "wind turbine syndrome" (which incidentally produces zero returns from the United States National Library of Medicine's 23 million research papers) is what we can call a "communicated" disease: it spreads via the "nocebo effect", by being talked about, and is thereby a strong candidate for being defined as a psychogenic condition.[1]

One prominent opponent of wind farms says he can hear them 35 kilometres away. Others talk about electricity from the turbines

---

1 A nocebo effect is the opposite of a placebo effect: instead of exposure to an inactive agent making people feel better becasue of their belief that it will, a nocebo effect is when a benign agent makes people feel worse because they have been told that it will.

"leaking" into the soil and causing deaths of hundreds of cattle and goats. Such catastrophic events would attract huge news attention. But try to find such coverage and instead you will only find website anecdotes about what happened on a neighbour's farm.

Opponents also say that only "susceptible" people are adversely affected by wind turbines. But they repeatedly say animals such as sheep, cattle, dogs and poultry are badly affected, with problems such as malformations, sudden death, sterility and yolkless eggs being common. Against this, on any trip to a wind farm region, one can find thousands of livestock grazing contentedly around the turbines. In Tasmania there is a poultry farm with a wind turbine at the front gate. Is the argument now that only some animals are "susceptible" too?

There have now been 17 reviews of the available evidence about wind farms and health, published internationally. These are reviews of all studies, not single pieces of research.[2] Each of these reviews have concluded that wind turbines can annoy a minority of people in their vicinity, but that there is no strong evidence that they make people ill. The reviews conclude that pre-existing negative attitudes to wind farms are generally stronger predictors of annoyance than residential distance to the turbines or recorded levels of noise. In other words, people who don't like wind farms can often be annoyed and worried by them: some might even worry themselves sick.

There are two main anti-wind-farm groups in Australia busily fomenting anxiety and opposition. One is the Waubra Foundation,[3] a group of mainly wealthy individuals, none of whom live in or near the town of Waubra, near Ballarat. Several of them, NIMBY-style, have opposed turbines near their own properties elsewhere. They are led by an unregistered doctor, Sarah Laurie, and a wealthy mining investor, Peter Mitchell, who also has connections to the Landscape Guardians.[4] Despite their name, the Guardians have never attempted to guard our landscape from overzealous residential developers, open-cut coal or coal-seam gas mining. They only target wind farm developments. All

---

2 Chapman and Simonetti 2015.
3 http://waubrafoundation.com.au/
4 Keane 2012.

three – Waubra, the Guardians and Mitchell's mining investment company – share a South Melbourne post office box.

Problems of falling and stagnant real-estate prices in many of Australia's rural areas are well known. When landowners with property that would be hard to sell see a wealthy energy company moving into an area and investing millions in turbines, it's not difficult to predict that some will see potential in being "bought out" by such companies. Mining companies do it regularly. When this has happened in some communities, word spreads fast. I have been given accounts of lavish renovation and relocation "shopping list" demands that have been given to some wind-energy companies by hopeful complainants. Tellingly, four allegedly unliveable houses near Waubra where complaining residents were bought out now house non-complaining occupants.

When anti-wind-farm leaders move around communities, sometimes with entrepreneurial lawyers, spreading anxiety that the turbines can harm heath, we can get a potent combination of poorly informed, worried and angry residents seeded with the idea that their protests might lead to a payout.

Other complainants appear to see the turbines as symbols of values and movements that they despise: totems of green politics, modernity and urban artifice. Almost daily, I receive a heated email suggesting I should host a turbine in my inner-city backyard. The irony is that for 22 years I've lived 300 metres below the main flight path into Sydney airport, 30 metres from a busy road and 200 metres from a railway line where the combined noise is incomparably louder than hundreds of wind turbines. I rather think I wear my fair share of community noise. But some in the bush believe that unlike city dwellers, it is their birthright to be sheltered from any intrusion in their pristine surrounds: the ultimate in NIMBYism.

Fortunately, anti-wind-farm voices in the bush are in a small minority, as this 2012 CSIRO study shows.[5]

---

5   Hall, Ashworth, Shaw 2012.

24
Questions a prominent wind farm critic needs to answer

In this piece, I examined public statements made by one of Australia's more public victims of health problems caused by wind turbines. I found a few problems with what he had been saying.

David Mortimer, who lives near Millicent in South Australia, is one of Australia's highest-profile critics of wind farms. Mortimer derives rental income from two turbines that are part of the Lake Bonney wind farm.

While the local Wattle Range Council that covers his property has never received a formal complaint from any resident about the wind farm, Mortimer has been a vocal critic for over 12 months, claiming that he and his wife are being made ill by their exposure to the turbines.

He has been interviewed on Sydney Radio 2GB by shock jocks Alan Jones (in November 2012)[1] and Steve Price (March 2013),[2] appeared on the national TV news magazine program *Today Tonight*,[3]

---

1 http://bit.ly/2cwXBIf.
2 http://bit.ly/2d0xoT4.
3 http://bit.ly/2cIupB8.

Originally published as Chapman, Simon (2013). Questions a prominent wind farm critic needs to answer. *Climate Spectator*, 8 November.

and has been covered extensively[4] by the anonymously authored *Stop These Things* website, where he says: "somewhere during the night it is going to wake me up and I am going to find myself half way down the passageway, trying to get away from scorpions and snakes and whatever the hell frightens the hell out of me".[5]

Mortimer is unique in Australia in being the only wind turbine host to have spoken out against wind farms. The Mortimers' claims are therefore of strategic importance to the anti-wind movement because they are being used to counter the argument that turbine hosts do not complain because the substantial rental money they earn acts as a kind of "preventive" to health complaints.

On 18 June 2013, Mortimer spoke at a poorly attended protest rally in the lawn in front of Parliament House in Canberra, chaired by Alan Jones. Here is part of what he said, with my emphasis in italics:

> Mary Morris was on recently . . . Now, not terribly long ago, earlier this year, we went for a bit of a tour up around North of Adelaide, etc., and *we happened to turn up at Mary's place, and we stayed the night there. Now we could look all around us, and we couldn't see a turbine within coo-ee, and so we thought there are no turbines around.* Now, we went to sleep about ten o'clock that night in our little camper, and we had been in bed for about ten minutes, I suppose, and I rolled over and said to my wife, and I said, "You know, you're not going to believe this," and she said, "Yeah, I can hear it too." Well, you know, I didn't prompt anything. In the back of our head we could feel it, the same pulsing sensation, the same deep rumbling, down inside our head, that disturbs our sleep. You can't block it out with earplugs or earmuffs.
>
> We had an absolute terrible night sleep. Now we expected to have a good night's sleep, as we always do when we go away from home. We can sleep next to a parking bay, as we did on Saturday night. Trucks going past all night. When the trucks are not there, the silence inside our head is absolutely like a vacuum. It is profound.

---

4   Stopthesethings 2013a.
5   Stopthesethings 2013b.

While we're home, it's just a constant pulsing turmoil. You don't get any sleep.

But anyway, we asked Mary next morning, "Are there any turbines around?" and she pointed up the range, she said, "Seventeen kilometres up that way." Seventeen kilometres, and we could still pick it up."[6]

Earlier in the year, Mortimer and his wife had travelled to King Island in Tasmania, where Mortimer spoke to a meeting of residents about a proposed development. The *King Island Courier* ran an account of his speech, in which he described his neighbours as "all being alcoholics", adding "if my neighbour's house was on fire and I wasn't threatened, I'd let them burn." In his Parliament House lawn speech Mortimer referred to this visit:

Now we went down to King Island, in Tasmania, to tell those poor silly fools down there that they're not going to have an island left to live on if they get these some 200 to 600 turbines on their place. We got taken to a little bed and breakfast that night, somewhere after midnight. We had no idea of our surroundings, and we had no idea what the island was like. We got into bed about – heading on towards midnight I suppose, and we once again had a terrible night's sleep, with this same pulsing, rumbling sensation inside our head, the same sense of anxiety in our chest.

We went for a drive the next morning, and on our way into Currie, the little town there, about 4 kilometres away from where we were staying, was five ruddy great big wind turbines. Part of their local wind, their local power plant. Now those were about 1-megawatt units. The next night the wind was blowing straight across those turbines and we had an absolute shit of a night's sleep. Now once again, we'd expected to have a damn good night's sleep. We were sleeping next to the coast, the ocean was calm, so there was no noise coming from there.

The owner of the guesthouse in which the Mortimers stayed has said: "We built the house in 2004 and lived there for a year before renting

---

6   http://bit.ly/2cAMKlQ.

it out as a tourist accommodation since then. No one else, apart from David Mortimer, has complained about any problems at the Ettrick house."

On 7 October this year, Mortimer posted a reply on an ABC blog,[7] in which he returned to the same issues. He wrote:

> neither my wife nor I have sleep problems when we are significantly removed from turbines but do so when we are home or in the vicinity of turbines such as we have been 17 km from Waterloo SA, 4 km from King Island and 12 km from Macarthur Vic. *With the exception of Macarthur, we had no idea until next day that there were turbines in our vicinity.* [My emphasis]

David Mortimer's public statements invite important questions.

1. He drove with his wife some 475 kilometres from his house near Millicent to near the town of Waterloo, where he "happened to turn up at Mary Morris' place". Mortimer and Mary Morris are known to each other as active opponents of the wind farms near where they live. By claiming to have asked Mary Morris the next morning, "Are there any turbines around?" and writing that he "had no idea until next day that there were turbines in our vicinity" he is suggesting that he was unaware that she lived in the vicinity of the Waterloo wind farm, when in fact she has often written and spoken about its effect on her family and others in the district. Is this "Well, I never!" account one that a reasonable person should accept?

2. Mortimer was invited to King Island to address a meeting of residents about the proposed new wind farm on that island. He suggests that in all his preparation for that visit, and in the time he spent in the company of those who brought him there before he slept at the guest house, he was completely unaware that the tiny community of King Island already had a wind farm in place, which had been operating for 15 years. It just never came up?

Please explain, Mr Mortimer?

---

7   Wilson 2013a.

25

Chilean earthquakes in Australia and other wacky myths from wind farm opponents

> In 2012 I began collecting examples of diseases and symptoms being attributed to wind farm exposure. Today the list includes a remarkable 247, including herpes, haemorrhoids and "disoriented echidnas".[1] In the piece below I spotlight some quite remarkable statements made by leading Australian wind farm opponents.

November has been another bad month for the efforts of Australia's most dogged opponent of wind farms, Sarah Laurie, to get her claims taken seriously by anyone other than her loyal flock. The high priestess of the concocted non-disease known as "wind turbine syndrome" had given evidence to South Australia's Environment, Resources and Development Court in a case brought by a wind farm developer, appealing a development refusal by a local government for the Stony Gap wind farm. In a judgement handed down on 4 November, the energy company won.[2] Laurie is the CEO of the Waubra Foundation, named after the Victorian town with an iconic wind farm. (Last year

---

1   Chapman 2016a.

Originally published as Chapman, Simon (2014). Chilean earthquakes in Australia and other wacky myths from wind farm opponents. *Crikey*, 17 November.

more than 300 members of the proud farming community petitioned the out-of-towners to stop using their name, a request the foundation rejected.[3]) In the recent South Australian case, Laurie gave evidence for the respondents, but, as has become a pattern, the court was unimpressed:

> Dr Laurie is not an expert in assessing whether there is a causal link between wind farm noise and health impacts. She has no relevant qualifications or experience in this kind of research.

But the court nonetheless apparently couldn't resist this priceless comment:

> Dr Laurie wishes to have investigated the theory that some people are "so exquisitely sensitised to certain frequencies that their perception of very, very low frequency is right off the shape of the bell curve", such that they can, for example, from Australia, perceive an earthquake in Chile.

Chile is a mere 11,365 kilometres from Australia's east coast. This is not the first bizarre claim Laurie has made. In 2012, she wrote to New South Wales' then-planning minister, Brad Hazzard,[4] advising him that claimed rapid fluctuations in barometric pressure around wind farms could sometimes "perceptibly rock stationary cars even further than a kilometre away from the nearest wind turbine". This was too much even for *Mythbusters* to investigate. Laurie may be a secret country and western fan, channelling the Patsy Kline and Kitty Wells duet "Talk back trembling lips" ("shaky legs, don't just stand there") when she told the South Australian court in 2011 that wind turbines can make people's lips vibrate[5] "from a distance of ten kilometres away". That's about the distance from the Sydney CBD to Chatswood.

---

2 *Tru Energy Renewable Developments PTY LTD v Regional Council of Coyder & Ors [2014] SAERDC 48* (2016).
3 Bray 2013.
4 Sarah Laurie to Brad Hazzard 2012.
5 Barnard 2012.

Indeed, these vibrations are "sufficient to knock them off their feet or bring some men to their knees when out working in their paddock," she added. A fellow traveller in the big-distance claims department is Yass pharmacist George Papadopoulos, who swears he can personally sense low-frequency noise up to 100 kilometres away from wind turbines under certain conditions.[6] That's about from downtown Sydney to Lithgow, as the crow flies.

Laurie and Papadopoulos are among 76 "professionals" whose names appeared on the Waubra Foundation's website supporting independent research. The list even includes two sociologists, a profession whose mention normally causes apoplexy among wind farm opponents, except when they join the true believers in opposition. But conspicuously absent from the list is medical practitioner and former federal health minister Michael Wooldridge, who as recently as 14 October[7] was presented as a director on the Waubra Foundation website, although interestingly he is today not listed. If he has resigned, the Australian Securities and Investments Commission hasn't yet taken his name off its database.

The Australian Charities and Not-for-profits Commission has the Waubra Foundation's status as a health promotion charity under active review,[8] with a decision expected by the end of the year. One of the main considerations in its decision will be its assessment of health authorities' conclusions about the evidence of harm from wind farms. There are now 22 published reviews of this evidence,[9] all of which reject the direct effects hypothesis, with most highlighting psychogenic and nocebo effects.[10]

No doubt news from Canada also contributed to Laurie's bad week. Health Canada published the results of a much-awaited $2.1 million investigation into wind farm health effects, in the sort of direct study that opponents have been demanding.[11] Again, they concluded there

---

6   Papadopoulos 2012.
7   http://bit.ly/2cAMh3f.
8   http://bit.ly/2cIv9WE.
9   Chapman and Simonetti 2015.
10   Crichton, Chapman, Cundy and Petrie 2014.
11   http://bit.ly/1wn3Joc.

was no reliable evidence of direct effects and yet again noted that "annoyance was significantly lower among the 110 participants who received personal benefit, which could include rent, payments or other indirect benefits of having wind turbines in the area".

Predictably, neither the Health Canada report nor the 22 reviews have dented the resolve of wind farm opponents. The controversy-laden Waubra Foundation is, and always has been, an elaborate campaign of well-connected landowners determined to use any means to keep wind farms away from the horizons of their bucolic weekend estates. With the medical evidence only going the other way, the courts ruling against them again and again, and the authorities closing in on their practices, is it the endgame for the Waubra Foundation? If, or when, they finally close their doors, rural citizens in wind farming areas will appreciate the peace and quiet.

26
Let's appoint a judge to investigate bizarre wind farm health claims

In 2015 a Senate Select Committee dominated by crossbench senators openly hostile to wind farms published its report on these "utterly offensive" monstrosities, as former treasurer Joe Hockey called them. I publicly suggested to the committee five questions they could settle by appointing an independent judge to investigate. Strangely, none of these were taken up . . .

On 30 April 2015, South Australian Family First Senator Bob Day published an opinion piece on his website titled "Wind turbines' inconvenient truth".[1] With gotcha-style exuberance, Senator Day noted that wind turbine motors incorporate rare earths, which are often sourced from heavily polluting mining in inner Mongolia. Highlighting in bold an excerpt from a 2011 *Daily Mail* report, Day emphasised: "Whenever we purchase products that contain rare earth metals, we are unknowingly taking part in massive environmental degradation and the destruction of communities." The subtext was plain: green wind energy supporters are indifferent to the environment and suffering and so are massive hypocrites.

---

1   Day 2015.

Originally published as Chapman, Simon (2015). Let's appoint a judge to investigate bizarre wind farm health claims. *The Conversation*, 14 May.

A small problem with this accusation is that by far the main use of rare earths is not in wind-turbine motors, but in a wide range of electronics that includes billions of mobile phones, computers, DVDs and fluorescent lights, all of which Senator Day uses himself.[2]

Senator Day, who has no training or experience in assessing medical evidence, also wrote to the *Australian* recently that he had heard "compelling" evidence about the adverse effects of wind turbines on humans and animals. Day is one of six senators currently conducting what is the third Senate enquiry into wind farms in four years. The committee is chaired by the ex-Democratic Labour Party senator John Madigan, a man who makes no secret of his loathing for wind farms and the industries which manufacturer and operate them ("I remain one of the wind industry's most stubborn and outspoken critics").[3] He is joined by four other like-minded senators (Day, Back,[4] Leyonhjelm,[5] and Canavan[6]) and a lone Labor senator, Anne Urquhardt, who must feel as lonely on the committee as a bastard on Father's Day.

Madigan is viewed as a hero by the anonymous authors of the virulently anti-wind-farm website Stop These Things,[7] a site which has over 15,000 Twitter followers, nearly all of which have been generated from "follow-back" bots.[8]

Against this background, here are some recommendations guaranteed to advance our knowledge about wind farms and health complainants, but which are highly unlikely to appear in the committee's report. Sitting astride them all is a proposal that a judicial investigator such as a retired judge should be appointed to investigate the evidence for the following claims by those strenuously insisting that their health is being affected by exposure to wind turbines. Specifically, such a judge should investigate the following:

---

2   King n.d.
3   http://bit.ly/2cT2nko at 8 minutes, 27 seconds.
4   Back 2012.
5   Parkinson 2014.
6   Vorrath 2015.
7   http://bit.ly/2dbRjBE.
8   http://bit.ly/2cREcoV.

"Abandoned homes?"

How many Australian families have really "abandoned" their homes near wind farms (meaning that they have not simply sold and moved, as many tens of thousands of Australian families do every year regardless of location)? I investigated claims about "more than 40" such families and concluded that the claim was a factoid.[9]

Senator Madigan claims he has confidential knowledge of many families who have abandoned their homes but that these people do not wish to go public. His claim is thus not open to any scrutiny. He could provide this information in confidence to the appointed judge, who could then investigate the veracity of these anonymous claims. Questions to be asked would include whether those who had moved had any other reasons for moving like seeking work, eviction from rented property or need to be near medical facilities. The judge could also investigate whether any complainants were property owners whose applications to host lucrative turbines were declined because of unsuitable topography, and who then began resenting neighbours whose land was suitable.

Those claiming to have to regularly leave their house for respite from the turbines would of course have no objection to making their home telephone records available to corroborate that no calls were made or taken in the many times when they claimed to have been away. They should also be willing to provide receipts for hotel accommodation or statutory declarations from family and friends who might have put them up on all these alleged many occasions.

Medical records

The judge should request the medical records of complainants from periods both before and after the operation of wind farms, to settle the matter of whether the complaints were sufficiently serious to have been given medical attention, and that they did not have these problems before the wind farm commenced operation. Problems like insomnia, headache and anxiety are very prevalent in all communities with and

---

9 Chapman 2014b.

without wind farms.[10] In Canada in 2012, the Ontario Environmental Review Tribunal called for such records from some "wind action" plaintiffs. Tellingly, they declined to produce them and their case fell over.[11] They then complained that these medical records would have been too onerous to obtain. This is an odd claim, because my GP can produce my records instantly on screen, going back nearly 20 years.

Has there ever been a wind disease diagnosis?

Next, public notices should be placed in the press and publicised in the attempt to find any medical practitioner who has ever diagnosed even a single case of "wind turbine syndrome" in Australia. If any such cases emerge, all relevant case notes should be made available to a panel of doctors appointed by the Royal Australasian College of Physicians. Consent would of course be needed from the patients concerned, but as they would be entirely confident that their diagnosis was real, they would surely leap at the opportunity to have this corroborated by an independent assessment process.

Experimental tests

Claims made by prominent opponents of wind farms that wind turbines can rock a stationary car from one kilometre away,[12] cause lips to vibrate ten kilometres away,[13] "bring some men to their knees when out working in their paddock near wind farms",[14] and be heard 100 kilometres away[15] could easily be subjected to tests under blinded experimental conditions. Wind farm operators would willingly co-operate in the experiment by powering turbines on and off unbeknown to the experimental subjects, and their lip trembling, their ability to

---

10 Petrie, Faasse, Crichton and Grey 2014.
11 Ontario 2012.
12 Sarah Laurie to Brad Hazzard 2012.
13 Barnard 2012.
14 http://bit.ly/2d4Fezz.
15 Papadopoulos 2012.

stand in paddocks and their claims about hearing turbines from massive distances all tested.

Magical mystery tour

Similarly, Senator Madigan may like to co-operate in organising an experiment where those claiming to be to be adversely affected by wind turbines at distances up to ten kilometres could have this claim experimentally tested. A bus could have its windows blackened and views out the front obstructed by a partition. Those alleging wind turbine impacts could then be driven through wind farm zones not knowing if the turbines were operating or not and their ability to discern operation tested. All mobile phones would be barred on the bus to prevent "phone a friend" assistance.

However, at least one serial-complaining Victorian couple would have an objection to this. Ann and Andrew Gardner have stated publicly that "Around the Macarthur wind farm, residents suffer from infrasound emitted by the turbines, even when they're not operating."[16] They believe that the stationary blades catch passing wind, vibrate and generate debilitating infrasound. They have not made similar claims about the impact of tall trees, buildings, mountains or any other tall objects.

While this inquisition rolls on in Australia, the rest of the world is powering away with growing wind energy. Leading nations are Denmark (where wind accounts for 34 percent of all electricity generated), Spain (21 percent), Portugal (more than 20 percent), Ireland (more than 16 percent) and Germany (9 percent).[17]

---

16   http://bit.ly/2cURmzL.
17   http://bit.ly/2cA8RXt.

27

Tragedy puts values at threat

Should those involved in tragedy financially profit from their experience? Stuart Diver was trapped in the 1997 avalanche at Thredbo beside his wife, Sally, who died. His experience raised challenging ethical issues.

Many readers will have watched with interest Stuart Diver's interview on Channel Seven's *Witness* program last night. Some may have felt uncomfortable with the arrangement between the Thredbo survivor and the channel. Diver had announced that "it would be completely inappropriate for any payment to be made" for his story, but he did accept a job as a full time "special commentator" with Seven. Here we can assume two things: that he will be being paid in his new job, and that, without his involvement in Thredbo, he would be still working as a ski instructor.

So why did Diver not simply sell his story to the highest bidder? In their eyes, he is a prize commodity because he promises huge riches in advertising dollars. In contrast to Diver's perceptions, Channel Seven has never doubted that it should profit from the tragedy. Doubtless the channel will promote Diver's forthcoming appearances. Doubtless,

Originally published as Chapman, Simon (1997). Tragedy puts values at threat. *Sydney Morning Herald*, 26 August.

too, advertisers wanting to secure advertising spots in the breaks will pay top dollar. And needless to say, Seven will syndicate its scoop for handsome dividends all around the world.

But it is Diver, not Seven, whom the nation's staffrooms and dinner tables have been discussing regarding the morality of taking the cash, however circuitously. There is nothing inappropriate at all, it seems, in the shareholders of Channel Seven and the advertisers attracted to the story's audience potential "profiting from a tragedy". Perhaps it's just a question of how well such players disguise their interests.

Diver, via his agent, Harry M. Miller, has found himself at centre stage as winner of a lottery he would have given everything to avoid entering. He is at once a highly marketable commodity and the centrepiece of one of the great contemporary Australian morality plays, which intertwines themes of selfless voluntarism and the behaviour expected of those who benefit from it. It is becoming an increasingly popular play and has many different endings (*vide* Tony Bullimore), because the tension between these two themes can be mediated by the nature of different tragedies and the roles available to those cast into them.

Generally speaking, Australians believe that it is morally wrong to profit out of tragedy. But there are interesting exceptions to this. Those who have endured pain and suffering can accept with impunity whatever money others raise on their behalf. Funds set up to support victims such as those bereaved at Port Arthur institutionalise this. No one condemns a family compensated for suffering a shocking crime or natural disaster. If the community offers large amounts, this is seen as testimony to its generosity and sense of caring, and the victims are seen to be deserving.

But if such victims were to engage in any entrepreneurial activity designed to maximise the amount the community donated, the community would see this as tacky and the victims as somehow less deserving. It is OK to benefit if you do not proclaim your own needs and if you do not appear to go on the front foot looking for reward or compensation. This is a phenomenon known well to the lawyers and the insurance industry: victims, frequently through survivor guilt, often fail to pursue compensation legally available to them and need to be goaded by those acting for them.

Had Diver been perceived as seeking overtly to maximise the return on his bad fortune, his value as a commodity may well have been considerably diminished. Significantly, a Seven spokeswoman said recently that Diver "has a real affinity with the Australian public". It better suits the story to have a young Australian wishing to reciprocate the spirit of voluntarism by speaking of his experiences and his gratitude than one shrouded in speculation about being paid stratospheric amounts for having the good fortune to survive.

After Thredbo, banners straddled highways and were unfurled at the football, proclaiming the rescue volunteers and paramedics as heroes. Unlike in the United States, we donate our blood rather than sell it. We have volunteer beach lifesavers, not paid ones. These reflect values that run deep and, at root, proclaim that helping others ennobles communities and should not be financially rewarded. These values venerate self-sacrifice and act as social glue, cementing communities.

The commodification of personal tragedies into stories to be auctioned off to the highest bidder places huge demands on those pushed involuntarily to centre stage. Faceless institutions are free to masquerade their venal interests as simply satisfying the community's appetite for information and vicarious experience. Yet Diver and others like him risk being judged for maximising benefits they never asked for in the first place, and which the community might well choose to shower on them anyway. While precarious, Diver's decision to minimise the perception that he is selling his story invites us to consider the important values behind why he and his agent are displaying such sensitivity.

Perhaps we should all be grateful that he turned away from the brazen take-the-cash alternative. To have done so would have inched us one step further towards the market-forces nirvana where the only measure of the value of anything is the money it commands.

28

Charities to be seen but no longer heard?

Conservative governments have form in trying to silence charities and the social agencies they help to fund when these charities challenge government policies that are relevant to the problems they try to alleviate. In 2001 the Howard government commenced a journey down this path to confine charities to the role of band-aid applicators.

Bill Crews' Exodus Foundation at Ashfield serves a relentless incoming tide of homeless and destitute visitors. Because of the high profile of Crews and his team in highlighting issues such as poverty, street kids, drugs and domestic abuse, thousands support Exodus with tax-deductible donations. So there's always a lot on the menu, and those going to the Foundation leave well fed. And if they come in ill, want to unburden themselves or have hit rock bottom with drugs, alcohol or money problems, they can see the foundation's doctor, counsellors or welfare workers.

But Bill Crews hands out more than soup and succour. Like a good many other active church people, he regularly dishes out far less palatable fare to those in political power.

Chapman, Simon (2001). Charities to be seen but no longer heard? *Sydney Morning Herald*, 26 February.

He has brought plain talk into arguments about the factors that perpetuate poverty. They include levels of social security, tenancy laws, policies that keep the poor "in their place", and social attitudes that kill people by placing the sensibilities of society ahead of life-saving programs such as safe injecting rooms and heroin prescription trials.

Last November, the prime minister announced an inquiry into the definition of charities and related organisations after a well-motivated Democrat initiative seeking to broaden "common law definitions [of charities] carried forward from 17th-century England". But the sometimes gormless Democrats had better watch themselves, lest the government blind-side them with its own agenda.

Announcing the inquiry, which reports next month, Howard said: "We need to ensure that the legislative framework in which [charities] operate is appropriate to the modern social and economic environment." Decoded, this may well be Howard-talk for applying the blowtorch to charities that step out of the government's Dickensian comfort zone.

The Dickensian image of charity is epitomised by the soup kitchen and workhouse. Charities were there to mop up human detritus from the streets and salve the disquiet of the comfortable classes: "There but for the grace of God . . ." For decades workhouses gave shelter and gruel in return for virtual slavery and scant hope of breaking out of poverty.

Meanwhile, the terms of reference for the inquiry suggest that Howard's reputed nostalgia for the past may involve a social vision much earlier than the 1950s. And the background issues paper to the inquiry provides loud hints of the government's agenda. The committee conducting the inquiry noted that charities are increasingly focusing on "advocacy activities" and that some engage in "activities that in isolation would not be defined as charitable, religious or community service . . . for example . . . lobbying on behalf of disadvantaged client groups". As plain as that.

The paper goes on to canvass whether charities that step out of the soup-and-shelter line of trade and have the temerity to suggest ways of preventing the revolving-door problems to which they minister, or criticise government inactivity, may lose their charitable status or have it downgraded.

Perhaps significantly, last November Tony Abbott, then employment services minister, told the St Vincent de Paul Society to pull its head in when it said Centrelink was trying to make the charity a de facto arm of government by referring thousands of people to it.

Also under fire could be groups such as the New South Wales Cancer Council, the largest charity in the state supporting research, patient support groups and efforts to prevent cancer. It has regularly got up the noses of different governments, lobbying forcefully for removing taxes on sunscreens, for the tax deductibility of outdoor workers' clothes and hats, for law and tax reform on tobacco, and for more public money for services such as radiotherapy. If the Abbott model triumphs through the inquiry, any charity lobbying for reform in this way could be cut off at the knees.

Crews has not put a submission to the inquiry. He didn't even know it was on. He has been too busy serving soup and fundraising, and talking about the jaws of poverty and what drives people into them. Many of those Crews assists are unable to fight their own battles. They're shattered by the devastation of poverty. Many can't read, let alone write letters to the minister. Marginalised, dirt poor and isolated, they can't rely on supportive social fabrics such as old-school-tie networks to get them through when their luck is down.

Any charity that were to lose its charitable tax status would close its doors within weeks. The Exodus Foundation, which survives entirely on tax-deductible and other donations from the community, may well be one if it continues to step outside the government's definition of charitable work. Tax deductibility is critical to the flow of public and particularly corporate benevolence.

There will be plenty of pragmatism in the boardrooms of the nation's charities if the government's goals are realised. Welfare charities, like the people they serve, will have to learn their place, button their mouths and be grateful for whatever role they can salvage. Acute problems such as feeding and housing the homeless will always take precedence over visionary concerns about ways of reducing poverty that involve structural reforms. Cancer research and support will be acceptable as long as they aren't backed by expressions of concern about shortfalls in government support or services. If it's a question of doing something or nothing, many will compromise and be cowed into submission.

Those within government departments cannot openly be critical of government policy. Likewise, policy advocacy by academics is often viewed with some suspicion, and considered of less importance than research and teaching. So it's often been down to non-government organisations (NGOs) working in health, welfare and human rights to provide the bulk of informed coalface criticism to governments of both stripes.

During the past two terms of the Howard government, NGOs have lost grants partly because of the government's Darwinian reverence for survival of the fittest but mostly because of a bulldozing contempt for any source of criticism. Now it seems charities risk being redefined as band-aids rather than being critical forces advocating on behalf of those often least able to fend for themselves.

There is no doubt that this will be one more blow against equity and justice and will have tragic repercussions in many areas of society.

29

Reflections on a 38-year career in public health advocacy: ten pieces of advice to early-career researchers and advocates

Near the end of my (salaried) career, I began to be asked to give talks on the lessons I'd learned. This one went down particularly well and as I write in July 2016, it has been downloaded some 25,000 times. My most recent book on public health advocacy is *Public health advocacy and tobacco control: making smoking history* (2007).

In the late 1970s, I worked with others to try to have the actor Paul Hogan removed from Winfield cigarette advertising.[1] It was, and remains, the most successful tobacco advertising campaign in Australian history. Hogan had immense appeal with teenagers. This made his role a clear breach of the voluntary code of advertising self-regulation that then operated.[2]

Our private, polite efforts to get something done about this through the complaints system were virtually ignored until we went public

---

1   Chapman 1980.
2   Chapman and Mackay 1984.

Originally published as Chapman, Simon (2015). Reflections on a 38-year career in public health advocacy: ten pieces of advice to early-career researchers and advocates. *Public Health Research and Practice* 25(2): e2521514.

through the media. Ten-thousand-watt lights tend to concentrate the attention of those with responsibilities to act. And so act they finally did. Hogan was removed 18 months after we started complaining.[3]

I learned a big lesson very quickly: sunlight makes a very strong antiseptic for malodorous health policy. And there is no sunlight stronger than major media attention.

I soon discovered there were remarkably few analytical histories of how either large or small public health advocacy campaigns and policy battles had been won or lost. So I set out to change that by writing books[4] and dozens of papers on the process I had often been part of. Today, on the eve of my retirement, I want to give you what I think are ten key lessons I've learned repeatedly throughout my career in public health advocacy. There are many, many more. But here are ten which are absolutely critical.

Lesson 1. Always respect evidence and if the evidence changes, so should you

The granite bedrock of all public health advocacy must always be evidence. Evidence evolves through stages. It starts with hypothesis-generating claims and observations and moves through to the gold standards of large-scale cohort epidemiology and randomised controlled trials in real-world settings. As evidence mounts, things that once looked true or effective can sometimes turn out not to be. We have seen the cancer screening and dietary areas slowly and sometimes reluctantly coming to terms with past doctrines being eroded by the tide of oncoming evidence.

Careers are often built on a lifetime commitment to particular phases of evidence. But if the evidence changes, it is absolutely critical for public trust in the integrity of public health, that we acknowledge – as the economist J. M. Keynes emphasised – that the facts have changed and that accordingly, we have changed our minds too.

---

3 Chapman 1980.
4 Chapman and Lupton 1994; Chapman 2013c; Chapman 2007; Chapman and Freeman 2014.

It is important to note here that the internet has changed forever the politics of expertise. For a long time, expertise was exercised in forums largely inaccessible to the public and then handed down to the populace in the form of advisories and campaigns. But today access to unprecedented amounts of research and to ways of disseminating it to millions has opened up a kind of anarchy of "expertise" that poses a massive threat to continuing public confidence in public health.

Two illustrations of the advance of junk and low quality science are the resilience and influence of climate-change denialism and the current efforts by e-cigarette interest groups to claim e-cigarettes are so revolutionary in their potential to make smoking history, that unlike all other therapeutic goods, foods or beverages, they should be allowed to stand on their own and totally avoid any form of regulatory oversight. The momentum that the interest groups behind these two major issues are succeeding in building may spread to challenge decades of public health and safety legislation.

Anyone embarking on a career in public health today faces unprecedented challenges to preserve and strengthen public and political confidence in the evidence base for public health policy. Challenging and confronting low-grade and self-interested evidence from such forces will never be more important. It is the very worst time to retreat into the unnoticed and inconsequential debates within the walls of academia. Today more than ever, we need far more of you out there promoting quality evidence and hammering rubbish.

Lesson 2. Be clear and concrete about what you want to change or support

I am often asked to speak to people who want advice on how to go about building momentum for their concerns. They say, "Tobacco control has done so well in changing policy that has reduced smoking ... what lessons do you have for our issue?" My first question to them is always what is it that they want to achieve. Almost invariably, they answer with a goal such as reducing obesity or problem drinking. Sometimes, they talk about some important but obtuse value like "reducing health inequalities" or "getting greater attention to the social determinants of health".

Talk about such complex and worthy abstractions is important and meaningful to small groups of specialists. But this is not how ordinary people talk. Public health is often mired in language that means little to those outside the cognoscenti. A "policy" to most people is what you get in the mail once a year from your house- or car-insurance company. Policy change may well be your goal, but policy will not change unless you can make it crystal clear exactly what you want from policy makers. That's exactly what we did with plain packaging. Every square centimetre of the pack, the fonts, the colours . . . everything . . . were specified following research with target groups. It could not have been more focused.

Take controls on alcohol advertising as an example. A colleague, Andrea Fogarty, interviewed 28 of Australia's leading alcohol-policy researchers for her PhD. All offered generalisations about the need for "controls" on alcohol promotion. But once she moved to the next stage and asked about precisely what sort of controls, there was very little consensus. There was no clear, sharp message for policy makers and the public to consider.[5]

I try to focus colleagues by asking them to pull their attention right into the foreground. What, precisely, needs to happen to reach the broad health goals that are so easily articulated? *Precisely* what policies, legislation or funding would they like the government to put in their Christmas stocking next year? Once that's decided, the meat and potatoes work of strategic, policy-relevant research can occur along with the precision "bombing" of false arguments from those opposed to change.

Lesson 3. "It's better to be looked over than overlooked" (Mae West)

I've never seen the sense in applying for grants, doing all the work with others for several years, and then parking it only in pay-walled journals where other academics are the only ones who can access it. The attitude

---

5   Fogarty and Chapman 2013.

that expertise carries no responsibilities to ensure that evidence reaches the public and policy makers is bizarre to me.

A few years ago, an NHMRC project I led with Wayne Hall and others interviewed 35 Australian public health researchers about why they were influential. They had been voted by their peers as Australia's most influential researchers working in six fields. Large majorities agreed or strongly agreed that researchers have a duty to increase policy and draw public attention to their work.[6]

We undertake research and systematically review it to provide evidence that can lever policy change or defend existing policies and practices. But there is only a small number of people who have the power to make action happen – to effect change or defend good policies. The most important of these are politicians. And guess what? They don't read research journals![7]

But over nearly 40 years, I have had countless occasions to speak to prime ministers and health ministers, their Cabinet colleagues, and thousands of influential people in every walk of life. I've done this as they lay in bed, as they ate breakfast, drove their cars, sat in their living rooms, and relaxed on their weekends or holidays in their shorts and T-shirts. By contrast, I have had face-to-face meetings with politicians perhaps 100 times in my life. Let me explain.

When I first met former federal health minister Nicola Roxon, many months after she commenced her ministry, we shook hands and I said I didn't think we had ever met. She replied she felt she had known me half her life. This could only have meant that she had often heard me and read of my work in the news media. She was one of the highly influential people I had spoken to, often without me even knowing. She was already very receptive to various issues I and my colleagues had been emphasising over the years. If you avoid the media, very few will ever learn about your work and what needs to be done because of what we know. You and your research are far less likely to be influential.

If you care about making a difference, you will put aside the regrettably still-prevalent attitude alive in some institutions that you should not "dally with the Delilah of the press."[8]

---

6 Chapman, Haynes, Derrick, Sturk, Hall and St George 2014.
7 Haynes, Derrick, Redman, Hall, Gillespie, Chapman and Sturk 2012.

Lesson 4. Study the media

If you want to be a potent media advocate for evidence and policy change, you need to know how it works and how you can best be part of it. Many of you will have taken days to prepare your 10- to 15-minute presentations for this conference. You may have rehearsed them in front of colleagues and finely manicured your sentences and slides. The really lucky ones will get to speak to 300 or so in a plenary session. Most, though, will address only 40 or 50 in a breakout session.

But a few will be tapped by journalists at the conference and even fewer will try to get in their faces through their own efforts. If you get interviewed for breakfast or drive-time radio, or evening TV news, your message might be heard by hundreds of thousands of people – sometimes millions. To maximise these unparalleled opportunities, you need to understand the medium and the programs on which you are about to appear. On Australian television news, the time that anyone gets to speak in a 90-second item averages 7.2 seconds, with an interquartile range of 4.8 to 9.2 seconds.[9] Knowing that, you can plan precisely what you are going to say and emphasise.

When print journalists request comments (and this increasingly will happen via email), I try to drop everything and send a selection of one or two sentence options. This makes journalists' jobs easier and they appreciate that. Again, knowing about length restrictions, you can shape a message with exact precision. Try to make every quote you send of potential "breakout box" quality rather than some anodyne, forgettable "memo to the public". This will mark you as someone they'll note is "good talent" and they'll contact you again and again.

Above all, be accessible. This should be so obvious. For seven years, I was a regular guest on Adam Spencer's Sydney ABC breakfast program with a listening audience of half a million. I was curious why and emailed him for this presentation. He told me immediately, "Because you always answer your phone. The number of people we rang

---

8   Osler 1904.
9   Chapman, Holding, Ellerm, Heenan, Fogarty, Imison, Mackenzie and McGeechan 2009.

and they missed out because they didn't realise tomorrow morning was their one shot, was incredibly frustrating."

Lesson 5: Use "killer facts"

Every year, people are exposed to thousands of facts, claims and narratives about many hundreds of health issues. Much of this is like informational wallpaper that is forgotten moments after it is encountered, contradicted by competing claims and washed away on the tide of tomorrow's more arresting news. Some issues rise above the rest and compel political action. Many issues plod along unchanging and others sink without trace.

A basic goal in advocacy is to have your definition of what is at issue in a policy debate become the dominant, top-of-mind way that people think about that issue.

Killer facts[10] are like musical earworms: once they get inside your head, it is difficult to get them out. They tend to kill off competing definitions of what is at issue. If they employ powerful and repeatable analogies, before and after comparisons, and humour if appropriate, this can really help. I heard one yesterday: "Public health is about saving lives . . . a million at a time".

Here are some examples:

- "The USA has 13.5 times Australia's population, 5.9 times Australia's rate per 100 gun ownership, and 305 times Australia's gun homicide rate. So more guns make a country safer?"
- "In the 18 years before Australia's 1996 gun-law reforms, there were 13 mass shootings (defined as shootings that involved five or more deaths, not including the perpetrator) in Australia. There have been precisely none in the 18 years since."
- "For four of the last five years, quad bikes have been the leading cause of non-intentional injury death on Australian farms. This is unique internationally as in all other Western nations, tractors continue to be the leading cause of injury deaths."

---

10   Bowen, Zwi, Sainsbury and Whitehead 2009.

Every advocate, for every issue, needs to stock up on killer facts for every sub-issue in their field. Plan to use at least one of them every time you are interviewed.

Lesson 6. Values are everything

I have said earlier that facts and evidence are the bedrock of public health advocacy. But unless those encountering this evidence *care* about it, they are highly unlikely to pay attention to it, let alone act on that evidence. Caring about something is *always* a necessary but not always a sufficient precondition for support and action.

Public health issues often feature in the news because they richly illustrate narratives about *values*: mini-dramas and secular parables about adversity and the solutions that are needed. These include the humane imperative to reduce early death and suffering; the injustice of inequitable distribution of disease and access to services; and stories about those who put financial gain ahead of population health.

So after you've filled your kit bag with killer facts, you need to take an inventory of the values which make these facts even more compelling. For example, killer facts about tobacco-industry expansion in nations with low literacy are powerful because they evoke eons of examples of the Pied Piper mythology: wolves in sheep's clothing who lead the vulnerable into illness and death. Your facts and evidence should be anchored firmly to the values that will make them resonate with what George Lakoff calls "moral politics".[11]

You also need to take an inventory of your vulnerability to opponents framing your position as embodying negative values and then seek strategically to reframe these as positives. The "nanny state"[12] epithet, for example, can be easily reframed positively by pointing out all the benefits caused by regulations and standards we all take for granted as we go about our daily lives. As I stood in my narrow hotel shower recess this morning, I whispered a silent "thank you" to the

---

11   Lakoff 2004.
12   Daube, Stafford and Laura 2008.

public health nannies who insured that if I slipped, the glass would not shatter and cut me to ribbons.

Lesson 7. Experts are fine, but they are not "a living thing"

A journalist once said this to me,[13] and I've never forgotten it. People who live with the diseases we try to prevent appear more often in news media coverage than experts or politicians ever do.[14]

When an expert speaks, we may admire their coherence, their grasp of the issues involved and their ability to explain complexity simply. But if a person suffering a problem speaks and does the same thing, it can be doubly powerful. Ordinary people can make amazing advocates and we should work with them far more. They bring a compelling authenticity to an issue.

Lesson 8. Use social media. A lot.

The internet has utterly revolutionised all our lives. And it has utterly transformed advocacy. There are simply massive global participation rates in social media. Anyone in public health who is not part of this, is the equivalent of a scholar in the Gutenberg era who declined to show interest in the potential of books.

I'm a heavy Twitter user. If you are like I used to be and thought that Twitter sounded like some sort of time-wasting indulgence for vapid twits, you may have already pulled the shutters down. But look what you are missing out on. Let me give you three examples.

The paper I published that has had the most downloads looked at the impact of the post–Port Arthur gun-law reforms on multiple killings and total gun deaths.[15] It has had 120,600 downloads since 1996, with 86,000 in December 2012 after I tweeted the link following the Sandy Hook massacre in the USA. It has been cited 102 times.

---

13 Chapman, McCarthy and Lupton 1995.
14 Chapman, Holding, Ellerm, Heenan, Fogarty, Imison, Mackenzie and McGeechan 2009.
15 Chapman, Alpers, Agho and Jones 2006.

A preprint of my much-tweeted paper on the nocebo effect and wind farm health complaints[16] is the most downloaded item in the entire University of Sydney's eScholarhip repository and featured in this video, which has been viewed 3.659 million times.[17]

My most retweeted tweet was one I sent after Treasurer Joe Hockey's public remark about wind turbines being an ugly blight on the landscape.[18] It has had 2,289 retweets, meaning that probably well over a million people have seen it.

Lesson 9. Successful advocacy takes time

Much public health research focuses on proximal associations[19] between interventions and outcomes – weeks, months, sometimes a year or two. But advocacy's dividends can often take decades to deliver their benefits.[20]

Smoking was first banned on public buses and trains in New South Wales in 1976. It took until 2006 – 30 years later – before such bans extended to the working environments where the problem was worst, and where in a totally rational world, smoke-free areas should have started. Even today, high-roller rooms in some casinos allow smoking. It's a little-known fact that second-hand smoke from wealthy gamblers is unique in not posing health risks to others.[21]

If you are serious about being a potent advocate, settle in for a long and often frustratingly slow, but immensely rewarding, career.

Lesson 10. Grow rhinoceros hide

Finally, unless you are an advocate for an utterly uncontroversial policy (I was going to say "for a mother's milk policy", but of course even

---

16 Chapman, St George, Waller and Cakic 2013.
17 See http://bit.ly/2ciSTSc.
18 See http://bit.ly/2cgLGgB.
19 McMichael 1999.
20 Chapman 1993.
21 Chapman 2013a.

breastfeeding still gets attacked in some contexts), as soon as you start to become a potent advocate and your work threatens any industry or ideological cabal, you will be attacked, sometimes unrelentingly and viciously.

I've been called a veritable sewer of names on social media, often by anonymous trolls and tobacco-industry-funded bloggers. I've also been attacked in the coward's castle of parliament under privilege, slandered on the Alan Jones radio program (and received a written apology and my legal costs paid), falsely accused of being an undeclared paid advocate for the wind and pharmaceutical industries, and sent white feathers each year on the anniversary of Port Arthur. My university administration is regularly deluged with orchestrated complaints. Yet I've had nothing but total support from my university and colleagues in the face of this. In all this nastiness, I take deep satisfaction and pride in having worked with colleagues who are lifetime friends to help make Australia's smoking rates the lowest in the world today.[22]

Many of you are doing fabulous work to achieve similar goals in your areas. Clinicians are thanked everyday by grateful patients and relatives for their skill in saving lives and limbs. In public health, we don't have people come up to us and say, "I've not been killed or injured because of your advocacy for road injury reduction policy", or "I've not got diabetes, and I put it down to you." But our achievements can be seen in many areas of declining incidence of disease and injury. We do fantastically important work and I've been blessed to be part of it for almost 40 years. Thank you for all you do.

---

22   Chapman and Freeman 2014.

30

Unravelling gossamer with boxing gloves: problems in explaining the decline in smoking

Many people in public health get their initial research training in experimental sciences conducted in laboratories, where all important experimental variables can generally be fully controlled and randomised. In real-world investigations such control can rarely if ever occur. I wrote this essay in 1993, trying to locate this problem in a day in the life of a smoker who quit and showing how insensitive it would be to try to attribute the decision to quit to one or even a few of the many influences that shape a smoker's decision. Over the years, many people have thanked me for writing what they often call a "penny-drop" explanation of something they had long felt was the case.

Between 1964 and 1991, per capita cigarette consumption among adults (aged 15 and older) in Australia fell by 33.3 percent, from 2,740 grams to 1,827.[1] For 13 years of this period (1964–76), consumption remained virtually unchanged. However from 1977, the year following a national

---

1   Department of Community Services and Health 1990.

Originally published as Chapman, Simon (1993). Unravelling gossamer with boxing gloves: problems in explaining the decline in smoking. *British Medical Journal* 307: 429–32.

ban on direct forms of radio and television cigarette advertising, the average annual fall has been 2.2 percent. And since 1983, the year when the first of a series of large-scale mass media campaigns commenced,[2] the fall increased still further to a mean 2.5 percent per year.

How do we explain this internationally acclaimed success story in modern public health? Is it reasonable to nominate, as implied above, particular policy or intervention landmarks such as advertising bans or large government campaigns as being more explanatory of the change than other less prominent and tangible but perhaps more pervasive influences barely deserving to be described as "interventions"? How can decisions be made about the success or failure of particular programs and policies intended to further this trend? What limitations are there on the ability of quantitative research methods to address these questions?

This paper explores these questions through consideration of some awkward problems raised by a case study. I argue that the ambition to attribute specific preventive or cessation effects to particular tobacco control interventions is highly problematic in any situation character-ised by the interplay of continuous, uncontrolled, unmeasured and sometimes unmeasurable variables intended to influence consumption. Such an ambition reflects a reductionist epistemology that is largely incapable of illuminating the complex nature of how it is that individuals either fail to take up smoking, quit, or reduce their consumption – when aggregated, the three determinants of falling per capita tobacco consumption. I will argue that attempts at attributing causal effects to specific interventions in situations characterised by multiple interventions and influences are invariably fraught with highly questionable assumptions that serve the interests of those requiring simplistic, quantified explanations of what are in fact highly complex phenomena. These explanations have more to do with the contexts in which attempts at explanation take place, and with the politics of program funding, than they do with any dedication to a full account of the changing phenomenon of smoking in cultures such as Australia.

---

2   Pierce, Dwyer, Frape, Chapman, Chamberlain and Burke 1986.

A day in the life of an Australian smoker

Consider a recent day in the life of an Australian smoker, John. As he wakes, John listens to a news item concerning a government decision to end all remaining forms of tobacco advertising.[3] Since the mid-1970s, he has woken to many similar announcements concerning various forms of tobacco advertising. These have occasioned discussions at his office and in social gatherings, where smoking has become a common and sometimes highly charged topic of conversation. Newspapers have also been thick with news about smoking. In 1988 for example, he might have read up to 1,600 separate items in newspapers alone, of which only 17 percent would have delivered even a vaguely comforting message.[4]

As John smokes at the breakfast table, his two children playfully chorus their usual anti-smoking slogans: "Smokers suck! But we get half the muck!" and "Kiss a non-smoker . . . taste the difference." It seem there have been dozens of these taunts over the years. Undoubtedly they have picked them up from school, where he knows that they are regularly given lessons about the health consequences of smoking.[5]

His wife, who doesn't smoke, has, like a lot of people, slowly turned into someone who actively dislikes smoking. She has recently begun seriously talking to him about whether he might go outside when he wants to smoke. In making this request, it seems to John that she is not really being overzealous.

On the way to the train station, he stops to buy a new pack. When he proffers $4.55 for his usual pack of 30s, the shop assistant reminds him that they have gone up by 20 cents a pack following the latest federal budget. John has calculated that by smoking a pack a day, he is spending $1,734 a year on cigarettes – the price of a ten-day holiday in a luxury hotel in Bali.

Boarding the train, he ponders that here is yet another place he can't smoke. Public transport went smoke-free in 1976, joined in 1990 by all domestic flights in Australia, and in 1992 by a ban on smoking on

---

3 Chapman and Woodward 1993.
4 Chapman 1989b.
5 White, Hill and Williams 1990.

an increasing number of some international routes and even a total ban inside Australian air terminals.

As he reads the morning newspaper, he notices how many of the "share accommodation" classified advertisements specify that only non-smokers need apply. Of 335 advertisements that day, 42 percent include this requirement[6] – a higher rate than any other quality sought by advertisers. He also notices that every government job advertisement, and a not inconsiderable number of private sector ads, states that "a smoke-free workplace is company policy". Browsing through the lonely-hearts advertisements he is again struck by how many of these people seek a partner who is a non-smoker. And then he is confronted by a full-page advertisement from a life-insurance company offering substantially reduced rates for non-smokers.[7]

Arriving at work, John stubs out what will be his last cigarette until lunchtime. In 1988, his office introduced a total smoking ban. Since then, there has been a virtual stampede throughout the Australian business world to do the same. By 1992, 58 percent of the top 139 companies in one state had total bans, with over half of these having introduced them in the previous 12 months.[8] A successful civil suit by a worker whose asthma was severely aggravated by passive smoking in her workplace seems certain to hasten this process.[9] The ban at work has certainly forced down John's own consumption. It has been estimated that the average smoking office-worker has reduced daily consumption by around 25 percent[10] and that the workplace bans will cost the Australian tobacco industry $73 million in lost sales a year.[11]

At lunchtime, John goes with some colleagues to a nearby Pizza Hut restaurant. The entire chain has recently gone smoke-free, reflecting an overwhelming community demand for smoke-free dining.[12] He then passes a street sign warning him that he could be fined for discarding his cigarette butt in the street[13] – the non-biodegradability of butts makes

---

6   Chapman 1992a.
7   Brackenridge 1985.
8   Mullins 1992.
9   Chesterfield-Evans 1992; Chapman, Borland, Hill, Owen and Woodward 1990.
10   Borland, Chapman, Owen and Hill 1990.
11   Chapman 1992.
12   Roberts, Algert, Chey, Capon and Gray 1992; Borland and Hill 1991.

them a major pollution problem, especially in a city where stormwater runs into the picturesque harbour around which the city is built. Being environmentally conscious, he feels awkward about his usual throw-away method of disposing of butts.

Home that evening, John relaxes in front of TV, where on the news he hears a report linking smoking with yet another dreaded disease – leukaemia.[14] "Is there *anything* that smoking doesn't cause?" he thinks to himself, reflecting on all the news reports he has heard about the subject over the years. Being a sports fan, he zaps his TV between channels showing the national soccer and basketball competitions. And there it is again: anti-smoking sponsorship messages on the sidelines and even on the players' clothing. And then to put the icing on the cake, a gory government advertisement showing how much black tar a smoker will inhale in a year is shown several times during commercial breaks.

The next day, John decides that he will finally quit. Over the next 12 months, he makes three or four unsuccessful attempts,[15] one inspired by a brief warning given to him by his doctor, and another being a period when he uses over-the-counter nicotine gum after prompting from his pharmacist. Eighteen months after his initial decision, he smokes what will be his last cigarette. In doing so, he joins approximately 3.8 million Australian adults who identify themselves as former smokers.[16]

Shortly after he finally stops smoking, he is phoned by a researcher working on the evaluation of a government media campaign to encourage people to quit smoking. John joins those respondents who say that they have seen the campaign, who strongly agree that it made them think about quitting, and who respond (unprompted) that "health reasons", "social unacceptability" and "cost" are the three main reasons they have stopped smoking.[17]

The researchers subsequently write a scientific article in which they claim that their state-wide media campaign is probably the factor

---

13   Anon 1992.
14   Brownson, Chang and Davis 1991.
15   Marlatt, Curry and Judith 1990.
16   Hill, White and Gray 1991.
17   Gilpin, Pierce, Goodman, Burns and Shopland 1992.

responsible for the state's higher than average quit-rate. This claim is based on extrapolations made from the aggregated sample of recent quitters like John.

Discussion

How do we explain John's decision to quit? What do we make of a community cessation rate extrapolated from data including John's responses and its partial attribution to the government campaign? And what should we make of John's own account of why he quit? In the evaluative research literature of tobacco control, such questions are seldom asked and even more seldom thoroughly pursued. Where questions of attribution are assessed, it is usual that the influence of a particular variable such as advertising or a health education campaign is examined using standard pre-post or intervention-control group designs. Occasionally, a limited number of potential confounders, like price changes, are incorporated into such studies. Control areas are seldom if ever matched with intervention areas for anything remotely like the range of variables described in the above scenario. Essentially qualitative variables such as tobacco advertising are conveniently homogenised into measurable units such as cost, as if all advertising campaigns could be considered of equal impact.[18] Such an assumption would be news indeed to many in the advertising industry, who know too well how many of their efforts seem to make little difference to brand sales.

Yet from the foregoing scenario, it is obvious that in the life of every smoker, there has been a plethora of interventions, campaigns and "influences" to which they have been exposed over many years. From John's perspective, these have not passed in front of him in any neat, sequential order, or in any way that would allow him to reliably quantify their respective influence on his gradually changing perception of his own smoking and the evolution of his decision to quit. Indeed, at many times in John's recent smoking history, it would have been quite impossible to isolate and quantify the effects of any one of up to a dozen

---

18   Chapman 1989a.

concurrent variables. Quantitative evaluative research processes avoid the methodological imbroglios that are inherent in accepting the reality of the dynamic interplay of the sort of factors described in the scenario above. There are at least four outstanding explanations for this.

1. Reductionist epistemology

Evaluative research in tobacco control is located almost entirely within the scientific tradition. This tradition assumes a reductionist epistemology whereby the task of science is to discover and quantify the exact relationship between variables. Any difficulties in assessing these relationships are assumed to lie with the imprecision of the methods used to assess them, and not with the very conception of the nature of how it is that a complex behaviour like smoking changes throughout a population or an individual's lifetime. The ambition to exactly quantify the assumed relationship is seen as a task worthy of pursuit, whereas consideration of the *gestalt* of how various cultural, economic, organisational and educational factors actually combine to influence smoking behaviour is viewed as messy and unscientific. The only manageable truths in this tradition are those that are simple and uncomplicated: advertising bans and price rises reduce aggregate demand, education programs decrease the incidence of uptake, and so on. The messy *gestalt* is entangled in the explanatory gossamer of a myriad of experiences, conversations, memories and exposures to interventions, but researchers bearing reductionist precepts and methods wear the equivalent of boxing gloves in their attempt to unravel these delicate threads.

2. The explanatory privileging of recent factors

It is not just *single* factors, but also *recent* factors that are privileged by reductionist explanations. The view seems to be that the effects of recent interventions and policy changes could be expected to be less confounded by the intrusion of other influences than policies and events enacted further in the past. This assumption is fuelled by attributions often given by individuals when they nominate specific events (e.g. recent illness or symptoms, the death of a relative, an intense period of haranguing from their children, a straw-that-broke-the-camel's-back price-rise) as "why" they quit. Such explanations may well represent accurate and heartfelt perceptions of the *precipitating* factors that prompted quitting, but reveal little of the complex historical precursors that may well have been necessary to predispose individuals to quit when finally subject to the precipitating event. For example, it may be the case that demand sensitivity to price rises is dependent on a widespread acceptance of the tobacco–disease nexus. Respect for the importance of such plausible predisposing factors is rare in evaluative studies about smoking control and was not raised in a recent expert consensus report on research priorities in tobacco pricing and taxation.[19]

3. Concern for policy tractable factors

In recent years, concern has been increasingly expressed that research should concentrate on better understanding how to influence so-called policy tractable factors that influence smoking. These are factors that are amenable to manipulation by government policies and include price, advertising, packaging, laws and regulations on smoking in public places, and school curricula. They stand in contrast to factors also said to be relevant to smoking that include age, sex and cultural proscriptions on smoking, social class, occupation, income, school performance, and smoking by parents, peers, siblings and workmates. None of these is as directly or even at all amenable to influence through government policy.

Pragmatic considerations of "What can we *directly* influence?", schooled from an "upstream" preventive analysis,[20] have directed research attention onto the role of precise factors such as price or large public information campaigns. Again, the problems arising from the reductionism involved here tend to be overlooked in the fervour to produce "action-oriented" research that can be fed into policy and political processes.

---

19 Sweanor, Ballin, Corcoran, Davis, Deasy, Ferrence, Lahey, Lucido, Nethery and Wasserman 1992.
20 Chapman and Bloch 1992.

4. Relationship of evaluation to funding

Health promotion campaigns that involve relatively large sums of money are generally subject to intensive scrutiny bred from the competitive funding climates in which they operate. Unlike "passive" preventive strategies like price controls and advertising restrictions, which require little or no money to implement, health promotion campaigns are continually called upon to justify their allocation of funds. Evaluation of the "effects" of funded health-education campaigns against smoking are thus partly inspired by a concern to be able to show that an intervention is effective or, better, cost-effective. Such considerations produce a highly selective orientation to evaluation driven by *a priori* concerns to assess interventions deemed worthy of evaluation, rather than an attitude toward explanation of the quitting process that is open to the possibility of a thoroughly "messy" account like the scenario above.

In many cases, these interventions have been organised, developed and run by the very people who either conduct or commission their evaluation. Often these people are employed on "soft" project funding which may cease should a political or administrative perception develop that the interventions "don't work". Such considerations raise more tangible concerns about the impartiality of the explanatory process.

Confounding run amok

Individual platforms of comprehensive tobacco control policy are seldom implemented by governments in isolation from others. Exceptions like Sudan, which banned tobacco advertising but has done virtually nothing else, simply prove the rule: that when a government is committed enough to introduce (say) bans on smoking on aircraft, it will have done this in a spirit of wanting to reduce the burden of death and illness caused by tobacco and accordingly will be predisposed to introduce other policies with similar intent. In practice this has meant that nearly all countries where evaluation studies of tobacco control policies and programs have been undertaken have been characterised by the coalescence of a multitude of these factors, much in the manner described in the scenario. Many of these factors will be introduced in an *ad hoc*, opportunistic way rather in any way remotely analogous to the timed and controlled drip-feeding of therapeutics in laboratory or clinical trials. Politicians and tobacco control advocates understandably have little to no regard for the violation of the sanctity of control groups, areas or periods so coveted by researchers hoping to conduct a neat study unconfounded by unexpected influences. Instead, they will have their noses constantly in the political wind for opportunities to engage in media advocacy, to lobby for price rises and further restrictions on advertising and so on. In large countries like the USA and Canada, where federal, state, provincial and local governments have jurisdiction over different elements of tobacco-control policy, it is often the case that at any given time, quite complex different configurations of tobacco-control activity will be being played out in different parts of the country. Some of these events will be newsworthy and picked up by national media networks, which will amplify a local issue into a national concern, thus further corrupting pristine research designs. Most evaluative studies simply pretend that all this does not occur and that the independent variables (policies and interventions) they are evaluating constitute the only players in the landscape.

Conclusions

What does this analysis suggest for the future of evaluation of tobacco-control policies and programs? The sort of methodological problems discussed above should not induce an evaluative paralysis in tobacco control researchers. They should not inspire any abandonment of the evaluation of outcomes in tobacco control nor any shying away from the challenges of the attribution problem. Continuing debate about ways of sampling and controlling for differing "micro climates" of influence and intervention between areas, states and nations will be very welcome. As well, though, a more open recognition of the limitations of reductionist thinking in considering the causes of declining tobacco-use throughout populations could redirect researchers into considering the potential of qualitative methods as important adjuncts in the explanatory process.

Mark Twain wrote that if your only tool is a hammer, then all your problems come to look like nails. And so it has largely been with the dominant explanatory paradigms in smoking-control research. Social scientists have long argued for multiple methods or *triangulation* in studying complex human phenomena.[21] Triangulated research can involve the use of different investigators, theories and methods to study the one phenomenon with the assumption that the weaknesses in each single method will be compensated for by the counter-balancing strengths of another. This is not to argue that triangulation can ever produce a single "true" reality beyond the frameworks and inter-pretations provided by each research approach.[22] Data collection methods and interpretive approaches drawn from ethnomethodology,[23] oral history and discourse analysis[24] hold promise as ways of rendering complex social processes like the natural history of smoking cessation more transparent. The products of such parallel research would doubtless be examples of what the anthropologist Clifford Geertz has called "thick description".[25] They would also frequently be culturally and historically specific: understanding the process and motivations of smoking cessation among septuagenarian men in cardiac wards in Cairo will throw up radically different insights than those provided by research into why Australian teenage girls in the age of Madonna are smoking more than their male counterparts.[26] Such hermeneutic characteristics would doubtless perplex and frustrate some number-bound readers hoping for simple, replicable truths and axioms about successful tobacco control. But just as it would be facile to attempt to describe the meaning of Da Vinci's *Mona Lisa* only in terms of paint and brush strokes, so too are tunnel-visioned truths tethered to the short leashes of quantifiable explanatory variables equally as frustrating.

---

21 Jick 1979; Brewer and Hunter 1989.
22 Jankowski and Wester 1991.
23 Garfinkel 1967.
24 Van Dijk 1985.
25 Geertz 1973.
26 Hill, White, Williams and Gardner 1993.

The degree of analytic sophistication possessed by most politicians and funding bureaucrats will rarely require any venturing into the complexities of the attribution problem. Such people invariably want two-paragraph answers to questions like "Do these school programs work?" or "Will banning advertising reduce demand?" They are slaves to entrenched, simplified decision-making processes that conspire against answers predicated on any honest admission of the highly intertwined nature of the relationships involved.

International tobacco control agencies and expert groups, in their wisdom, have long called for comprehensive policies to turn the public tide against tobacco.[27] They have also been dismissive of efforts by the tobacco industry to attribute population-wide trends in tobacco consumption to the presence or absence of single variables (e.g. the industry's frequent insistence that the absence of tobacco advertising and the high smoking rates in the former Soviet Union *proved* that advertising bans did not reduce demand).[28] The rationale for comprehensive policies lies not in any belief that the individual platforms of such policy (advertising bans, price increases, clean indoor air policy, mandated school health education, strong health warnings and so on) simply have incremental, additive effects on demand. Rather, it lies in the recognition that each of these platforms are nurtured by the others, creating a synergism which produces slides in demands apparent in countries including Canada, New Zealand and Singapore. Probing the dynamics of this synergism using the wider range of research and analytic methods proposed above is long overdue in the professional literature of tobacco control. *Tobacco Control*, the *BMJ*'s new specialist journal in this area, will welcome reports and analysis that attempt to do this.

27 Gray and Daube 1980; World Health Organization 1979.
28 Chapman 1992a.

31
The banality of tobacco deaths

Smoking causes very large numbers of people to die: currently about 6 million a year, with an estimated 1 billion forecast to die this century, on present trends. The 11 September 2001 terrorist attacks caused the deaths of 2,996 people, and a colleague and I wrote the piece below, reflecting on why tobacco-caused deaths seem so unremarkable by comparison.

The attacks on 11 September 2001 and the subsequent anthrax scare have provided twin lessons in the perils and possibilities of tragedy.

> Thrift, thrift, Horatio! The funeral baked meats
> Did coldly furnish forth the marriage tables
> > William Shakespeare, *Hamlet*, Act I, Scene ii

The king dies and his son Hamlet mourns. Hamlet's grief is increased by his mother's unseemly haste to marry her late husband's brother. She has calculated too coldly. Health advocates are not evil plotters, but their motives and actions have sometimes been likened to those of Queen Gertrude and King Claudius. The question arises: should

---

Originally published as Shatenstein, Stan, and Chapman (2002). The banality of tobacco deaths. *Tobacco Control* 11: 1–2.

they profit from tragedy? And can the tobacco-control community appropriate dramatic images for its denormalisation campaigns and not alienate the public?

The 11 September attacks in New York and Washington, and the subsequent anthrax scare, have provided twin lessons in the perils and possibilities of tragedy. The bonds of faith, family and community can be shattered or strengthened in suffering's wake. In similar fashion, tobacco control advocates' messages can be emboldened, weakened or even repudiated by their proximity to disaster.

Tobacco control has had the dismal luxury of unimaginably "great" statistics to make its case. Globally, an estimated 4 million people die each year from tobacco-related illness,[1] compared to 2.7 million from malaria[2] and 2.8 million from AIDS.[3] After deaths from malnutrition (5.9 million in 1990)[4] and violence and injury (5.8 million),[5] tobacco claims more deaths than any other single cause. Between 1950 and 2000, it was estimated that smoking caused about 62 million deaths in developed countries (12.5 percent of all deaths: 20 percent of male deaths and 4 percent of female deaths). More than half of these deaths (38 million) will have occurred between the ages of 35 and 69. Currently, smoking is the cause of more than one in three (36 percent) male deaths in middle age, and about one in eight (13 percent) of female deaths. Each smoker who dies in this age group loses, on average, 22 years of life compared with average life expectancy.[6] By 2020, the World Health Organization estimates that "the burden of disease attributable to tobacco will outweigh that caused by any single disease".[7]

Those are numbers, well, to die for, but they fail to create a sense of urgency in the media, nor among policy makers or the public. As Joseph Stalin argued, "A single death is a tragedy, a million deaths are a statistic." Beatle George Harrison's death on 29 November 2001 from smoking-induced cancer was noted as much as if he had died from

---

1   Murray and Lopez 1996.
2   Breman, Egan and Keusch 2001.
3   UNAIDS 2000, 6.
4   Murray and Lopez 1996.
5   World Health Organization (n.d.b). Violence and injury prevention.
6   Peto, Lopez, Boreham, Thun and Heath 1992.
7   World Health Organization (n.d.a). The global burden of disease.

any other cause, despite losing more than 20 years off the average life expectancy of a 58-year-old man. Indeed the ABC network in the USA went so far as to note that unlike many other rock stars (Hendrix, Joplin, Morrison) Harrison had died of "natural causes". Eighteen years ago, Alan Blum reflected on community and political complacency about tobacco's death toll in an editorial titled "If smoking killed baby seals . . ."[8] Smokers are not, by and large, cuddly little things with plaintive round eyes. Their deaths, by cancer, heart disease and respiratory distress, tend to be quietly painful affairs, remarked only by those who knew and loved them.

Tobacco-control advocates have long tried to make smoking statistics resonate with a public numbed by endless quantification rhetoric advanced by myriad interest groups. Annual tobacco deaths in different nations have been routinely compared with deaths from so many jumbo jet crashes, the loss of football-stadium crowds, and the obliteration of entire medium-sized cities. Conferences and shopping centres display digital death-clocks for tobacco where audiences and shoppers transfix on the ever-mounting toll.

But, for all this, community concern about health problems can reach its zenith over low-probability threats that barely rate an asterisk on national cause-of-death tables. Risk-communication research shows that exotic, involuntary, catastrophic and sudden risks strike fear into the heart far easier than chronic, day-in-day-out dangers like smoking.[9] Folk wisdom tells us that a small sum spent on prevention is worth a fortune spent on cures, but cancer charities know which emphasis will see larger banknotes flow into collection buckets. Governments, with eyes firmly trained on the next electoral cycle, continue to give budgetary priority to acute health problems. Politicians wish to cast themselves in rescue fantasies in which grateful patients and their families form the backdrop to photo opportunities. And the news media are generally happy to perpetuate these myopic myths. One person killed after ingesting the contents of a contaminated tin of food can be more newsworthy than 4 million dying the world over, each and every year, from consuming tobacco products bought off the same store shelves.

---

8   Blum 1985.
9   Slovic 2000.

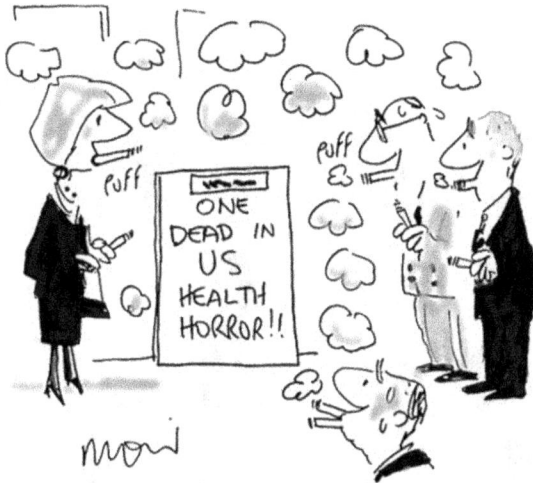

Figure 31.1 A cartoon by Alan Moir, published during the
2001 anthrax scare. Courtesy of the artist.

Alan Moir published a cartoon in the *Sydney Morning Herald*
in the first days of the anthrax mailings in the USA (Figure 31.1). It
showed a group of smokers reading the banner coverage of a single
death attributed to anthrax. As we go to press, five people have died
as a result of anthrax inhalation. An anti-smoking poster plainly
appropriating the New York twin towers outrage featured a simple call
for "No more killing", and showed two upturned cigarettes burning
in the shape of the World Trade Center before their collapse (Figure
31.2). Produced in Hong Kong by graphic artist Michael Miller Yu
and designer Eric Chan, tobacco-control groups there and elsewhere
refused to endorse it, branding it as gratuitous, "cheap, sensationalist
and 100 percent exploitative".[10] The chair of the Hong Kong Council
on Smoking and Health (COSH), Professor Tony Hedley, with an
understandable eye toward such sentiments, said, "We want people to
look at tobacco deaths on their own merits".[11]

---

10   Nichols 2001.

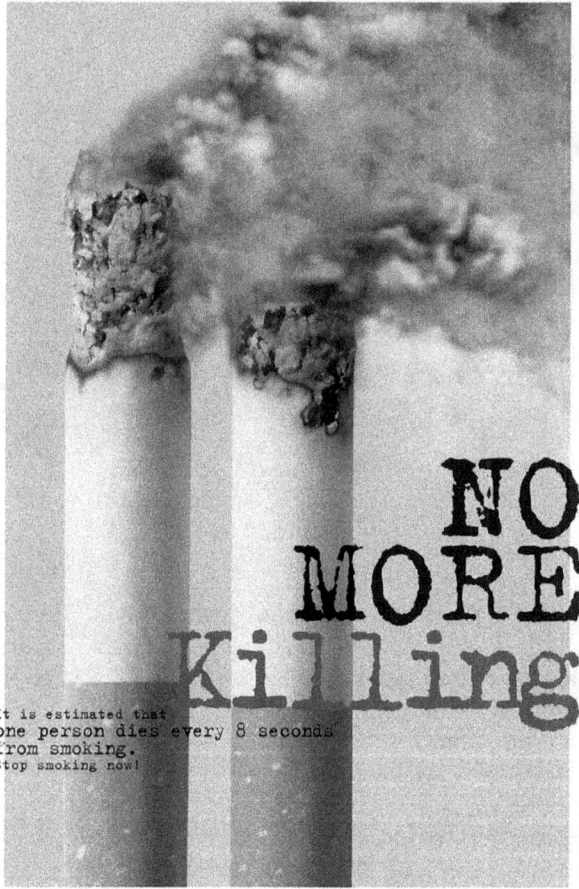

Figure 31.2 Anti-smoking poster by Hong Kong graphic artist
Michael Miller Yu and designer Eric Chan. Local tobacco control
groups refused to endorse it. Courtesy of the artist.

---

11   S. Schwartz 2001.

However, just three weeks later, former US surgeon-general C. Everett Koop translated tobacco's toll into a "Trade Tower fiasco" equation.[12] There is a saying that tragedy plus time equals comedy. Hitler was not the best subject for comedy right after the Second World War, but the Third Reich eventually became the subject of the movie and stage comedy *The Producers*, and an American TV sitcom, *Hogan's Heroes*. Perhaps Dr Koop has signalled that the time for a changed sensitivity about terrorism versus tobacco has come already.

It is a journalistic maxim to declare that "if it bleeds, it leads". Tobacco-control advocates don't have the sanguinary "luxury" of bold headlines to make their case, but they are not evil plotters. Their cause is relatively simple: smoking kills an obscenely large number of people, about half in middle age. But while smoking kills in large numbers, it does so one quiet, private death at a time. A single jumbo-jet crash that kills 300 people makes the front pages for days. The towers' collapse and anthrax deaths have created a climate of fear that will forever mark the generations that have been through it "live". The "excess mortality" deaths of 300, 3,000 or 30,000 tobacco users go relatively unnoticed, except by the smokers' grieving relatives. Hannah Arendt wrote of the banality of evil among the very "ordinary" men who perpetrated the Nazi atrocities.[13] Tobacco deaths have their own banality in desperate need of redefinition so that communities may become outraged in the face of industry misconduct and government inaction.

Whatever we think of the tobacco industry, it would be unfair to claim that, like terrorists, they hope their victims will die. However, the industry certainly knows that up to 50 percent of its users will, in fact, die as a result of using its products. It has spent decades knowingly and falsely reassuring smokers that they should not worry too much about "statistics" while also opposing every serious tobacco control measure in all global jurisdictions. This is not called terrorism, because the tobacco industry does not intend to strike fear and horror into people's hearts. But its behaviour is undeniably, appallingly criminal, on both the corporate and individual levels.

---

12   Koop 2001.
13   Arendt 1963.

The tobacco industry does not slow its rapacious campaigns to recruit and sustain its customer base, and the resistance may need to be just as muscular. From Australia's aorta TV ad to Canada's diseased gums package warning label, it's already taken some loud, even shocking images[14] to steal a march on the industry. There is a constant need to be forcefully creative while avoiding insensitivity.

The twin towers have fallen, the clean-up continues. The anthrax spores leave the mail system, but the investigation proceeds. And tobacco's toll grows higher, but the battle against the industry progresses slowly and fitfully. "It is estimated that one person dies every eight seconds from smoking", reads the fine print on the Hong Kong poster. Can any presentation of that message be more shocking than the number itself?

---

14   Mahood 1999.

32

Smokers spend, then pay with their lives

The late John Button was a senator in the Hawke government and after retiring from politics wrote opinion pieces for newspapers, including one in 1994 in which he let fly at tobacco control and stuck up for smokers' "rights". I returned serve with a few comparisons.

Last century, before John Button was a little boy, many pubs and shops scattered sawdust all over their floors. This helped absorb mud, and blood and vomit in some of the more exuberant establishments. But the sawdust was also very handy for soaking up the constant gobs of phlegm that people would unblinkingly spit when and where it pleased them.

Clearing one's throat and nose is undeniably pleasurable, as is farting – the indelicate subject raised by the dinner guest in John Button's article. In Elizabethan England, flatulence was considered normal and not proscribed by considerations of politeness or offensiveness. There seems to be no history written on the cause of the demise of public farting, but public expectoration went by the boards when its role in spreading tuberculosis was suspected.

Originally published as Chapman, Simon (1994). Smokers spend, then pay with their lives. *Age*, 24 March.

There are interesting similarities between spitting, farting and smoking in enclosed public spaces. Each is essentially personal and capable of being exercised in both private and in public. All three behaviours have emerged as the focus of social ostracism and, in the case of spitting and smoking, legal sanctions.

The pleasure these behaviours give to their perpetrators also causes unpleasant, and in the case of spitting and smoking, potentially harmful results to those exposed. In 1992 Mrs Liesel Scholem successfully sued her employer for $85,000 for the exacerbation of her asthma caused by occupational passive smoking. The US Environmental Protection Agency last year categorised cigarette smoke as a class-A carcinogen – meaning there was no safe level of exposure.

So where are the records of the spitters' and farters' rights groups? Did last century's spitters howl about being labelled social pariahs when asked to go to the bathroom to clear their throats? Was there a Farters' Rights Institute that sponsored tame ear, nose and throat specialists and gastroenterologists to correct misinformation being spread by those who like their air fresh? The critical difference between the three is that it is only smoking that involves a purchased commodity. With nothing to sell, there's no financial gain to be made by a group like the tobacco industry in promoting social acceptability. Talk today of spitters' rights might be appropriate to the clauses of a footballer's code on on-field conduct, but greeted with derision anywhere else. Yet John Button alluded to the plight of smokers' rights using language about Stalinism that insults everyone in medicine and public health who tries (and succeeds) now to prevent lung cancer.

When someone dies after a road crash, after eating a can of contaminated salmon or after an industrial accident, the death has a visibility that largely determines both private and public perceptions of what sort of death it was – whether it was avoidable, and the speed and style of response from government to prevent further similar deaths. The authority by which officials act to prevent further avoidable sudden deaths is testimony to the broad horror that we share about dying unexpectedly and to the unchallenged assumption that preventive action in such cases is a good thing.

Deaths caused by smoking tend to be quite different. In 1991, 1,739 men and 623 women in New South Wales died from lung cancer.

Deaths caused by smoking almost always occur away from the public gaze. A death from lung cancer or heart disease in a smoker will often occur following a decline in health or previous attacks. Lung cancer deaths, while often taking only a few months from diagnosis to grave, conclude in hospitals and hospices, settings where deaths are expected.

Again unlike dramatic deaths, where the causal agent (like a speeding car) or environment (like a drunken party before a road crash) is obvious to all, smoking deaths can tend to perplex others. The person smoked all their life, and there at the funeral stand several others who have also smoked all their lives. Consequently, there is widespread incredulity at statements that smoking is the leading cause of death in industrialised countries.

Australian tobacco consumption has declined by more than a third since 1976, the year John Button's Stalinists banned direct tobacco advertising on radio and television. Last year, sales were down by a record 6 percent in one year. Much of this is the flow-on from passive smoking: if people can't smoke at work, they not only reduce the risk to non-smokers but reduce their own consumption. In 1978, William Hobbs, a president of the tobacco multinational R.J. Reynolds, said about anti-smoking measures: "If they caused every smoker to smoke just one less cigarette a day, our company would stand to lose $92 million in sales annually. I assure you that we don't intend to let that happen without a fight."

Part of this fight has been the astute cultivation of the civil liberties causes by the tobacco industry, replete with the sort of gratuitous name-calling that John Button exemplified. People who save one person from drowning or rescue another from a burning building are rewarded for bravery. Transplant surgeons like Victor Chang are valorised as secular saints. Yet by public health standards, Chang saved a tiny number of lives in a highly dramatic fashion, compared to the less obvious results of preventive health endeavours like those John Button so demeans.

The National Heart Foundation estimates that between 1968 and 1988, the falling death rate from heart disease in Australia has "saved" 115,144 lives. Analysis of the equally dramatic decline in coronary heart disease mortality in the United States between 1968 and 1976 attributes 54 percent of the decline to lifestyle changes (principally the reduction in smoking) and only 3.5 percent to bypass surgery.

Cancer and heart disease charities know that if they talk about breakthroughs in treatment when they shake their collection tins, the public digs deeper. If they ask for money to help fund large passive-smoking prevention campaigns, far fewer feel disposed to be generous. John Button's views seem certain to perpetuate this futile outlook.

33

Death of a Fat Lady

When smokers die at "a certain age" there's often a tendency to shrug and feel that they were . . . well . . . old enough, and so what? But such subtle ageism that dismisses people who lose a decade or so off normal life expectancy, and often live in poor health before they die, is worth examining.

When Jennifer Paterson, half of the culinarily "incorrect" British TV cookery program *Two Fat Ladies*, recently died of lung cancer at 71, she lost eight years off the normal life expectancy of a British woman. If she started smoking at 18 years old, and smoked an average of 20 a day, she would have inhaled 387,165 cigarettes. At 12 puffs per cigarette, that is 4.65 million point-blank curings of the once-pristine pink linings of her lungs. With one cigarette taking an average of 5.6 minutes to smoke, she would have puffed continuously for 4.12 years. Put another way, for each cigarette she smoked, she lost nearly twice the time it took to smoke it.

Paterson lost a tenth of the life she might have otherwise lived. She enriched the lives of the viewers of her hugely popular program for only a short time, in what might otherwise have continued for years as one

Originally published as Chapman, Simon (1999). Death of a Fat Lady. *Tobacco Control* 8: 443.

of the most rewarding periods of her life. Some commentators waved this away with the condolence that she had a good innings and lived her eccentric life to the fullest. In doing so, they reveal an interesting ageism not unrelated to a whole raft of social policy that implies older people are not really worth bothering about. Yet how would these people feel if someone offered to remove the decade of their 20s or 30s? The absurdity of such an offer contrasted with the apparent acceptability to these commentators of such an early death says much about attitudes toward the aged.

Several years ago, the conservative British columnist Auberon Waugh wrote a small book, *Crash the ash: joy for the beleaguered smoker* (see *Tobacco Control* 4 [1995], 198). The intent of the book was to reclaim smoking from the clutches of the health fanatics and restore it to its former glories, before all this tiresome business about it killing people got about. Not unlike the "good on her" obituaries for Jennifer Paterson, Waugh argued that smokers should be seen as heroes because they have the decency to die early:

> smokers are heroes because they do . . . die, if indeed they do, on average two or three years younger. They do not then clutter up the welfare services, nor put a terrible burden on their children, nor spend everything they have to leave on nursing home fees. Longevity is becoming the great curse of Western civilisation. At its worst manifestation, there are wards and wards where old people lie in semi-coma, usually on a drip, recognising nobody, understanding nothing, being turned three times a day like damp hay.

The view of the aged as decrepit, and of tobacco as a laudable, deadly pleasure that can hurry them along, contrasts with the reality of ageing in many countries. In Australia, for example, 19 out of 20 people aged over 65 years do not live in hospitals or nursing homes. Even in those aged over 75, the figure is still nine in ten living in the community, often in good health. Lifetime tobacco-use contributes to unparalleled cardiovascular and respiratory morbidity in the aged, which, with the reduction in smoking, is being "compressed" into fewer years of disability.

Writing of Paterson's death, long-time tobacco-control cynic and Sydney columnist Paddy McGuinness claimed that "everyone" knows the risks of smoking, which have been "adequately conveyed" to the public, and that the tobacco industry did not knowingly conspire to addict, harm or kill people. I wonder if Jennifer Paterson had the remotest idea that she had a fourfold risk over non-smokers of going blind? Or that one in two smokers will die from a tobacco-caused disease, on average 12 years early, meaning that the average smoker will lose six years of life? Or that more than 80 percent of people first diagnosed with lung cancer will be dead within five years, one of the worst prognoses for any disease? How informed was her "choice" to smoke, and how much was it a lifetime of stoking her body's need for the next nicotine fix?

Jennifer Paterson perhaps sensibly told her surgeon to disappear when he suggested she quit after her diagnosis. What would have been the point when she was to die weeks later? The widespread mythologising of her smoking as another welcome nail in the coffin of political correctness will warm the hearts of the tobacco industry. Too bad, though, for the millions of anonymous victims around the world whose similar bleak demise each year passes unsung.

34

Stop-smoking clinics: a case for their abandonment

Very early in my career, I saw a major roadblock in tobacco control. This was the complete mismatch between the effort put into individually focused quit-smoking strategies and the sheer number of smokers in the population. The "reach" of these small efforts could never hope to make anything but a tiny and inconsequential impact on population-wide smoking. So I took courage and pointed this out in one of my first pieces of heretical writing on tobacco control. The article below, published in *The Lancet*, nearly caused me to be lynched by English quit-smoking leaders, some of whom were actively promoting quit-smoking clinics. But as we shall see in the next three pieces, I've felt it important to keep this perspective under active consideration over the next 30 years.

Health agencies seeking to maximise the number of people stopping smoking must consider two broad questions. The first concerns effectiveness: is one approach more effective than another in helping smokers stop; do different methods work better with different smokers? Questions of effectiveness are asked by academics and therapists with

Originally published as Chapman, Simon (1985). Stop-smoking clinics: a case for their abandonment. *The Lancet* 1(8434): 918–20.

professional interest in the intrinsic merits of various approaches. The second question asks whether interventions can be applied throughout a community: has an approach the potential to meet the mass demand its successful operation would imply; what staffing levels are necessary to penetrate a target group; are these levels realistic in times of economic recession? If these questions are asked at all, they are asked by health administrators, funding agencies, politicians, and above all by the tobacco industry. The industry's opposition can be thought of as the litmus test of a method's likely impact. The industry has gone on record as "fully supporting sensible and effective public education"[1] about smoking and only the naive could see such a statement as anything less than encouragement for orthodox smoking-control activities. The industry has never opposed stop-smoking groups and therapies, but it has actively fought mass health-promotion programs[2] and legislative proposals.[3] In 1982, 38 percent of men and 33 percent of women smoked in the UK[4] – a formidable number of people. All cessation approaches need to be evaluated in relation to this second goal of mass application before they are assessed in terms of their effectiveness. A 5 percent success rate among 10,000 people is over 333 times more efficient than the 30 percent success rate achieved by group work involving only 50 subjects. It is this latter sort of activity, however, that occupies nearly everyone involved in smoking cessation.

Most of the people working in the field are psychologists and the literature is dominated by therapeutic approaches based on individual and small-group techniques. A randomly chosen year of the annual bibliography[5] from the US Office on Smoking and Health, which abstracts all research and commentary connected with the subject, was surveyed to establish this domination. The 1981 volume contained 2,055 abstracts. One hundred and twenty-eight concerned research and descriptions of cessation techniques, but only four of these described mass-reach programs and a further four described strategies that might

---

1   Wood 1983.
2   Egger, Fitzgerald, Frape, Monaem, Rubinstein, Tyler and McKay 1983.
3   Peachment 1984.
4   Office of Population Censuses and Surveys 1982.
5   Shopland 1981.

be adopted by general practitioners and other health workers. Of the 128 abstracts, 33 were doctoral dissertations that included such esoteric procedures as "subliminal stimulation of symbiotic fantasies", "contingency contracting", and "griefwork". The study groups of the reports seldom exceeded 100 self-selected subjects. The literature on smoking cessation is biased towards therapeutic interventions modelled on psychological concepts of smoking as a behavioural or dependency problem.

Smoking cessation groups and clinics: their contribution to reducing smoking prevalence

Raw and Heller reviewed[6] the functioning of all 55 stop-smoking clinics in the UK in 1983. There are considerable difficulties in estimating the precise contribution of these clinics to a national reduction in smoking prevalence. Only 19 (36 percent) of the clinics had usable data and none had kept records of follow-up essential for determining the permanency of cessation. These 19 had a total annual throughput of 2,390 smokers and a total abstinent population after one year of 560 (mean 23 percent and a range of 14 to 43 percent). If this figure were trebled to account for success rates from the remaining 36 clinics (probably a very liberal assumption), a total emerges of approximately 1,680 people who appear to have stopped smoking following attendance at cessation clinics and groups in one year. How does this figure compare with the potential number of smokers who might be described as ripe to stop? When 1,711 British smokers were asked "How determined are you to try and give up smoking?", 42 percent answered positively.[7] If this figure were at all indicative of the proportion of smokers actively thinking of stopping, then 8.3 million (of Britain's 19.8 million adult smokers) represents the number of potential ex-smokers. In contrast, organised stop-smoking groups and clinics benefit 0.2 percent, or one in every 5,000 smokers currently wanting to stop. Levitt reached similar conclusions about the role of

---

6   Raw and Heller 1984.
7   Marsh and Matheson 1983.

clinics in the USA, where, in 1975, 2,176 reached less than 0.1 percent of smokers.[8] At that rate, 200,000 clinics would be required just to keep the proportion of smokers at the present level. As can be seen from a comparison with the rate at which people are stopping smoking unaided, clinics make an utterly insignificant contribution to the overall pattern of smoking cessation. In Britain in 1982, 30 percent of men and 16 percent of women were ex-smokers, proportions that had risen from 23 percent and 10 percent respectively in 1972.[9] This trend corresponds to the decline in smoking prevalence over the same decade (down from 53 to 38 percent in men and from 41 to 33 percent in women). Evidence suggests that the decline in smoking prevalence is a result of people giving up smoking rather than fewer young people taking up the habit. Marsh suggests:

> Smokers do give up. Many relapse but try again. So much so that it is increasingly difficult to see "smokers" and "ex-smokers" as discrete categories. There is heavy traffic in both directions but the aggregate flow is constantly swelling the numbers of enduring ex-smokers.[10]

How then have therapeutic, small-scale approaches come to dominate worldwide cessation efforts when simple arithmetic points to the futility of group-based approaches? One answer is that clinical psychologists have long had a professional interest in dependency problems. It was natural for them to apply their training and skills to programs of smoking cessation. Psychologists view themselves as assisting individuals. Criticism that their aggregated efforts do not reduce smoking prevalence is misplaced, since that was never their aim. Raw and Heller also found that 62 percent of clinics were run by health-education officers, whose work is normally of neither an individual nor therapeutic nature.

---

8 Levitt 1983.
9 Office of Population Censuses and Surveys 1982.
10 Marsh 1983.

Public demand for clinics

People who work in smoking control receive enquiries every day from smokers wanting to join a stop-smoking group. The frequency of these inquiries has led health workers to establish groups in response to demand. Potential ex-smokers hold media-fanned preconceptions about what they need and what they will experience, particularly in connection with group work. The reflex action of health workers to provide these groups clouds perspective: how representative of smokers are these people, and is the time and labour investment appropriate as a long-term strategy? There are many benefits associated with cessation clinics that have nothing to do with reducing smoking prevalence, but which are nonetheless real. Stopping smoking is seen as a cure, and if smoking needs to be cured, then the magical, laying-on-of-hands accoutrements of curing must parallel those of medicine in general. Clinics and groups are tangible entities, located in buildings with staff who have concrete, comprehensible tasks, unlike most health-education work, which sounds vague and has imperceptible effects in the short term. Public expectation that stopping smoking involves some sort of supervised therapeutic process has probably been amplified by media interest in the more exotic forms of cessation. The mystique and paraphernalia of popular notions of psychology, acupuncture and hypnotism are infinitely more newsworthy than the fact that most people stop smoking unspectacularly and alone. There is the expectation that stopping is extremely difficult and that one should place oneself passively in the hands of a healer.

Lehrer has described a quasi-sick role in group attenders, suggesting that their motivation includes a need to define themselves as ill, as much as a desire to stop smoking.[11] Smoking-cessation groups are often used as a pretext for unburdening wider psychosocial difficulties. Apologists for the clinics report attenders to be hardcore heavy smokers, whose habit is so entrenched that it is unlikely to be broken unaided. However, there is no evidence of such a difference between clinic attendees and those who stop smoking on their own in terms of smoking habit, smoking history, number of attempts to stop or

---

11   Lehrer 1978.

personality.[12] A second view current in the professional community is that stopping smoking is so difficult that not to provide assistance to people wishing to give up is victim-blaming at best and sadistic at worst. The argument runs that mass-media campaigns that persuade and frighten people into wanting to stop smoking must include some sort of program of help. Clinics are often described as support services for clients, with no objective of reducing smoking prevalence in the community. However, among people who stopped smoking unaided, the picture is somewhat different. Only 19 percent of British ex-smokers report stopping as very difficult, 27 percent as fairly difficult, while a majority of 53 percent remember stopping as not at all difficult. Fifteen percent reported stopping as harder than expected, 38 percent as expected, and 41 percent as easier than expected.[13] It should be remembered that these figures are obtained from successful ex-smokers. Those who found it impossible are not included. This unsuccessful group remains substantial and cannot realistically be treated in therapeutic settings.

A case against providing support for smoking cessation

It seems likely that there will always be a small proportion of dissonant smokers (who may appear quite large in number) who genuinely seem unable to quit unaided, and who seek help from groups and therapists. Ideally, this tail-end of the smoking population should be catered for in ways that are effective, non-exploitative and above all not disproportionately demanding of scarce capital and staff. Since health-service resources exist in a far from ideal world, priorities for the allocation of staff funding must be determined in the light of reducing total smoking prevalence. Provision of cessation clinics and groups perpetuates the idea that smoking has to be cured, so inhibiting the growth of confidence in self-directed cessation. A spirit of comprehensiveness sometimes motivates the establishment of a two-tiered system of help: self-help materials and a group or clinic. Self-help

---

12   Pederson and Lefcoe 1976; DiClemente and Prochaska 1982.
13   Lehrer 1978.

then becomes a second-rate option: why just get a kit when you can get the full treatment? The provision and publicity of group treatment can only cast a shadow over self-help. Most smokers attracted to self-help campaigns will have tried several times to stop smoking. People who view the prospect of stopping as easy will be unlikely to seek out any form of assistance. Those who do probably view themselves as failures. The task facing campaign planners is to instil confidence in such people. If intensive therapy, with its aura of psychology and cure, is on offer, how much more difficult does it become to help people to motivate themselves?

There is one vitally important exception to the argument that labour-intensive cessation programs are a waste of time: the daily contact of thousands of smokers with their doctors. Russell's study of general practitioners' advice to smoking patients suggested that a GP could expect about 25 long-term successes a year. If all GPs in the UK participated, the yield would exceed half a million ex-smokers a year, a target that could not be matched by increasing the present 50 or so clinics to 10,000! Obvious potential exists for involving dentists, health visitors, physiotherapists and nurses in similar schemes. A cardinal emphasis throughout this paper has been that if smoking prevalence is to decline significantly throughout a population, then efforts must be made to induce mass numbers of people not to smoke. Techniques pursued face-to-face or in small groups may occasionally produce impressive success rates, but they are insufficiently broad-based to achieve impressive numbers. The most widely acclaimed smoking cessation programs remain in the worst traditions of inconsequential research if they are incapable of becoming incorporated into a delivery system involving significant numbers of the smoking community.

35
The inverse impact law of smoking cessation

In 1971, Welsh GP Julian Tudor Hart wrote a seminal essay in *The Lancet* on what he termed the "inverse care law". He postulated that "The availability of good medical care tends to vary inversely with the need for it in the population served." Twenty-three years after I wrote the previous essay in *The Lancet*, I revisited the issue with my twist on Tudor Hart's observation, this time applied to the back-to-front concentration of research and effort in smoking cessation on individuals rather than on populations.

In 1985 I argued for the abandonment of smoking cessation clinics,[1] which make an inconsequential contribution to reducing smoking in whole populations[2] – the test of their public health significance. Their labour intensity devours resources that could be better used in mass campaigns[3] to motivate cessation in far more smokers than the best

---

1 Chapman 1985.
2 Milne 2005; Bauld, Judge and Platt 2007.
3 Wakefield, Durkin, Spittal, Siahpush, Scollo, Simpson, Chapman, White and Hill 2008.

Originally published as Chapman, Simon (2008). The inverse impact law of smoking cessation. *The Lancet* 373: 701–3.

evidence shows are interested in attending clinics, let alone benefiting from them.

But the most powerful argument against a frontline role for clinics is their reiterating message that "You need help and are unlikely to succeed alone." Over 25 years, with the advent of nicotine-replacement therapy (NRT), buproprion and varenicline, this arguably misleading message has been turbocharged through heavy pharmaceutical advertising directed at both consumers and physicians. Whilst legions of clinical trials[4] and more equivocal real-world evaluations[5] show that assistance improves cessation, unassisted cessation remains the preferred and most successful method used by most ex-smokers.

Today's sustained medicalisation of cessation epitomises Ivan Illich's concept of a disabling profession.[6] It purposefully erodes smokers' confidence in taking control of a process that hundreds of millions of ex-smokers globally have demonstrated works better for more than any other. Typical of this medicalisation, a recent *Lancet* seminar on tobacco addiction[7] devoted just half a sentence in ten pages to the rhinoceros in the living room: that some 25 years after the advent of NRT, there remains daylight between unassisted cessation and the population cessation-yield obtained by all other methods combined.[8][9]

Acknowledging Julian Tudor Hart,[10] I propose the inverse impact law of smoking cessation. This law states that the volume of research and effort devoted to professionally and pharmacologically mediated cessation is in inverse proportion to that examining how ex-smokers actually quit. Research on cessation is dominated by ever-more-finely tuned accounts of how smokers can be encouraged to do anything but go it alone when trying to quit – exactly the opposite of how a very large majority of ex-smokers succeeded. The virtual silence about this undeniably positive news reflects the dominance of those whose careers depend on continuing to offer and evaluate labour-intensive regimens

---

4 Silagy, Lancaster, Stead, Mant and Fowler 2006.
5 Walsh 2008.
6 Illich 1977.
7 Hatsukami, Stead and Gupta 2008.
8 Biener, Reimer, Wakefield, Szczypka, Rigotti and Connolly 2006.
9 Doran, Valenti, Robinson, Britt and Mattick 2006.
10 Hart 1971.

and the influence of the drug industry, which has a vested interest in prolonging cessation and in repeat attempts after relapse. Those impertinent enough to note the continuing dominance of unassisted cessation among ex-smokers and to encourage smokers to go it alone are regarded as heretical, so pervasive is the inverse impact law of smoking cessation I describe and the imperatives for researchers to inhabit its doctrine. Disciples of the law are preoccupied with success rates, when success numbers are what really matter in public health. Extrapolating from Californian data for 1996,[11] of 1 million smokers attempting to quit, I calculate that nearly twice as many smokers (60,999) quit unaided than with any form of help (33,014), despite many years of NRT availability.[12] I know of no population data from any nation since that shows otherwise.

Cold turkey is routinely framed as the enemy of effective smoking cessation, a kind of amateur half-hearted approach to cessation, when it ought to be embraced as the first-choice method that over decades has consistently assisted far more than any other approach. Failed quit attempts (the average ex-smoker can experience up to 14 of these[13]) should be redefined as normal rehearsals for success, the unassisted quitting experience demystified as how most people actually quit, and pharmacotherapy restored to the perspective it deserves.

The English approach to cessation epitomises the legacy of the law I propose. There, tobacco-control expenditure has been heavily focussed on dedicated smoking-cessation services, requiring attendance at individual or group counselling sessions with emphasis on NRT. A 2005 report that examined the contribution of this program to reaching a national smoking prevalence target of 21 percent by 2010 stated:

Nationally, stop smoking achieved a reduction in prevalence of 0.51 percent in 2003/04. If persisting up to 2010, this success rate would lead to a reduction in prevalence of 3.6 percent – i.e. from the current level of 26 percent to 22.4 percent. For stop smoking services alone

---

11   Zhu, Melcer, Sun, Rosbrook and Pierce 2000.
12   Biener, Reimer, Wakefield, Szczypka, Rigotti and Connolly 2006; Zhu, Melcer, Sun, Rosbrook and Pierce 2000.
13   Hughes, Keely and Naud 2004.

to meet the target of 21 percent, in England the number of successful quitters each year would need to be 50 percent greater.

However, in a remarkably understated next paragraph, the report continues:

since successful quitting [in these calculations] is measured by a self-report at 4 weeks and only 25 percent of smokers remain quit at 12 months . . . all the estimates of reduction in prevalence calculated in this report could legitimately be divided by four – producing an overall reduction of 0.13 percent per year or around 1 percent (from 26 percent to 25 percent) by 2010 for England.[14]

Australia, by contrast, has negligible cessation services and since 1997 has run large scare-based[15] campaigns to motivate quit attempts. Daily smoking prevalence in those aged 14 years and older has fallen by 30.2 percent, from 23.8 percent in 1995 to 16.6 percent in 2007,[16] with only 3.6 percent of adult smokers having ever even called the Quitline.[17] While pharmaceutical advertisers coattail the governmental campaign, the latter has never given centre stage to messages implying that smokers need help. We need to restore smokers' confidence in their ability to do what literally millions of smokers have done for many decades without having to rely on help.

14   Tocque, Barker and Fullard 2005.
15   Hill, Chapman and Donovan 1998.
16   Australian Institute of Health and Welfare 2008.
17   Miller, Wakefield and Roberts 2008.

36

Quitting unassisted: the 50-year neglect of a major health phenomenon

In this essay, my colleague Andrea Smith and I elaborated on the theme of the previous article in this book, after an invitation from the editor of *JAMA* to reflect on what we had learned (or forgotten) about an important issue in the last 50 years of tobacco control.

Smoking-cessation research today is dominated by the development and evaluation of interventions to improve the odds of quitting successfully. Yet little attention has been paid to the large majority of ex-smokers who quit without recourse to any formal assistance. To many, these unassisted quitters are of little interest other than as a comparator population against which to test the efficacy or effectiveness of pharmaceutical or behavioural interventions. The impact of this neglect is compounded by the preference for reporting intervention success as *rates* rather than as the *numbers* of ex-smokers generated across populations through such interventions. In so doing, researchers have insulated those in policy and practice from the importance of

Originally published as Smith, Andrea L. and Simon Chapman (2014). Quitting unassisted: the 50-year neglect of a major health phenomenon. *The Journal of the American Medical Association* 311(2): 137–8.

unassisted cessation and the unparalleled contribution it has and will continue to make to reducing smoking prevalence.

In 1955, five years after Wynder and Graham's historic study of smokers and lung cancer was published in the *Journal of the American Medical Association*,[1] 7.7 million Americans (6.4 percent of the population) were former smokers. Ten years later, following widespread publicity surrounding the 1964 US surgeon-general's report, this had ballooned to 19.2 million (13.5 percent) ex-smokers. By 1975, 32.6 million Americans (19.4 percent) had stopped smoking.[2] In 1978, the then-director of the US Office on Smoking and Health noted in a National Institute of Drug Abuse monograph: "In the past 15 years, 30 million smokers have quit the habit, almost all of them on their own."[3] Many of these quitters had been very heavy smokers.

In the same monograph another commentator continued: "longitudinal studies should be designed to investigate the natural history of spontaneous quitters . . . We know virtually nothing about such people or their success at achieving and maintaining abstinence."[4] Thirty-five years later, very little has changed about that ignorance: knowledge of mass smoking cessation across 50 years reflects the "inverse impact law of smoking cessation".[5] Far more is known about the "tail" of people who quit via pharmacological and professionally mediated interventions than about the mass "dog" of ex-smokers who continue to quit unassisted.

Yet smoking-cessation research has its roots in unassisted cessation. In the 1970s and 1980s, those grappling with why success rates for therapy seekers were no better than those for self-quitters turned their attention to study those who quit on their own.[6] As a population, self-quitters were thought to hold the answers to the problem of smoking cessation. Studies throughout the 1970s and 1980s led to the identification of strategies that successful self-quitters

---

1 Wynder and Graham 1950.
2 Horn 1978.
3 Krasnegor 1979.
4 Krasnegor 1979.
5 Chapman 2009.
6 Prochaska, DiClemente and Norcross 1992.

employed, and these occasionally informed the design of both individual and mass-reach interventions.

In 1988, understanding of the effects of nicotine on the central nervous system and on the ability of nicotine replacement therapy (NRT) to mitigate withdrawal prompted the widespread belief that moderating withdrawal reactions would facilitate quitting. Four years later, a review of smoking cessation concluded that in light of this new knowledge, "What is required is a broader perspective and greater respect for the limited role of individual and even small-group interventions. Over the past decade we have witnessed a sometimes grudging acknowledgement of and interest in the pharmacological aspects and addictive properties of tobacco."[7] Psychologists wedded to clinical models were making way for what they saw as the first potentially mass-reach effective approach to cessation.

Twenty-five years after tobacco use was officially labelled an addiction and NRT heralded as the first big hope for smoking cessation, it is time to take stock of cessation pharmacotherapy. It appears that this "treatable condition" is not responding as hoped either to NRT or to the prescription stop-smoking medications bupropion or varenicline that followed.[8] Sadly, it remains the case that by far the most common outcome at 6 to 12 months after using such medication in real-world settings is continuing smoking. Undoubtedly, much smoker resistance to using cessation medication is because many smokers learn from other smokers that real-world experience of using these drugs does not produce outcomes that remotely compare with benchmarks for other drugs they use for other purposes. Few if any other drugs for any purpose with such records would ever be prescribed.

Despite massive publicity and (in some nations) subsidies given to NRT, bupropion and varenicline during these decades, the additional tens of millions (or hundreds of millions globally) who quit smoking in this time continued to be dominated by those who quit without pharmacological or professional assistance.[9] For the congenitally

---

7   Lichtenstein and Glasgow 1992.
8   Walsh 2011.
9   Fiore, Novotny, Pierce, Giovino, Hatziandreu, Newcomb, Surawicz and Davis 1990; Pierce, Cummins, White, Humphrey and Messer 2012.

optimistic this is perennially explained as sub-optimal reach or dissemination, with the solution being facilitating greater access to assistance, improving smoker knowledge about the benefits of assistance, or further individualising treatment. But after nearly three decades of turbo-charged effort by the pharmaceutical industry to increase physician engagement and erode population resistance to pharmaceutical cessation, can there be any more serious rabbits left in that hat?

It has been argued that NRT and stop-smoking medications are less effective under "real-world" conditions than in research trials.[10] In Australia, data on the real-world experiences of varenicline indicate stark differences from experiences under research conditions.[11] For example, compliance is far lower: in Australia, 44 to 50 percent of patients who received subsidised prescriptions for varenicline failed to commence the last eight weeks of treatment (no data were available to indicate what proportion of the remainder completed the last eight weeks of treatment), in contrast to 12-week completion rates of 68 to 76 percent in clinical trials. Yet between January 2008 and October 2009, the Australian government spent $93 million on varenicline prescriptions. This compares with $59 million allocated over four years to social marketing campaigns designed to promote quit attempts in Australia. Given this relatively high spend on pharmacotherapy, it is essential that we are realistic about its potential impact on population smoking prevalence and whether attention would be better focused on boosting the campaigns known to stimulate mass cessation.[12]

It may be time to place greater value on the lived experiences of the millions of ex-smokers who have successfully quit smoking, particularly in recent years. A 2013 national Gallup Poll reported only 8 percent of ex-smokers attributed their success to NRT patches, gum or prescribed drugs.[13] In contrast, 48 percent attributed their success to cold turkey and 8 percent to willpower, commitment or "mind over

---

10   Walsh 2011.
11   Walsh 2011.
12   Wakefield, Durkin, Spittal, Siahpush, Scollo, Simpson, Chapman, White and Hill 2008.
13   Newport 2013.

matter". Nearly 40 years earlier, Gallup reported that most smokers would not attend formal cessation programs and preferred to quit on their own.[14] Unassisted cessation has always been both the most preferred way of quitting and the method used by most ex-smokers on their final, successful quit attempt, yet quitting unassisted is routinely denigrated as being not "evidence-based".

The 1964 US surgeon-general's report kick-started the first significant and sustained period of anti-smoking activity and public consciousness of smoking and health issues. Compared with today's plethora of comprehensive tobacco-control policies, the subsequent smoking exodus was driven by only a handful of anti-smoking policies. For many smokers, having a reason to quit (a *why*) was more important than having a method to quit (a *how*). The key may therefore be to focus on motivating more smokers to try to quit and to try to quit more frequently, regardless of whether these quit attempts are assisted or unassisted.

A recent review attempting to shed light on the apparent failure of contemporary obesity-prevention policy and practice concluded that the fundamental flaw in obesity research is that "medicine today is taught untethered from its history".[15] Smoking cessation, in looking to its future, should not forget the ever-repeated important lessons from its past.

---

14   Lichtenstein and Glasgow 1992.
15   Taubes 2013.

37

Is it time to stop subsidising nicotine replacement therapies?

Nicotine replacement therapy used without expert "supervision" is now acknowledged as almost useless, even by those who championed it for many years.[1] When it is used in conjunction with professional support, it does better. But the problem here is that only a tiny proportion of smokers have any interest in going along to such support. And after some 30 years of it being available, no one knows how to change this lack of interest. In this piece, I asked whether it might be time that the government pulled the plug on subsidising it.

Nicotine replacement therapy (NRT) became available in Australia in 1984 (gum) and 1993 (patches), first as prescription-only items. From 1988, they started becoming available over the counter, with patches available without prescription from 1997. Today, some forms of NRT can even be bought in supermarkets.

If prescribed, NRT attracts a government subsidy. In the 17 months from July 2013 to December 2014, data provided by the Department of

---

1 See Kotz, Brown and West 2014.

Originally published as Chapman, Simon (2015). Is it time to stop subsidising nicotine replacement therapies? *The Conversation*, 27 January.

Health show 199,818 NRT scripts cost the government $8,617,804. But 31 years later, what should governments do if data show that NRT is little better, or even a good deal worse, at helping smokers quit than if they try to do it cold turkey?

Globally, the pharmaceutical industry understandably wants to convince quitters to use their products as much as possible. The smoking-cessation field has long been dominated[2] by research and promotional activity on how to deter smokers from ever attempting to quit without pharmacological or behavioural assistance, despite this being the way that most smokers have always quit.

Claims have abounded for years that NRT can significantly increase a smoker's chance of quitting compared to placebo. These claims have overwhelmingly derived from clinical trials. But clinical trials differ markedly from real-world use of NRT:

- Clinical trials exclude many people who might purchase NRT, such as those with any mental illness.[3]
- There are major problems with blindness integrity (unsurprisingly, many smokers pickled in nicotine for years can guess if they have been allocated to the placebo arm of the trial).[4]
- Trialists are contacted an average of 7.6 times by eager and supportive research staff trained to maximise retention of participants in the study.[5]
- Trialists are often paid for their participation.
- The drugs participants get are always free.

All this combines to produce an unreal situation in which trial participants do not represent all smokers and can be highly motivated to complete the trial to "please" the researchers.

So, 31 years on, how does NRT perform away from clinical trials in the real world?

---

2 Chapman and MacKenzie 2010.
3 Le Strat, Rehm and Le Foll 2011.
4 Mooney, White and Hatsukami 2004.
5 Walsh 2008.

One of the world's most rigorous and important data sets on smoking cessation comes from the Smoking in England study.[6] A recent paper from that project casts a pall over any impact of NRT, other than generating more expensive urine in most of those who use it. The paper reported on 1,560 English smokers who had made at least one recent and serious quit attempt.[7] At six months, 23 percent were not smoking on the day they completed the questionnaire.

Several things stand out from this important study. First, smokers who used NRT obtained over the counter had by far the worst quit rate (15.4 percent) of any of the methods used. Even quitting unassisted (without using any medication or professional support), much denigrated by the makers of NRT and many smoking-cessation professionals, saw 24.2 percent taking this approach quit: a rate 57 percent higher than in those using NRT obtained over the counter. The authors of the paper speculate that this low rate of success for NRT users may be explained by "inappropriate usage and low adherence in the real world".

Over the past three decades, NRT has been massively promoted via advertising and by pharmacists and doctors who have been heavily targeted by visiting sales reps. Doctors have been deluged with reprints of scientific articles on the virtues of NRT, and many have attended often lavishly catered educational meetings. Today, undying optimists still flying a flag for NRT still think there is hope that its users might one day start using NRT properly. Meanwhile, most who buy it keep smoking.

Second, the "most effective" method of quitting was also by far the least popular and acceptable. Using a prescribed medication (including NRT) and receiving specialised support for "at least six sessions" from one of England's dedicated smoking-cessation services saw 38.7 percent quit. But while the authors emphasised this throughout the paper, they were silent on how this best rate multiplied by the relatively small numbers availing themselves of these services would make much impression on the national goal of significantly boosting England's quit rate at the population level. Any "most effective" way of quitting

---

6   http://www.smokinginengland.info/.
7   Kotz, Brown and West 2014.

radically reduces in importance if few people are prepared to use it. Only 4.8 percent of people attempting to quit were prepared to avail themselves of the "full monty" specialist cessation centres. These, even with the best success rate, contributed just 29 of the 359 who had quit using any method (8 percent of all quitters). This compared with 168 who had quit unassisted (a rate of 24.2 percent), yielding in this study nearly six times as many quitters as the specialist centres.

Third, having doctors write prescriptions for NRT or other prescribed cessation medications, and offering brief advice on quitting, produced a success rate only marginally higher than unassisted cessation (27.8 percent v 24.2 percent).

The fourth stand-out message is what was *not* emphasised in the paper. If over-the-counter NRT (as it is mostly used), produces a far worse quit rate than smokers going cold turkey, where is the chorus of smoking-cessation experts telegraphing this message to the community? How much worse would the data have to be before cessation experts declare its use-by date has arrived? If the focus is on methods that yield high numbers of quitters throughout a population, this paper shows – as have many others – that cold turkey produced nearly 90 percent as many quitters (168) as all other methods combined (191). Yet cold turkey is denigrated in pharmaceutical industry messaging like Pfizer's "Don't go cold turkey" campaign.[8] The neglect[9] of serious study of the way most smokers actually quit may be keeping us from gaining important insights that could be useful in campaign messaging.

Important questions also need to be asked about whether continuing the substantial government investment in subsidised NRT is sensible. In the six months from July to December 2012 (the latest available data), the Commonwealth spent $8.7 million on media placement of anti-smoking messages, trying to stimulate smokers to make quit attempts.[10] How many more attempts might have been made had that figure been able to draw on the money being allocated to

---

8   http://bit.ly/2cA8TP1
9   Smith, Chapman and Dunlop 2015.
10 *Campaign Advertising by Australian Government Departments and Agencies* 2013.

subsidised NRT? Two studies of various Australian policies and programs' impact on declining smoking prevalence between 1995 and 2011 found no evidence[11] of impact by NRT sales or advertising volume.[12]

---

11   Wakefield, Durkin, Spittal, Siahpush, Scollo, Simpson, Chapman, White and Hill 2008.
12   Wakefield, Coomber, Durkin, Scollo, Bayly, Spittal, Simpson and Hill 2014.

38

The ethics of the cash register: taking tobacco industry research dollars

In "It's alright, ma (I'm only bleeding)", Bob Dylan sang that "money doesn't talk, it swears". The influence of the tobacco industry via its financial support to political parties, sport, culture, charities and research over decades has bought it many favours and slowed progress in global tobacco control. In 2002, British American Tobacco funded the International Centre for Corporate Social Responsibility at Nottingham University. Stan Shatenstein and I drew a few analogies and considered the ethics involved.

A dictator plunders billions from his nation's treasury. Soon for exile, he offers some ill-gotten millions to one of his land's universities, insisting that it fund a new school of social welfare studies that will bear his name.

For years, an oil baron has traded petroleum products for weapons, fuelling a lengthy, futile regional conflict. Sensitive to international criticism, he promises a few million pounds to a prestigious European university, to create a chair in "peace studies".

Originally published as Chapman, Simon and Stan Shatenstein (2001). The ethics of the cash register: taking tobacco industry research dollars. *Tobacco Control* 10: 1–2.

A pornographer makes millions from films employing, on miserable wages, illiterate men and women from slums and villages of Asian nations. Now the subject of international vilification in the Western media, he offers a fraction of his riches to his alma mater. The caveat? The money must establish a chair in erotic literature.

An unrepentant Nazi officer amassed fabulous wealth by selling possessions of concentration camp victims. Grateful to the country that provided him refuge from judgement at Nuremberg, he expresses appreciation on his death bed by donating his fortune to the nation's leading school, insisting that it be used to teach "a critical history of the Holocaust".

A leading tobacco company controls over 15 percent of the global market,[1] making it responsible, annually, for more than 600,000 deaths worldwide.[2] The company promises millions of pounds to create an International Centre for Corporate Social Responsibility, where students may learn of the "social and environmental responsibilities of multinational companies".[3]

The above suggestions are in lurid, poor taste. Surely, no academic institution would risk international opprobrium by accepting such a scheme? Yet, that is precisely what has happened this past December.

For the sobering sum of £3.8 million (around $5.7 million), British American Tobacco (BAT) announced that it would fund an International Centre for Corporate Social Responsibility at Britain's Nottingham University. As one television reporter succinctly asked: "Ever heard the joke about the cigarette salesman and social responsibility? Well, it turns out this is no cheap gag."[4]

Two things should immediately be clear here: first, a university not hungry for money is a fiction; second, there are few universities that would not draw a line *somewhere* about the appropriateness of taking money from disreputable sources. Apparently, Nottingham University is one of the unhappy few that would seem to have no such qualms.

---

1 British American Tobacco.
2 Action on Smoking and Health n.d.
3 Rushe 2000.
4 Thomson 2000.

BAT's gift comes at a time when the company is being investigated by the UK Department of Trade and Industry over allegations of involvement in international tobacco smuggling[5] and in the still-churning wake of revelations concerning what is, undeniably, the world's largest, longest running and most mendacious consumer fraud ever perpetrated.[6]

We wrote to Nottingham's vice-chancellor, Sir Colin Campbell, asking him if he would also be willing to accept money for university purposes from the above interest groups. No reply was received. Like the tobacco industry, our list of benefactors above are all either purveyors of perfectly "legal products" or people who have mostly escaped prosecution for their reviled conduct. Like the barons of the tobacco industry, the world's disgraced dictators, arms dealers, war criminals and pornographers display pathological disregard for their victims. But, unlike the tobacco industry, our cast has mostly spared the world's universities a goring on the horns of such funding dilemmas. The tobacco industry, however, has hung about university research funding corridors like a wheel of ripe cheese in a sunbaked phone booth, provoking strenuous protest, particularly in universities in the USA,[7] Canada,[8] the UK,[9] Australia,[10] Israel[11] and South Africa.[12]

Academic institutions must adhere to certain core principles. Among the highest is a commitment to open scientific enquiry. The tobacco industry is institutionally allergic to this central tenet, preferring to bury incriminating data and to obfuscate emerging truths about the toxicity of its products. The story of how Philip Morris treated the work of its own scientists, particularly Victor DeNoble and Paul

---

5   Department of Trade and Industry 2000.
6   International Consortium of Investigative Journalists 2000; Action on Smoking and Health 1988.
7   Ruter 1996.
8   Sibbald 2000.
9   Maguire 2000.
10   Walsh and Sanson-Fisher 1994.
11   Siegel 2000.
12   Anon 1996.

C. Mele,[13] is staggering proof of the industry's incompatibility for partnership with universities.

For decades, the tobacco industry's seductive international program of research benefaction masqueraded behind the legitimising language of independence, dispassionate enquiry and respect for scholarship. But, as revealed in the avalanche of internal industry documents now available on the worldwide web, the industry was peerless in its proclivity for cultivating venal or naive scientists into a massively funded public relations campaign. The sole purpose of the exercise was to sow doubt among the public.[14]

Tobacco industry grant recipients often unwittingly reinforced the industry argument that it was genuinely seeking to define more precisely the relation between smoking and illness. "If only we could do this, we might then be prepared to agree that our tobacco kills and is addictive," their rhetoric pleaded in the days before it publicly agreed that the "C" and "A" words (cancer and addiction) properly applied to their products. Such collusion was utterly naive and served to perpetuate the industry's intent – that the issue of smoking and disease needed to be seen as wide open, therefore allowing the industry to remain blameless and unfettered in promoting its products.

But what can we make of the Nottingham case? We can imagine titles of seminar programs: "Deceiving your customers: is it *always* wrong?"; "Early death as moral virtue: a communitarian view"; "Burying discomfiting research: don't publish and don't perish"; "When good science goes bad". Fact is, the truth would be stranger than fiction. Tobacco ethics is a grotesque oxymoron and has all the ethical weight of a cash register. John Toy, the Imperial Cancer Research Fund's medical director, put it simply and eloquently: "If you accept money from the tobacco industry you are partly in cahoots with them. For me, it's a simple division of black and white. I think it's a great shame that Nottingham University has agreed to accept this money."[15] A chair in corporate responsibility, funded by tobacco money, can only collapse under the weight of its own shame.

---

13 *County of Los Angles, Plaintiff, v R.J. Reynolds Tobacco Company et al.* 1996.
14 Boyse 1988; Peto and Lopez 2000.
15 Maguire 2000.

Taking tobacco dollars tends to induce timidity among scholars who might otherwise trumpet the implications of their research in policy forums: why bite the hand that feeds so well? Tobacco-funded scientists seldom, if ever, promote their findings in arenas that might influence health policy or publicly criticise the tobacco industry. Indeed, there are several examples of funded scientists actively doing the industry's bidding in policy areas that threaten the tobacco cartel's future.[16]

Of course, many tobacco research questions can only be fully elucidated by medical research. Tobacco money has enabled some to remain employed, with undeniable benefits to colleagues and dependants. But the worthiness of research and the desirability of employment ought not to be evaluated apart from the means by which they are achieved and the wider agenda behind the industry's benefaction. Tobacco-grant money derives directly from the sale of tobacco. Researchers with industry grants benefit directly from the sale of tobacco products, suffering the attendant ethical considerations about ghoulishly profiting from industry-induced death and disease.

A common rejoinder to this argues that there is no such thing as clean money. Isn't anyone in a government's employ getting a salary that derives partly from tobacco excise receipts? But, here, one might as well argue that an automobile driver is in the same position because the state pays for roads: by this argument, no one can avoid "benefiting" from smoking. Those who might not want to profit from tobacco money in such indirect ways are still, in effect, compelled to do so. The governmental practice of placing all forms of tax and excise into consolidated revenue, rather than hypothecation in the manner of, say, petrol tax for road programs, prevents individuals exercising such choice. But, in the case of tobacco research grants, recipients actively choose to obtain the money and so should be prepared to defend their decisions.

Industry-funded scientists have employed crude rationalisation to defend themselves: "There is money on the table, and someone is going to pick it up, so it might as well be us." Another tendentious argument claims that researchers have a moral duty to apply their knowledge

---

16   Philip Morris Tobacco Company Document Site 1988.

and skills, striking a balance between the implications of accepting the money and a neglect of important health and medical research. This would elicit sympathy if it were true that other funding sources were simply unavailable. The present state of non-industry-sponsored research into tobacco and health shows this is not the case.

It is difficult to imagine a more calculated cynical gesture than the Nottingham incident. The tobacco industry's sponsorship of sports, fashion and motor racing, and its funding of schools, youth groups and hospitals, all merit condemnation. But, even by industry standards, the marriage of tobacco and university ethics would make more than just the bride blush.

While defending the Nottingham deal, John Carlisle, of the Tobacco Manufacturers' Association, was asked directly, "Do you accept that this [tobacco use] is a threat to health, and that you're killing people?" His reply? "I accept that this is a controversial product . . . We would expect, obviously, some hard discussion would go on within that university as elsewhere."[17] Carlisle's non-answer neatly encapsulates the reasons for categorical rejection of the industry's "blood money".[18]

In announcing the Nottingham donation, Michael Prideaux, corporate affairs director for BAT, said, "We are very serious about demonstrating responsible behaviour in an industry seen as controversial."[19] But, if BAT cannot admit that its products are lethal, then it is the antithesis of a responsible corporation. How, then, can it help Nottingham University answer subtle questions about ethical business practice?

BAT can provide the funds, but it cannot deliver the truth. Nottingham can take the money, but it cannot run from the truth.

17　Channel 4 News 2000.
18　Maguire 2000.
19　Nottingham University 2000.

39

Smoke screen

In "The banality of tobacco deaths" (see Chapter 31 of this volume) Stan Shatenstein and I wrote about the statistics that flow all over the smoking and health issue. But each one of those statistics is a person: the victims, and those who love them and who live through their decline, death and beyond. Rolah McCabe took up smoking in her teens and was diagnosed with lung cancer in her early 50s. She sued British American Tobacco for negligence. In this piece, I explored why she did that.

The toxic sludge that percolates through talkback radio has had a vintage year, with litigants who "got lucky" in court coming in for particularly vicious criticism. Two cases provide telling contrasts. Marlene Sharp, the non-smoking Port Kembla barmaid who was awarded half a million dollars in 2001, was seen to be deserving: she didn't bring it on herself. It probably helped that she looked like everyone's favourite aunt. But 51-year-old smoker Rolah McCabe, who got $710,000 in April this year, had to run the shock-jock gauntlet. "No one forced her to smoke." "Hello! Has she been living on Mars for the last 40 years? Everyone knows smoking is dangerous, so those who

Originally published as Chapman, Simon (2002). Smoke screen. *Good Weekend*, 6 July.

smoke voluntarily assume the risks." And what about the millions of ex-smokers who have quit unaided – the subtext being that those who whine that they can't stop didn't really try. Parents of children suffering from horrendous idiopathic diseases like childhood cancers noted that they couldn't sue anyone, so why should someone who consciously elected to smoke and was too indifferent to quit be "rewarded" when their unlucky number is drawn in this voluntary lottery?

Justice Jeffrey Eames' judgement in the Supreme Court of Victoria in April against British American Tobacco (Australia) seems destined to become a landmark in the pursuit of justice by the tobacco industry's millions of victims. Eames found extensive evidence of BAT's 17-year program of systematic document shredding and that this had denied McCabe a fair trial. The legal implications of the case are momentous, but its public discussion has provided sobering reminders of the propensity for victim-blaming in our community.

Rolah McCabe is in every respect a typical tobacco victim. Like tens of thousands before her, she commenced smoking at 12, rapidly developed a dependency on nicotine that took her to a pack a day, and by middle age was diagnosed with lung cancer. If she dies within the next year as predicted, she will lose 30 years off the lifespan that the average Australian woman can expect today. Over 4,200 Australians aged below 65 die each year from tobacco-caused disease.[1] About half of those who smoke long term will die from a tobacco-caused disease, on average losing about 12 years. Each cigarette they smoke takes about double the time it took to smoke it off the end of their lives. There is no cause of death that even comes close to this.

People who sue tobacco companies find themselves the focus of wider public discourses about the intertwined themes of personal responsibility and the spectre of the sort of bleak society that wraps its citizens in cotton wool in the slavish pursuit of zero risk. Throw in anti-lawyer venom and you have a potent mixture. These discourses reach out to us all, including citizens who might be selected for jury duty in such trials. Two recent cases widely ridiculed by the public have included a man who became a quadriplegic after diving into a sandbank at Bondi. He sued Sydney's Waverley Council for failure to

---

1   Australian Institute of Health and Welfare 2001.

warn him about the dangers of diving into waves and was awarded $3.75 million. Public comment went ballistic about what was seen as bordering on the idea that life itself should carry a health warning. Weeks later, a boy injured in a rock fight while playing truant from school successfully sued his school for negligence in failing to supervise him and was awarded $221,079. Such cases receive massive negative prominence and can infect all litigation involving any volitional activity as being all about rewarding the sort of people who blame others for their own misdeeds.

Get them young

So why should juries give smokers the time of day? The sport of blaming smokers for their fate falls at a trifecta of interlinked hurdles. The first is the tobacco industry's deep and abiding interest in children. In 1998, under the weight of the disclosures among 40 million pages of internal documents made public via US court action, the world's tobacco companies opted for global rebirthing. After decades in denial, they announced that they had suddenly decided that smoking really did *cause* diseases like lung cancer and that nicotine was addictive. The name of the game from now on was informed consent by adult smokers. It wasn't just the government saying tobacco killed; Philip Morris et al. now agreed it did. The line would be that smokers should be regarded like motorcyclists or hang-gliders: informed, sentient and consenting participants in a dangerous activity with only themselves to blame if things went wrong.

In all this, however, it is significant that the industry has clung resolutely to its mantra that it doesn't want children to smoke. It knows that all societies revile those who would seduce and harm children, exploiting their innocence. It is thus inconceivable that the industry might ever swallow a truth serum powerful enough to cause it to confess, "We *love* it when children smoke! As our shareholders know, their money is as good as any adult's. The earlier they start, the more money we get." With tobacco, the script for the Pied Piper metaphor could have been written in Business Studies 101. As one 1973 document put it, "Realistically, if our company is to survive and prosper . . . we must get our share of the youth market".[2] No amount of denial and sugar-coated earnestness about "adult choice" can ever make this bottom line go away. Thanks again to the revelations in their own documents, robotic denials about industry designs on children may now be comprehensively matched with dozens of gloating sales forecasts about the contributions of new smokers from the teenage market and focus group research on how children might use different brands to badge themselves in their relentless pursuit of teenage tribal identity. A market analysis for 1994 showed that across all three companies then operating in Australia, brand switching between companies totalled 1.6 percent of overall market share, but new smokers that year (almost all children) constituted 2.3 percent – 43 percent times more important to the companies than gaining customers from other brands. But of course, the big earner – brand-loyal smokers, representing 96.1 percent of sales – are nearly all smokers who started smoking as kids.[3]

If the global tobacco industry was sincere in its sanctimonious loathing for teenage smoking, it could hand back its billions in ill-gained profits – with interest – from teenage smoking gained since it first commenced this rhetoric in the 1970s. Don't hold your breath.

Everyone knows it's harmful

When victim-blamers grudgingly concede that the tobacco industry invested millions in teenage-friendly campaigns, this is waved away by arguing that once kids mature, they are free to stop taking the risks they can now appreciate as sovereign, fully informed adult consumers. Just as nearly everyone has heard of Santa Claus, so has everyone heard the proposition that smoking is harmful. But how many believe it? And moreover, what are we to make of a 40-year exercise the industry called its "smoker reassurance" program?

The sordid 40-year history now being painstakingly unearthed by tobacco control's document archaeologists reveals pharaohs' tombs full of private acknowledgement in the industry that tobacco causes disease,

---

2 Teague 1973.
3 Barber and Sharrock 1994.

overlain by massive international programs of public obfuscation and reassurance, and tame-scientist dissembling. For every newspaper report that smoking was harmful, there were dozens of advertisements whose entire choreography said, "Forget all that! *This* is what smoking means!" And sprinkled liberally throughout the bad news on smoking were hundreds of carefully orchestrated stories placed by the industry's PR machine about air pollution causing all the cancer, confounders like diet and pet bird keeping, and apparent anomalies of low lung cancer rates in high-smoking populations. The industry built lists of everyday agents and practices said to be dangerous which had ever been the subject of news reports, and distributed these to its spokespeople so that they could put it to audiences that "scientists" warned us that brussels sprouts, bubble baths and books were dangerous too.[4] So what were we to make of their claims that smoking was harmful? Stock phrases like "The jury is still out" and "Only a statistical association" that fed the ordinary person's scepticism about science were grist to the same mill.

Commencing in 1969, the Australian tobacco industry acted like the Michael Edgley of travelling scientists. Its documents show at least 12 heavily promoted media tours between 1969 and 1988, many focused on promoting the ideas that scientists were divided about smoking being harmful and that it was air pollution, not smoking, that caused lung cancer (the rather unfortunate argument here is that lung cancer rates per head of population are currently the highest in Australia's remotest and most unpolluted areas, the difference being almost entirely explained by the higher proportion of smokers in the bush).[5]

In 1978 Philip Morris, Rothmans, and W.D. & H.O. Wills set up the Tobacco Institute. Its main role was to attack each and every proposal with the slightest potential to impact on sales, and to implement the companies' international programs of misinformation. In 1984, Ita Buttrose interviewed me with the head of the Tobacco Institute, John Dollisson, on her 2UE radio program. After ten minutes, Ita turned the program over to talkback. A woman named Pat called in said:

---

4   Brown & Williamson.
5   Jong et al. 2002.

I'd just like to give my opinion. I've been a smoker for many years and I have lung cancer. I gave this a lot of thought when I found out that I had the tumour. I thought, is it the smoking or is it not? In our days we weren't educated to know about cigarettes and all the smoking and nicotine and whatever. I have given it a lot of thought and I'm a highly nervous person and with my smoking, if I was to stop now I might even die sooner. I have the cancer and I really and truly believe that I got it from stress and stress will give you cancer. If you have an air conditioner open it up and see the dust and dirt in the filter. It's not smoke, it's what we breathe in the air . . . I think it depends on the individual.

I replied, "Diseases like lung cancer occur far, far more in smokers than they do in non-smokers. It's not the only thing that causes lung cancer. Asbestos and all sorts of other agents can cause cancers in the body and so can smoking." Then, in what I count as one of the more chilling moments of my career, Dollisson took his turn:

Let me say firstly that I'm sorry to hear that you have lung cancer. It's good to see that you've taken an objective assessment as to why you have lung cancer. It's interesting to note that factors like stress, genetics, heredity, indoor/outdoor pollution are taken into consideration. The so-called statistical association is virtually removed, that Simon talks about. It's good to see that you've taken an objective assessment of that and not believed the rhetoric that is being put around today.

Such statements were commonplace for several decades. Retail magazines distributed to tobacconists are filled with material described as "convincing arguments to pass back to nervous customers". In 1987, a Sydney study of smokers reported that 59 percent of smokers agreed that "everything causes cancer these days". Another in 1992 found that 42 percent of smokers agreed with the statement, "Most lung cancer is caused by air pollution, petrol fumes, etc." and 45 percent believed that "the medical evidence that smoking causes cancer is not convincing".

Addiction

The victim-blamers' final *bête noir* is addiction. A 1980 Tobacco Institute memo expressed the problem plainly: "Shook, Hardy and Bacon [the tobacco industry's lawyers] remind us ... that the entire matter of addiction is the most potent weapon a prosecuting attorney can have in a lung cancer/cigarette case. We can't defend continued smoking as 'free choice' if the person was 'addicted.'"[6] Behind closed doors, the addictiveness of nicotine was a commonplace to the industry (BAT in 1978 noted that "very few consumers are aware of the effects of nicotine i.e.: its addictive nature and that nicotine is a poison"). But in public, it constantly denied nicotine was addictive and succeeded in keeping the dreaded word off pack warnings for over a decade. The acres of documentary evidence now available on industry nicotine manipulation evoke nothing less than imagery of scheming industrial chemists setting out to maximise addiction. Australian Bill Webb, now one of the most senior people in Philip Morris in the USA, wrote to head office to arrange to have Marlboro reformulated in Australia: "our aim is to make Red and Special Mild as close as possible to the USA blend and thus make it harder for existing smokers to leave the product".[7] When such material is set next to the industry's blue-in-the-face denials on addiction, its desperate efforts to resist "addiction" on pack warnings and its trivialisation via comparisons with chewing-gum, chocolate and television viewing, recourse to glib talk about free choice sounds simply puerile.

The victim-blamers would have it that if, like Rolah McCabe, you were a 12-year-old girl, awkward about your identity, and reassured by advertising that promised friendship and togetherness from smoking (Rolah McCabe smoked *Escort*, advertised with the cheery ditty "Join the club"), you were to blame. If the nicotine receptors in your brain became rapidly primed via the best nicotine pharmacology that the industry's scientists could secrete, without any advice or warning into their chemical cocktails, again, it was your fault that you became addicted. And if you were stupid enough ever to have fallen for any of

---

6   Knopik 1980.
7   Webb 1984.

the scientific denials peddled by credentialed industry scientific stooges ("Light up, drink up and stay healthy! That's the good news from American expert Dr Carl Seltzer who claims that smoking is not related to heart disease . . . The Harvard University lecturer says he's never been challenged by the medical profession . . . Dr Seltzer's word must be taken very seriously. After all, he *is* the doctor of Harvard University"[8]) then you deserved what was coming to you.

All over the world, smoking and the diseases it causes are increasingly becoming the providence of nations' poorest and least educated sub-populations. Such people are the least able to assess the complexities of conflicting epidemiological evidence. These are also the often dirt-poor people for whom aspirational brand names like Winfield, Holiday and Longbeach and the ad campaigns that accompany them are named by the cynical and well-paid interpreters of tobacco-industry smoker focus groups.

The mass document-shredding uncovered in the McCabe case adds another potent element to the discourse about tobacco-industry culpability. It is difficult to conceive of any industry other than a crime syndicate that would feel so ashamed or vulnerable about their work as to systematically destroy evidence about their core activity. Ordinary people, like the citizens who make up juries, know that this is what the guilty do when they know they are in the wrong. While the evidence from undestroyed internal documents is damning enough, one can only begin to imagine the contents of the material that went into the shredders. And the view from those at the top? Nick Greiner, BAT's chairman, put it neatly in 1997:

It's all a charade isn't it? You read the packet, everyone else's packet, it tells you that the government health officers, who are not stupid, assert that smoking causes cancer and so on. I am prepared to assume that they haven't made it up. But I am here to do a job. I took the job knowing what I was involving myself in. I am not heavily into hypocrisy. We are all lightly into it.

---

8   Interview with Carl Seltzer 1979.

40

It's smokers, better still those trying to quit, who should benefit

Whenever tobacco companies get hammered by the courts, I'm delighted at the news. But in the case below, my reading was that the beneficiaries of the case should have been smokers, not tobacco retailers. The case was settled out of court in 2011.[1]

Hands up, shopkeepers who want $10,000? The Sydney law firm Maurice Blackburn Cashman has a deal for you. If you were selling tobacco between 1 July and 5 August 1997, you would have paid the tobacco companies a "state licence fee", plus the money for the cigarettes.

The trouble was, the fee was abolished as unconstitutional by the High Court, so the tax should never have been charged. But the tobacco companies hung onto the money – $250 million plus interest. The law firm, with a company called Feesback formed to represent tobacco retailers, has launched a class action. According to the Feesback website, it is generously offering to return 60 percent of the booty if it wins.

---

1   See http://bit.ly/2cn2DYW.

Originally published as Chapman, Simon (2002). It's smokers, better still those trying to quit, who should benefit. *Sydney Morning Herald*, 28 June.

If all eligible tobacconists signed on, that's $150 million plus interest for the retailers, with the $100 million remaining going to the backers of the Feesback proposal after costs. Nice work if you can get it. But should they? Remember, it was smokers who first got dudded by the imposition of the licence fee. The retailers added the tax to the retail price, passed it to the manufacturers and now want something back to which they have no moral claim.

At a press conference last week the Feesback people said that there was no way of identifying which smokers bought cigarettes in the period in question. How about just lowering the price for a month, then? This would still leave the $250 million in the undeserving hands of the manufacturers.

So what would be a decent way of using the $250 million? The premier, Bob Carr, has written to the prime minister, John Howard, suggesting that a 100 percent tax be put on the money to pay for a $250 million national quit campaign, which could boost the pathetic level of funding allocated to tobacco control in Australia (the federal government allocates $2 million a year for tobacco, while reaping $5 billion from tobacco tax and spending more than $600 million a year on illicit drug control).

The Commonwealth created a similar fund to allow Howard to keep an election promise that the price of beer would not rise after the GST. When it did, rather than keep the money, a bill was introduced to ensure that the full equivalent of the increase in excise collected on draught beer since 1 July 2000 was allocated to the Alcohol Education and Rehabilitation Foundation. The alcohol field is swimming in money, while tobacco control lives hand-to-mouth despite smoking being, in the government's own words, the single largest cause of premature death and disease in the country.

A window of opportunity has been opened and it will close very quickly. If the state Labor governments sit on their hands and don't add leverage to Carr's initiative, they will miss an opportunity to do more to boost tobacco control than has ever been done before. They acted quickly to set up a co-operative scheme between the states and territories over failed travel agents. They could also consider intervening as interested parties in the court case.

41

Corporate responsibility is fast becoming a smoke-free zone

The tobacco industry's core business is selling a product that will cause the death of two in three of those who use it over many years. Yet it has the effrontery to take the stage at "corporate social responsibility" conferences, where it talks about anything but this core business.

This month in Sydney, the Australian public relations industry is holding a summit on corporate communication. Spin doctors for rugby and apologists for late trains will swap war stories about clothing naked emperors, turning frogs into princes and the art of the extreme corporate makeover.

Until this week, the meeting was to feature Philip Morris' manager of communications, listed to give an anodyne talk about "aligning corporate social responsibility with business objectives". After the Cancer Council wrote to all speakers urging them to reconsider sharing the stage with a tobacco company, at least two key speakers threatened to withdraw if Philip Morris was represented. The conference organisers now agree they misread the corporate mood and have "uninvited" Philip Morris to speak.

Originally published as Chapman, Simon (2004). Corporate responsibility is fast becoming a smoke-free zone. *Sydney Morning Herald*, 5 August.

This is the second recent occasion tobacco companies have been shown the back door by their colleagues in the corporate world. In October, *Ethical Corporation* magazine is running a conference on corporate responsibility in Hong Kong. After others speakers protested, organisers removed Philip Morris and British American Tobacco from the program. A petition signed by about 80 global ethicists also condemned their participation.

So why the fuss? Philip Morris' core business objective is to get as many people as possible to smoke as much as possible of the company's brands. As the world's largest multinational tobacco company, it now blithely admits that its products kill. But as if nothing had changed, it hoped to schmooze on stage at such meetings next to the Red Cross, the Sydney Children's Hospital and other last-word-in-decency agencies.

Curiously, the company's state-of-the-art website omits to provide any estimate of how many of its best customers around the world die because they smoked the company's products. Let me assist. With 17 percent of global tobacco sales, and 4.9 million annual tobacco deaths, an approximate figure of 8.3 million deaths over ten years might be a place to open the bidding. Smoking kills 19,000 Australians a year, more than 4,000 before retirement age, more than those who die from breast, cervical and skin cancer, AIDS, suicide, alcohol and road crashes combined.

But the soothing rhetoric of "corporate responsibility" hasn't got time for such detail. The spin today is all about people knowingly taking risks, or perhaps something even more noble. As a tobacco strategist put it more than 25 years ago: "With the general lengthening of the expectation of life, we really need something for people to die from. Cancer may have some predestined part to play."

The conference program promised that the man from Philip Morris would enlighten his audience on "choosing, and prioritising, which societal expectations to address". Here, the audience could have anticipated some pearls about its global program to prevent children from smoking, with details of how many governments have twigged that here's another example of public-private partnerships: get the tobacco industry to run your youth anti-smoking program.

But would he have been as candid as one of his colleagues who noted in a now public internal document: "This is one of the proposals that we shall initiate to show that we as an industry are doing something about discouraging young people to smoke. This, of course, is a phoney way of showing sincerity as we all well know." If the tobacco industry was sincere about not wanting children smoking, it could start by funding an independent foundation appointed by cancer councils, representing the millions it rakes in each year from underage sales.

The conference organisers were giving a stage to a tobacco company to gloat to the PR industry about its "strategies" and to portray itself in a good light. Philip Morris has been engaging in a global program of spending vast sums of money to publicise its support for programs such as domestic violence awareness, carefully selected to ensure that it is largely immune from criticism. Who could attack anyone helping to reduce domestic violence? In Australia it has even funded an Aboriginal health promotion campaign, knowing our Indigenous populations have among the highest smoking rates.

When the tobacco industry succeeds in positioning itself as just another ordinary industry, it is halfway home in its normalisation strategy, designed to soften government and community attitudes. Conference participants would be unlikely to extend the same inclusiveness to arms dealers. Or mercenary recruitment agencies. Or the PR agency of a despotic nation with a taste for torturing its opposition. Or the gun lobby. Or a racist political party. Each of these organisations is, like tobacco companies, also "legal". The PR industry has drawn a low-water mark, below which the tobacco industry occupies bottom-feeder status.

42

The problem with selling a lethal product: you just can't get the staff

Across nearly 40 years of observing tobacco industry spokespeople, I've often been struck by how dreadfully mediocre most of them are when they try to answer questions from interviewers. When you think about it, when considering who to target for job applications, the best and the brightest graduating from business or marketing schools would have just about any other industry than Big Tobacco as top-of-mind. Big Tobacco pays its staff well, but for most, that's apparently not inducement enough to work for a company where improvements in your key performance indicators are all ultimately going to mean the deaths of more of your best customers.

In this paper Mike Daube and I looked at what some of the companies had to say about their staff in their recent risk reporting to the United States Securities and Exchange Commission.

Tobacco causes 6 million deaths a year, and Big Tobacco was recently described in a British High Court judgement[1] as an industry "which facilitates and furthers, quite deliberately, a health epidemic".

Originally published as Daube, Mike and Simon Chapman (2016). The problem with selling a lethal product: you just can't get the staff. *Guardian*, 14 July.

But it's a great place to work. Just look at the company tweets. Imperial Tobacco "is once again named as @TopEmployer in Poland".[2]

Imperial Brands PLC is "thrilled to be a winner at the CIPR #InsideStory Awards for our global employee magazine".[3]

British American Peru and BAT Central America and Caribbean are "recognised . . . amongst top employers in LatAm 2016",[4] while BAT South Africa "unlocks leadership potential of their talent".[5] BAT Mexico has been recognised as the "#OneEmployer in Mexico in 2016"[6] and BAT West Africa "wins awards for outstanding employee engagement strategies".[7] Meanwhile, at Japan Tobacco International: "We did it again! JTI ranked #One employer in French-speaking #Switzerland".[8] And Philip Morris International "actually has proof" that it is one of the best employers around.[9]

So it goes. Great employers doing great things for their employees.

But what do these lethal companies say about their employees when they report on the risks their industry faces? Reports to the United States Securities and Exchange Commission seem to tell a different story about the calibre of people in the tobacco industry.

Altria (Philip Morris USA's parent company) recently reported that "Altria Group, Inc. may be unable to attract and retain the best talent due to the impact of decreasing social acceptance of tobacco usage and tobacco control actions . . . our strategy of attracting and retaining the best talent may be impaired by the impact of decreasing social acceptance of tobacco usage".[10]

1 *British American Tobacco & others v Department of Health* (2016) EWHC 1169, http://bit.ly/2cSkGKs.
2 http://bit.ly/2cEVRy6.
3 http://bit.ly/2cT5Grv.
4 http://bit.ly/2cEWfwK.
5 http://bit.ly/2cA94K9.
6 http://bit.ly/2c71QOA.
7 http://bit.ly/2cSlFdA.
8 http://bit.ly/2cEVtQw.
9 http://bit.ly/2c71Vlm.
10 http://bit.ly/2crZgBO.

The Lorillard Tobacco Company report that "As a tobacco company, we may experience difficulty in identifying and hiring qualified executives and other personnel in some areas of our business. This difficulty is primarily attributable to the health and social issues associated with the tobacco industry".[11]

Philip Morris International report "We may be unable to attract and retain the best global talent",[12] while Reynolds American Inc. report that "Recruiting and retaining qualified personnel may be difficult given the health and social issues associated with the tobacco industry".[13]

And it affects the bottom line. According to Lorillard, these risks "could have a material adverse effect on our results of operations and financial condition",[14] or, as R.J. Reynolds put it, "could have an adverse effect on the results of operations cash flows and financial position of these companies".[15]

These concerns are of course global. The UK-based British American Tobacco reported in 2015 to its shareholders that, "the Board has considered the risks associated with the inability to recruit required talent and the loss of existing talent.[16] The impact of the risks has increased to reflect the challenge posed by negative perceptions of the sustainability and corporate reputation of a tobacco business and is now listed as a principal risk facing the business."

The evidence that smoking kills has been overwhelming since 1950. It is understandable that tobacco company leaders were slow to accept the magnitude of the problem. But six decades on, anybody working for tobacco companies has come into this industry knowing that they are selling and promoting a product that is lethal when used precisely as intended.

Even the once-supportive alcohol industry wants to distance itself from Big Tobacco. According to the UK Scotch Whisky Association's

---

11 http://bit.ly/2cITObt.
12 http://bit.ly/2chb2B7.
13 http://bit.ly/2cADayr.
14 http://bit.ly/2cITObt.
15 http://bit.ly/2cADayr.
16 BAT *Delivering Today, Investing in Tomorrow: Annual Report 2015*, at www.bat.com/annualreport.

Chief Executive, David Frost, "there is a fundamental difference between tobacco and alcohol, which is that alcohol, when consumed responsibly and in moderation, can be part of a normal healthy lifestyle",[17] while the Sales Director for Australia's Carlton United Breweries, Peter Filipovic put it even more starkly: "Tobacco kills you when you use tobacco as it is intended and beer doesn't".[18]

Small wonder that, as Philip Morris delicately note, "We tend to reward our employees more than other companies do".[19]

Small wonder that the industry's leaders stay out of the spotlight, and are reduced to deceitful PR, lobbying, political donations, legal threats and processes, and working through front groups.

Small wonder too that tobacco companies are finding new names – Philip Morris changed to Altria,[20] Imperial Tobacco is now Imperial Brands,[21] while British American Tobacco has established "consumer healthcare" and "consumer focused"[22] companies under the names of Nicoventures[23] and Nicovations.[24]

Money still talks, and the tobacco companies have a lot of it. But the global campaign to reduce tobacco's massive death toll is gaining momentum, and the industry is losing crucial battles in both the law courts and the court of public opinion.

It must be good news that fewer than ever job applicants with good intellects and decent values want to sell their souls for the glistening salary packages at Big Tobacco – and that those who work for Big Tobacco know their own employers worry that they are second-rate.

Maybe the recruitment tweets should read, "we know you're not very good, but we're getting desperate".

---

17 Frost 2014.
18 Wells 2012.
19 http://bit.ly/2c71Vlm.
20 J. Schwartz 2001.
21 Ruddick 2015.
22 http://bit.ly/2cSkKdh.
23 http://bit.ly/2cVnEfV.
24 http://bit.ly/2cT7EbE.

43

International tobacco control should repudiate Jekyll and Hyde health philanthropy

What should we make of the world's richest man throwing much appreciated money at health, education and poverty charities while at the same time sitting on the board of a global tobacco company and presumably taking his fiduciary duties there very seriously?

The founder of the Salvation Army, William Booth, famously said, "Take the Devil's money, wash it in the Blood of the Lamb, and use it to save a dying world". Booth thus opened the door for people of goodwill to take money for noble works from assorted devils. Today it is commonplace, for example, for religious charities to accept money from gambling taxes. The gratitude of the poor, the sick and the needy can quietly usher aside impertinent considerations about where the money came from. When the sums offered are modest, the high moral ground of principled refusal is more easily climbed. But the devil can have all the best tunes when it comes to Faustian temptations.

So what should global tobacco-control workers make of the world's richest man,[1] Mexican billionaire Carlos Slim Helú, pouring rivers of money into health, education and poverty charities in Latin America?

Originally published as Chapman, Simon (2008). International tobacco control should repudiate Jekyll and Hyde health philanthropy. *Tobacco Control* 17:1.

Slim announced this year that he will expand the endowment of his foundations, such as the Carso Foundation, to US$10 billion over the next four years, up from US$4 billion, and will dedicate himself more to philanthropy. Slim set up the Carso Health Institute, initially endowed with US$500 million, and nominated Dr Julio Frenk (former minister of health in Mexico and former candidate for WHO's director-general position) for the institute's executive-director position.[2]

Although most known for his telecommunications business, Group Carso, which he controls, Slim owns many other businesses, including until recently a majority ownership of Cigatam, Mexico's largest tobacco company. Cigarros la Tabacalera Mexicana (Cigatam) was majority owned by the Carso Group (Philip Morris Mexico owns the other 49.9 percent). In July 2007 Philip Morris International announced an agreement to buy an additional 30 percent of shares from the joint venture with Group Carso (which would keep 20 percent of shares). The acquisition is valued at US$1.1 billion. PMI's press release on the deal quoted Miroslaw Zielinski, president for the PMI Latin America and Canada region: "Our relationship with Grupo Carso and its founder, Carlos Slim Helú, has proven to be extremely successful and we look forward to further growth of our business in Mexico." The release continued: "Carlos Slim Helú will continue to serve as an advisor to Philip Morris Mexico, S.A. de C.V. and will remain an active partner in our Mexican tobacco business."[3]

"Extremely successful" business for a tobacco company is none-too-subtle code for maintaining and increasing smoking in populations. It means seeing new generations of young smokers commence smoking, slowing cessation and maximising the retention of smoking opportunities by opposing smoke-free policies. Unavoidably, it means that your core business causes unparalleled numbers of preventable, often early and hideously wretched deaths, increasingly among smokers who are the least educated and most economically disadvantaged in the population. It means publicly posturing about informing smokers about health risk and addiction while "maintaining

---

1   Mehta 2007.
2   Associated Press 2006.
3   Philip Morris International 2007.

in a litigation setting its former position that it cannot be proved that smoking causes disease or is addictive".[4] It means embracing tokenistic and ineffectual tobacco control programs[5] while opposing effective tobacco control policies known to seriously harm tobacco sales. In summary, it means having all the ethics of a cash register.[6]

Slim's efforts to improve the health of Latin Americans while continuing to profit from tobacco sales is nothing but the latest episode in Jekyll and Hyde duplicity. His continuing "active partnership" with Philip Morris invites consideration of what advice he might be giving them. What will he suggest about compensating the families of tens of thousands of Mexican smokers who died early from smoking Cigatam products? What will he advise that they do with their earnings from underage smokers each year? Will he urge that Mexico move all retailed tobacco under the counter as happens in Thailand, significantly raise tobacco tax and be the first nation to introduce plain packaging? Will he fund mass reach, effective graphic campaigns known to reduce sales or support PM's tepid, feel-good and ineffectual youth smoking prevention campaigns?

There is now a conga line of health and poverty-relief agencies and researchers applauding Slim's philanthropy and hoping to get in on the action. Business philanthropy is to be applauded, but when a philanthropist's day job is a major contributor to the death and disease that his generosity in part seeks to redress, it is time for all self-respecting agencies to make a stand and refuse to have anything to do with it.

---

4 Friedman 2007.
5 Wakefield, Terry-McElrath, Emery, Saffer, Chaloupka, Szczypka, Flay, O'Malley and Johnston 2006.
6 Chapman and Shatenstein 2001.

44

When will the tobacco industry apologise for its galactic harms?

Every parent, school teacher and friend knows what's expected after someone does something egregious. The expectations about acknowledgement, contrition, and how those who have done something wrong can turn the page on what they have done are well known. The tobacco industry has apparently found it impossible to work its way through these steps.

Last week, four US tobacco companies finally reached agreement with the US Department of Justice to fund large-scale corrective advertising about five areas of tobacco control. Each advertisement will include the statement that the companies "deliberately deceived the American public."

The case against the companies commenced in 1999 and saw a 2006 judgement by US District Court Judge Gladys Kessler that the companies had misled the public across decades. Judge Kessler's orders came in a judgement in a lawsuit brought by the US Department of Justice alleging that the companies had violated the Racketeer Influence and Corrupt Organizations Act (RICO), an anti-racketeering statute. The companies dragged out the case for nearly 15 years. Further appeals

Originally published as Chapman, Simon (2014). When will the tobacco industry apologise for its galactic harms? *British Medical Journal Blogs*, 21 January.

are now possible on the wording of the correctives that they will be required to pay for. These will appear in newspapers and on prime-time television for a year.

Since the public release of some 80 million pages of previously internal and often highly explicit documents after the 1998 Master Settlement Agreement, the conventional wisdom has been that the tobacco industry was forced to publicly drink gallons of truth serum. Because of the revelations in the documents, it was thought that it could no longer engage in its standard denials of health effects and addiction, and would be scrupulous in hiding its intense interest in how to ensure as many children as possible were beguiled by smoking. Unctuous, weasel-worded statements followed the settlement on company websites that smokers should be aware that medical scientists had found smoking to be a serious health hazard. Earnest requests intensified to be allowed to be seen as "stakeholders" in public health efforts. Watch us reduce the harms from smoking through product innovation, they promised, as they had for decades previously.

But as snakes shed their skins only to replace them with more of the same, the global tobacco industry continues its business as usual. A friend teaching in Myanmar emailed me last week describing sales promotion staff for foreign brands openly handing out free cigarettes to children. Indonesia, the world's fourth-largest nation, where smoking by men is almost compulsory and tobacco control policies almost non-existent, is a transnational tobacco industry paradise wallpapered with tobacco advertising by BAT, Philip Morris and local companies. The industry says ad nauseam that it supports "effective" tobacco control, while continuing to lobby – as if its economic life depended on it – against any law or policy like plain packaging that threatens its bottom line.

Tobacco companies are widely regarded as corporate pariahs whose conduct over many decades has set the ethical bottom-feeder benchmark. If you google "just like the tobacco industry", thousands of examples cascade down the screen of writers reaching for the tobacco industry as a way of calibrating the deceitful, duplicitous, irresponsible venality of a large variety of industries. It is not difficult to explain why such a reputation is so deserved.

The obvious starting point is its peerless record in sending its best customers to early graves: 100 million last century, and a forecast 1 billion this century. But as I wrote this week,[1] Stalin's observation that "one death is a tragedy, a million deaths is a statistic" tends to inure many from the realities of the suffering that precedes many of these early deaths.

My wife is a primary school teacher with 35 years' experience. She has often described incidents where five- to nine-year-olds with poorly developed moral compasses have been caught red-handed bullying, stealing, cheating or lying, but unblinkingly deny it regardless of the evidence in front of them. More than once, she's suggested that such a child might one day make an ideal applicant for a job in a tobacco company.

Globally, different legal, moral and religious codes tend to share basic principles when it comes to how to deal with those who have done serious wrong. Sentencing often takes note of evidence of contrition, and civilised societies and judiciaries tend to look for five broad preconditions in considering punishment:

- Full public acknowledgement of the misdeeds and harms caused
- Apologising for these harms
- Promising never to repeat them
- Making good the damage done, and
- Undertaking some form of public penance to symbolise your changed moral status.

Like many caught-out five-year-olds and recidivist adult sociopaths, the tobacco industry has done none of these things. Its corrective advertising is being done reluctantly after 15 years of legal kicking and screaming. While schmoozing with the global corporate social responsibility movement and publicising its donations to carefully selected charities, the industry gets on with trying to sell as much tobacco as possible, regardless of the misery it causes.

It has all the ethics of a cash register.

---

1 Chapman 2014b.

45

Smoking bastions set to crumble

Smoking has long been banned in all indoor public areas. It started with smoke-free buses and trains and then moved to cinemas, workplaces, restaurants and finally bars and pubs. Each time, there was talk about sacred cultural bastions crumbling. By the time smoking was banned in restaurants (in 2000 in New South Wales), the "last bastion" rhetoric itself was looking threadbare, as life continued but we all breathed easier.

Last night I ate the best pizza in Sydney. I was in an unfashionable Calabrian restaurant in the suburbs, where boomboxed cars burned donuts in the street outside.

Since six weeks before the Olympics, the law in New South Wales has said that people can't smoke inside restaurants.

Every few minutes, a tattooed player at the pool table, or a burly tradesman in his working clothes wolfing pizza, or a tizzed-up, bare-midriffed 18-year-old would go out to the footpath to smoke. It was as if it had always been this way. There were no smoking police tapping them on the shoulder to move outdoors. There were no complaints from management run off their feet trying to control people who didn't know

Originally published as Chapman, Simon (2001). Smoking bastions set to crumble. *Newcastle Herald*, 4 May.

about the law. And there were certainly none from the many family groups and stray yuppies eating inside.

Wednesday's historic jury verdict in the Supreme Court, where a former Wollongong bar worker, Marlene Sharp, was awarded $450,000 in compensation for having acquired throat cancer from passive smoking, has catapulted the debate into pubs and clubs, romanticised as the so-called last bastions for smokers.

The gradual creep of smoking bans into hospitality venues has sadly left those most vulnerable to last in their search for a healthy working environment. Can there be any occupational setting anywhere in the world where workers are more exposed to passive smoking than bar workers? What sort of half-pregnant logic allows us to accept that the public (the least exposed) should be protected from passive smoking? So should restaurant workers, people who travel on public transport and those who go to the movies. But if you work an eight-hour shift in an atmosphere thick with tobacco smoke in a bar or club, like it or lump it.

Marlene Sharp didn't like it and her brave action, following that of Liesel Scholem in 1992, whose successful court action accelerated smoke bans in offices, will almost certainly pave the way for a return to the Victorian days of the "smoking room". Here, people retired temporarily to a room where they could smoke, before rejoining those who didn't want to be forced to smoke involuntarily.

We see the equivalent of this today in airports, where separately ventilated rooms cater for smokers to feed their addiction and enjoy the gothic ambiance of overflowing filthy ashtrays and the company of glum fellow-addicts, counting the seconds before they can leave the fog themselves. Provided such rooms were genuinely separately ventilated, doors were not left open and cleaners could enter during intervals when the occupants were not allowed inside, everyone's civil liberties would be protected, while sane occupational health principles would finally be enacted.

So why hasn't this happened long ago?

When smoking was allowed in the back sections of airlines, many smokers actually preferred to sit in non-smoking seats rather than endure the unpleasantness. Over the years as community attitudes changed, preferences for smoking seats became so marginal that the airlines lobbied governments to introduce a ban to set a level playing field across all airlines. People haven't stopped flying. Restaurants are not closing. Cinemas aren't empty. The TAB is doing a roaring trade. McDonalds and Pizza Hut, two of the first to go smoke free, are not exactly doing badly.

The big losers in all this are, of course, the tobacco companies. Workplace smoking bans cut 24-hour smoking by 20 percent, which translates into hundreds of million of dollars foregone and reduced smoking unparalleled by any other strategy. For more than 20 years the tobacco industry and its mates in the hotel trade have put it about that smoking bans ruin businesses. Yet a 1994 Philip Morris internal document states:

> the economic arguments often used by the industry to scare off smoking ban activity were no longer working, if indeed they ever did. These arguments simply had no credibility with the public, which isn't surprising when you consider that our dire predictions in the past rarely came true.

Tobacco companies oppose smoking bans because they eat away seriously at the number of cigarettes consumed. Their arguments about lost business for others are, by their own internal admissions, absolute nonsense. Marlene Sharp's bravery in going to court to face the formidable prospect of the legal costs of losing will be an important milestone in the historic erosion of public smoking.

NSW health minister Craig Knowles and premier Bob Carr have been a breath of fresh air in introducing the ban on smoking in restaurants. It now seems certain that they will write the final chapter in this saga. The myopic, ill-informed and self-interested lobbying of the Australian Hotels Association to exempt bars from these bans is one of the most contemptible chapters in Australia's occupational health history.

46
Why even "wowsers" argue about smoke bans

I've long broken ranks with many colleagues in public health who take the view that smoking should be banned from any public space, no matter how fleeting and homeopathic the exposure to tobacco smoke might be. This argument is most exercised when it comes to banning smoking in wide open, outdoor settings like parks. I first wrote about this in 2000[1] and again in 2008.[2]

The state government's proposed raft of smoking restrictions is generating debate, even among anti-smoking campaigners. The ethical basis for restricting others' smoking rests on the 19th century philosopher John Stuart Mill, who famously wrote: "The only purpose for which power can be rightfully exercised over any member of a civilised community, against his will, is to prevent harm to others. Over himself, over his own body and mind, the individual is sovereign."

---

1   Chapman 2000.
2   Chapman 2008a.

Originally published as Chapman, Simon (2012). Why even "wowsers" argue about smoke bans. *Sydney Morning Herald*, 23 February.

There is now a large body of evidence dating from the early 1970s that being exposed to others' tobacco smoke can cause serious disease. But this evidence is nearly all about chronic exposure over many years, experienced by the families of smokers and by workers such as airline crew and bar staff who got concentrated lungfuls of it every day. Their occupational health rights to a safe workplace were shredded by neo-Dickensian assumptions that they should just have to put up with it.

Children are particularly vulnerable, with the earliest studies showing increased respiratory problems in infants living in smoky homes. Acute exposure to cigarette smoke produces measurable but temporary bodily changes, and in some people with diseases such as cystic fibrosis, even short exposures can be very distressing and dangerous.

Public health policy, though, is rarely set on the basis of the vulnerabilities of small groups of exquisitely sensitive people. Rather, it is done by balancing population-wide liberties against net harms. So outdoor smoking bans struggle for justification.

Last year, my university debated the introduction of a ban on smoking on all areas of its campuses, after the senate alumni representative and *Sydney Morning Herald* columnist Peter FitzSimons led the charge. To the surprise of some, I spoke against banning it entirely. I supported bans near buildings, because of significant smoke drift into offices, and in outdoor eating areas, because of the sardine-like proximities and the easy option for smokers to move away. But I wanted nothing of banning it on the big campus boulevards or lawn areas. I know of no evidence that the fleeting encounters you can get from walking past a smoker in a wide-open space can cause any disease. The campus is now smoke-free, save for four outdoor smoking zones.

While it is true that there is "no safe level of exposure to tobacco smoke", it is also true that to set public policy aiming for zero risk would cause mayhem and a good bit of duplicity. Tobacco smoke contains many carcinogens and irritants, but so does smoke from any source. I didn't hear any calls around the university to ban rugby-club barbecues, exhaust from motor vehicles or Indigenous smoking ceremonies.

Where the ethics get interesting, though, is when the smoking argument shifts from harm-to-others to amenity, or "I don't like it" arguments. I was comfortable with supporting smoke-free outdoor coffee tables, for the same reason I support outdoor stadium smoking bans. Someone smoking next to me while I eat lunch outdoors is not going to really harm me, but the imposition is unpleasant in the same way as loud music away from music venues or dog faeces underfoot.

Some of my colleagues believe that it's OK to ban smoking in public spaces because it denormalises smoking by driving it out of sight. Some argued at my university that banning smoking altogether would promote non-smoking as the norm, and that we should all feel comfortable with coercing smokers to stop smoking publicly, to set a good example to children. The government's ban on smoking on suburban playing fields and playgrounds, and the long-standing ban on smoking by teachers on school premises, are all about reducing adverse role-modelling.

On balance, the New South Wales government has got it just about right. There are no bans planned on park, beach or wide-open-space smoking, other than in child-dense areas. With only 15 percent of adults now smoking daily, and many of these considerate of others, those who couldn't give a stuff about others can move away from the rest of us. But the decision by the health minister, Jillian Skinner, to honour the ill-conceived memorandum of understanding with clubs and pubs and put the reform back to 2015 is disappointing and will only engender cynicism. Bob Carr's pre-Olympics ban on smoking inside restaurants gave six months' notice, and restaurateurs coped just fine with the change.

47

How Santa and the Tooth Fairy collaborated to allow smoking at casino

If you ever needed a perfect example of how the influence of money can override even established occupational health and safety legislation, you need go no further than this case study.

It is now official that the casino at Barangaroo will be open slather for smoking. Casino patrons and staff will enter a public health Tardis and travel back to the 1980s, when Australian workplaces last fully allowed smoking.

This week I tried to explain this anomaly to some of my international students who asked why, if all workplaces in Australia have long been smoke-free, the new casino would allow smoking. Wouldn't it have any staff, they asked?

I explained to them that the New South Wales government, like the governments of 177 nations around the world that have signed the legally binding World Health Organization's Framework Convention on Tobacco Control, agrees that exposure to secondhand smoke in indoor areas both causes and exacerbates serious respiratory and cardiovascular diseases, and lung cancer. The New South Wales government was one of the first to ban smoking in its own offices in the

Originally published as Chapman, Simon (2013). How Santa and the Tooth Fairy collaborated to allow smoking at casino. *Sydney Morning Herald*, 29 November.

1980s. New South Wales was the first Australian state to get smoking out of restaurants just before the 2000 Olympics. And after a decade of futile efforts to convince recalcitrant tobacco smoke that it just must not drift over the five-metre magic line from bar-serving areas, it also banned smoking in all pubs and bars. This year it has even led the nation by extending smoking bans to bus shelters, which are open-air but tend to get pretty crowded, particularly on wet days.

I then explained that the New South Wales government can only have obtained secret scientific information that it has so far suppressed, showing that when very wealthy people smoke, their smoke is harmless to others. Perhaps the very wealthy have such highly evolved airways or buy such advanced cigarettes that the sidestream and exhaled mainstream smoke they exude into casinos is totally harmless.

My students looked incredulous. But how, I asked, could it be otherwise? Occupational health law in the case of every other toxic pollutant has nothing to say about rules for the rich and rules for the rest of us. Wealthy restaurateurs or entertainment-venue owners are not exempt from laws requiring adherence to noise regulations. We don't allow ear-bleeding-decibel rock concerts to break maximum noise laws just because the very wealthy might want to pay top dollar for the privilege. We don't look the other way on air-conditioning standards, toxic gases, dusts or chemical because wealthy factory owners might argue that they would set up their business in countries still operating with Dickensian occupational health laws. We don't tell schools to just forget the asbestos removal because it might cost too much. But smoking in the casino is apparently quite OK.

Apparently, industrial-strength ventilation equipment will be installed that will pull all the nasty stuff out of the air. That tactic was a tobacco industry favourite in the years leading up to the eventual ban on smoking in pubs. It was abandoned when it was revealed that such ventilation would need to be so powerful that it would suck the beer out of a glass.

I haven't heard the argument yet, but I expect to soon, that casino staff "don't have to work there", or that many of them smoke themselves, so hey, what's the problem? If this principle was accepted across occupational health law, many possibilities would open up. Desperate workers would need only to be advised of the risks, told to sign away their rights to compensation and led back to the occupational health landscape of 19th-century England.

The acquiescence of the O'Farrell government to this ludicrous exception sets a dangerous precedent that occupational health standards can be negotiated. Last month I flew Korean Air. South Korea has one of the highest smoking rates in the world, yet all passengers have to go without lighting up for ten hours on long-haul flights. The arguments that hotels, restaurants and tourism would collapse when smoking was banned in restaurants and pubs came to nothing in the many countries in which they were repeatedly threatened.

The same would happen in casinos. This is quite disgraceful.

48

Is a smoking ban in UK parks and outdoor spaces a good idea?

I returned to the ethics of banning smoking outdoors for a debate in the *British Medical Journal*, after moves to ban smoking in London's parks.

Smoking restrictions began being introduced when the weight of evidence consolidated about the harms of chronic exposure to secondhand smoke. This evidence was almost exclusively obtained from indoor domestic and occupational exposures, where non-smokers – including infants[1] – spent hours on most days exposed to others' tobacco smoke, sometimes for decades in small enclosed conditions. Notwithstanding slogans about "no safe level of exposure", as with active smoking, the harms of exposure to secondhand tobacco smoke arise from chronic exposure, not occasional fleeting encounters with single plumes.

With almost all indoor public spaces now smoke-free in nations with comprehensive tobacco control policies, some are now

---

1   Colley, Holland and Corkhill 1974.

Originally published as Chapman, Simon (2015). Is a smoking ban in UK parks and outdoor spaces a good idea? *British Medical Journal* 350, 25 February.

emboldened to turn the attention onto outdoor spaces like parks and beaches. One such proposal comes from Lord Ara Darzi's London Health Commission report.

The ethical justification for restricting where smoking can occur derives entirely from the Millsian precept of preventing harm to others.[2] Evidence soon also mounted about important collateral benefits of banning smoking in workplaces: smokers reduce their daily consumption by about 21 percent,[3] and more importantly many quit, welcoming the bans as a form of imposed self-discipline on a behaviour that 90 percent of smokers regret ever starting.[4] Smoking bans fomented a rapid denormalisation of smoking:[5] venues associated with relaxation, pleasure and conviviality like restaurants, bars and cinemas have no smoking, while smokers excuse themselves to go outside to footpaths in any weather or sit morosely in the fug of smoke in those desperate airport smoking rooms, wondering about how much they really enjoy smoking.

The proliferation of smoke-free areas certainly contributes to reducing both the frequency of smoking and the proportion of people who smoke. But so would forced incarceration, forfeiting smokers' rights to healthcare or other draconian strategies too tame for the Ottoman Sultan Murad IV, who had smokers executed. The ethical test of any policy is plainly not just its efficiency in achieving outcomes.

Since I last contributed to this then-nascent debate in the *British Medical Journal* in 2008,[6] the evidence base about the risks of outdoor smoking has grown. Our 2012 review[7] found only studies of real world or simulated outdoor exposure in crowded cheek-by-jowl settings like bar patios, beer gardens and bus shelters. No studies looked at exposures in parks or beaches, almost certainly because researchers with any knowledge of airborne exposures would appreciate that such exposures would be so small, dissipated and transitory as to be of no concern.

---

2   Mill 1975.
3   Chapman, Borland, Brownson, Scollo, Dominello and Woodward 1999.
4   Fong, Hammond, Laux, Zanna, Cummings, Borland and Ross 2004.
5   Chapman and Freeman 2008.
6   Chapman 2008c.
7   Licht, Hyland, Travers and Chapman 2013.

The momentum to outdoor bans has incorporated three arguments that go well beyond direct health effects. First, large majorities of the population do not like being exposed to tobacco smoke. Outdoor bans premised on communities' amenity preferences are not about public health but akin to ordinances about playing music in parks, bans on public nudity and littering. Outdoor smoking bans based on amenity should not be dressed up in the language of public health. Second, cigarette butts and packaging constitute a significant proportion of litter. Local governments wanting to abate this relentless source again should not appropriate public health arguments in justifying their decisions but be upfront about the litter problem.

Third, some have invoked the virtues of shielding children from the sight of smoking as worthy evidence in this debate.[8] They may concede that smoking in wide open spaces like parks and beaches poses near homeopathic levels of risk to others, but point to indirect negative impact from the mere sight of smoking. This line of reasoning is pernicious and redolent of the worst excesses of totalitarian regimes' penchants for repressing various liberties, communication and cultural expression not sanctioned by the state. North Koreans are routinely subjected to such fiats, but many would recoil at the advance of such reasoning elsewhere. If it is fine to tell smokers that they cannot smoke anywhere in public, why not extend the same reasoning to drinkers or people wolfing supersized orders in fast food outlets?

Coercing smokers to stop smoking in settings where their smoking poses negligible risk to others is openly paternalistic. Well-intentioned advocates for such policies argue, as paternalists always do, that such actions are for smokers' own good, that many will be sooner or later grateful (which is often true). Paternalistic for-you-own-good laws about seats belts and motorcycle helmets involve trivial restrictions on liberty. Telling smokers they cannot smoke in public sight is a restriction of a different magnitude.

Last weekend I attended a twilight rock concert at Sydney's Taronga Zoo. Announcements were repeatedly made that the open air event was non-smoking, but that smoking areas were available on the periphery of the crowd area. This arrangement struck me as totally civilised. Most,

---

8   Thomson, Wilson, Edwards and Woodward 2008.

like me, don't want to spend a few hours jammed up next to smokers. We all hope that smokers will quit, particularly those we love or care for. But when they don't, we should not cross a very sacrosanct line and force them not to smoke if they are adults.

In Australia, daily smoking prevalence is now only 12.8 percent[9] and highly likely to keep falling. This has been achieved without the unethical coercion of smokers. Those of us who have resolutely refused to cross that line, even knowing that it would likely bring public health benefit, have won the respect of a wide cross section of the community. Political support for dissuasive but not coercive policies like plain packaging and high tobacco tax rates has been bipartisan from the left and right of politics. That would almost certainly not have happened had we abandoned the ethical concerns that some are urging should occur.

---

9   Australian Institute of Health and Welfare 2014b.

49
Are today's smokers really more "hardened"?

Today's smokers are all "hardcore" heavily addicted smokers. All the policies and campaigns that have been tried just haven't worked for them, right? Actually, not right at all. If anything, many of today's smokers are "softening" rather than hardening.

As smoking continues its inexorable southward journey toward single-digit percentages of populations being smokers, it's common to hear people say that the smokers who remain are all "hardcore", heavily dependent smokers, impervious to policies and campaigns.

The argument runs that the ripe fruit of less addicted smokers have long fallen from the tree, and that today anyone still smoking will be unresponsive to the traditional suite of policies and motivational appeals. This argument is known as the "hardening hypothesis".

The hardening hypothesis is predictably most often used by pharmaceutical companies; those who are making a living out of promoting the idea that smokers are foolish to try and quit on their own and need professional help; and most recently by promoters of electronic cigarettes, who often highlight the idea of smokers who

---

Originally published as Chapman, Simon (2015). Are today's smokers really more "hardened"? *The Conversation*, 14 October.

"can't" or won't quit but want to switch to less dangerous ways of dosing themselves with nicotine every day.

Hardening adherents argue that ex-smokers are dominated by those who were not heavily addicted and so who were better able to quit unaided, and that a greater proportion of today's smokers, said to be more addicted, cannot succeed alone and need help.

A study of smokers in 18 European nations has just been published in *Preventive Medicine*[1] that provides important data of direct relevance to the hardening hypothesis.

The most recognised way of measuring the "hardness" of smoking is the Heaviness of Smoking Index (HSI). This scores smokers out of a maximum of six, comprising a score of one to three for number of cigarettes smoked each day, and one to three on the time taken to lighting up the first cigarette of the day.

The study, involving 5,136 smokers drawn from a total 18-country sample of more than 18,000 people, found that across the 18 nations, there was no statistically significant relationship between a nation's smoking prevalence and the HSI.

If the hardening hypothesis had been confirmed, nations with low smoking prevalence would have had higher HSI scores in the remaining smokers. They would have been smoking more cigarettes and lighting up earlier in the morning in nations with low smoking prevalence than in those with high. But they weren't.

Similar findings have been reported for the United States. Data on smokingin 50 US states for 2006–2007 indicate that the mean number of cigarettes smoked daily, the percentage of cigarette smokers who smoke within 30 minutes of waking, and the percentage who smoke daily are all significantly lower in US states with low smoking prevalence.[2] This provides compelling evidence against the hardening hypothesis.

In Australia, a 2012 paper in the *Australian and New Zealand Journal of Psychiatry*[3] examined three series of Australian surveys of smoking – the National Drug Strategy Household Survey (NDSHS),

---

1   Fernández, Lugod, Clancye, Matsuof, La Vecchiad and Gallusg 2015.
2   Giovino, Chaloupka, Hartman et al 2009.
3   Mathews, Hall and Gartner 2010.

National Health Survey (NHS) and National Survey of Mental Health and Well-being (NSMHW) – that spanned seven to ten years. The authors found that in two of the surveys (NDSHS and NHS), while smoking fell across the population, there was no change in the proportion of smokers who smoked less than daily. While in the NSMHW survey, that proportion increased from 6.9 percent in 1997 to 17.4 percent in 2007.

The authors concluded that the evidence presented "weak evidence that the population of Australian smokers hardened as smoking prevalence declined".

Those arguing that today's smokers are more and more heavily addicted and unable to quit have poor evidence supporting their case. Many thousands stop and reduce their smoking every year.

We also forget what happened when the bad news on smoking first became "official" with the two historic reports of the Royal College of Physicians of London (1962) and the US Surgeon-General's first report on smoking (1964). In the decade that followed, there was nothing remotely approximating today's suite of tobacco-control policies that have driven down smoking in countries such as Australia to only 12.8 percent smoking daily.

There were no tobacco advertising bans, cigarettes were dirt cheap, there were no sustained mass-reach anti-smoking campaigns. Smoking was allowed everywhere and pack warnings, where they even existed, were tiny and timid.

In 1955, five years after Ernest Wynder and Evarts Graham's historic study of smokers and lung cancer was published in the *Journal of the American Medical Association*,[4] 7.7 million Americans (6.4 percent of the population) were former smokers. Ten years later, following widespread publicity surrounding the 1964 US Surgeon-General's Report, this had ballooned to 19.2 million (13.5 percent) ex-smokers. By 1975, 32.6 million Americans (19.4 percent) had stopped smoking.

In 1978, the then director of the US Office on Smoking and Health noted in a National Institute of Drug Abuse Monograph, "In the past 15 years, 30 million smokers have quit the habit, almost all of them on their own." Many of these quitters had been very heavy smokers.

---

4   Wynder and Graham 1950.

Quitting unaided (going cold turkey) remains the most common way that most ex-smokers have quit, despite more than 20 years of the availability and heavy promotion of nicotine-replacement therapy and other drugs. We need to be very circumspect about voices trying to downplay this major and enduring phenomenon.

50
Light cigarettes – deadly despite the name

In April 2005, the Australian Consumer and Competition Commission made it illegal for tobacco companies and importers to use the words "light" or "mild" as variant descriptors. Some 80 percent of Australian smokers were choosing brands with these descriptors, so successful had the marketing of these products as harm reducing. In this piece, written before the announcement of the ruling, I explain why the ACCC ruled that these descriptors were misleading and deceptive. True to form, the companies simply switched to other descriptors (like "smooth" and "fine"), presumably gleaned from market research to convey the same false implications.

Next time you hear a smoker ask a shopkeeper for the "mild" brand, reflect on what that smoker thinks he or she is getting. The competition tsar the Australian Competition and Consumer Commission has been pondering this for nearly four years and has now told the government there is a strong case that the decades-long practice of the tobacco industry labelling products "mild" and "light" is seriously misleading.

Originally published as Chapman, Simon (2005). Light cigarettes – deadly despite the name. *Sydney Morning Herald*, 24 February.

So-called light cigarettes are largely a result of the industry successfully selling the idea that machine-testing of tar and nicotine is a reliable basis for consumers to differentiate brands. The problem is that people do not smoke like machines. Smoke-testing machines do not get addicted to nicotine and so, unlike humans, do not take more and deeper puffs, smoke light cigarettes down further, or smoke more cigarettes to get the nicotine that their brain cries out for hundreds of times a day.

So what is a light cigarette? Basically, it's much the same as a regular cigarette except for one vital little matter that the industry fails to tell its customers about. Mild and light cigarettes are perforated with microscopically small air holes just in front of the filter. When the mouth of the smoking machine grips the cigarette, air rushes in through the holes and dilutes the smoke, causing lower tar and nicotine readings. Smokers don't know about the holes, but their brains do.

They quickly learn to compensate by either smoking more, more deeply, or by unconsciously blocking some of the holes with their lips and fingers, giving them an intake that machine-testing would never record. This is bad news for the health of smokers who buy these products and, to date, good news for companies that saw light cigarettes as a life raft, for them, which they could throw to desperate consumers thinking of quitting.

Evidence presented to the commission by health groups was undeniable. Much of it came from the industry's internal documents. These documents show the industry nakedly exploited smokers' health concerns. As far back as 1983 British American Tobacco (BAT) knew Australian "smokers of the ultra-low-tar brands are very conscious of the smoking and health controversy, but that smokers of 6- to 9-mg tar brands split between those wanting mildness per se and those wanting smoker reassurance".

In 1994 BAT knew that 16 percent of smokers in Australia believed "lights would be safer for health reasons", with a "key finding" that lights were "perceived as a clever psychological ruse intimating that the smoker was indulging in a low tar content cigarette, an innocuous cigarette". Philip Morris, which, after a corporate makeover, calls itself Altria, owes most of its US$131 billion ($170 billion) global value to its cigarette division. It also owns Kraft, maker of Vegemite and peanut butter, one version of which is labelled "light". Altria's Kraft division knows that "light" means "healthier". But down the corporate corridor in the tobacco division, executives want to tell us that it doesn't mean that at all. It means "light taste", and has nothing to do with promoting a health message.

The ACCC's call has come as no surprise to the local industry, whose overseas parents have been prevented from using such words in the European Union since 2003. But the Australian divisions were happy to continue to exploit this outrageous fraud for as long as it took for local regulators to wise up.

Industry sources insist that "descriptors" would still be needed to differentiate varieties of the same brand, repeating the line about the differences being all about taste, not health. According to one report, the ACCC may accept smooth and fresh as substitutes. Fresh carcinogens? A smooth journey to emphysema, lung cancer or heart disease for one in two long-term users?

The consequences of this conduct are more serious than a telco diddling consumers out of a few hundred dollars with some misleading small contract print or a bait-and-lure ad for sale goods that mysteriously were sold out before the doors opened. These are the sort of cases where we have become used to seeing the commission chesting companies in court, or negotiating a few days of corrective advertising. Here, we have a very big, deadly fish on the line with fearsome financial teeth, and in the case of one company, a former state Liberal premier as chairman. Its behaviour in this decades-long fraud has misled countless Australian smokers into thinking they are reducing their health risks. Many have and will die early as a result. This looms as the biggest test yet of the ACCC's importance.

Please, Mr Samuel, keep your nerve.

51

Matter of smoke and hire

The World Health Organization asks all its prospective employees if they smoke and explains that its policy is to not hire smokers. I think the policy raises unsupportable ethical problems.

The World Health Organization has announced it will no longer hire smokers. At least two cancer-control agencies in Australia have obtained exemptions from anti-discrimination authorities to do the same. Is this policy just?

I once taunted Nick Greiner, then chairman of British American Tobacco Australia, in a letter to the *Herald* because he had let it be known he did not smoke. While the man in charge of a lingerie company would not be expected to "choose" to wear women's underwear, smoking is a choice open to all. It is scarcely imaginable that the chairman of Ford would drive a Toyota or that the head of the meat marketing board would be a vegetarian. Such lack of confidence in their products would probably ensure they didn't last long in their jobs. The tobacco industry does not seem to mind such a paradox.

Originally published as Chapman, Simon (2005). Matter of smoke and hire. *Sydney Morning Herald*, 10 December.

Some jest that smoking should be compulsory for all tobacco industry executives, but should the reverse be applied: that employers could choose to insist on smoker-free workplaces? Employers can oblige staff to wear uniforms or conform to dress codes, and to address customers with repeated inanities such as "Not a problem". Occupational health law has stopped smoking in indoor workplaces, except in bars, where staff are effectively defined as unworthy of such protection. But should employers be able to insist that a worker cannot be a smoker, even if they smoke only after hours? Smokers have repeatedly been shown to have higher workplace absenteeism than non-smokers. In many workplaces, smokers take additional breaks to smoke outside and there is no evidence that these breaks somehow supercharge their subsequent productivity. Smoking breaks can also cause deep resentment among non-smokers, who see them as rewards for smoking.

Against this background, policies to allow employers to discriminate against the hiring of smokers are understandable. But is it justifiable? The World Health Organization will not hire smokers, reasoning that a smoking cancer-control advocate walks the thin ice of public hypocrisy, and that could undermine the agency's reputation. A cancer-control body would presumably have the same reservations in hiring a deeply tanned Caucasian to work in skin-cancer education, or having mammogram and Pap-smear refusniks spearheading these campaigns.

So I would support the World Health Organization in its policy of not hiring smokers in cancer control. But I am convinced that to extend such a policy to the wider community – into jobs where the issue of smoking is quite irrelevant – would be unethical.

Two arguments are typically advanced: employers' rights to optimise their selection of staff (smokers are likely to take more sick leave and breaks) and enlightened paternalism. The first argument fails because, while it is true that smokers, as a class, are less productive through their absences, many smokers do not take extra sick leave or smoking breaks. By the same logic, employers might just as well refuse to hire younger women because they might get pregnant and take maternity leave, and might later take more time off than men to look after sick children.

But what about paternalism? There are some acts where governments decide that the exercise of free will is so dangerous that individuals should be protected from their poor judgements. Mandatory use of seatbelts and motorcycle helmets are good examples. We do not allow someone to knowingly drink a glass of cholera-infected water, assuming such behaviour must indicate mental incapacity.

The World Health Organization would argue that its policy of quit or reduce your chances of employment is founded on similar enlightened paternalism. The comparisons are questionable. Seatbelt and helmet laws represent trivial intrusions on liberty and cannot be compared with demands to stop smoking – something that about 20 percent of smokers want to continue doing.

By the same paternalistic precepts, employers might consult their insurance companies about dangerous leisure activities and interrogate employees as to whether they engage in risky sports, ride motorcycles or like lone ocean sailing. Many would find this an odious development that diminished tolerance. There is not much of a step from arguing, out of paternalism, that smokers should not be employed (in anything but tobacco companies), to arguing that they should be prosecuted for their own good. We don't need this.

52
Butt clean-up campaigns: wolves in sheep's clothing?

We've all seen footpaths, parks and beaches strewn with cigarette butts, which take many years to biodegrade. So when the tobacco industry starts a nifty campaign to try and help smokers remember that they shouldn't litter, we should all give them a collective pat on the back, right? Wrong.

In 2005, matches and lighters were struck under an estimated 5.494 trillion cigarettes consumed by the world's 1.3 billion smokers. The great majority of their non-biodegradable butts are thrown on the ground. Butts are easily the single most common form of litter, with one analysis showing they constitute 39 percent by weight of all litter.[1] For many smokers, the world is their ashtray.

There is growing concern about this form of unsightly and dangerous[2] pollution. Google shows 63,500 hits for "cigarette butt" and "litter" and the international tobacco industry has got a nasty lungful of

---

1   EPR Expert Reference Group 2015: 5.
2   Chapman and Balmain 2004.

Originally published as Chapman, Simon (2006). Butt clean-up campaigns: wolves in sheep's clothing? *Tobacco Control* 15: 273.

this new ill-wind and may be coming soon with a big environmentally friendly smile to run a publicity campaign near you. In Australia, British American Tobacco has set up the Butt Littering Trust, with $2.8 million allocated over four years. Philip Morris has spent $331,775 on butt-litter reduction in one Australian state.[3] Cheery staff hand thoughtful smokers a little film canister to store their butts, and suburbs get awards for running local awareness campaigns. The Butt Littering Trust website gushes that by April 2006, three years after the program commenced, 12,000 Australians smokers have "signed the pledge" not to discard butts. This leaves around 2,880,000 who haven't signed and provides insight into a recent government assessment that these campaigns "have not translated into widespread reduction of cigarette butt litter. The impact of current activities funded by cigarette manufacturers is clearly unsatisfactory."[4]

The Butt Littering Trust is wholly supported by BAT, who sit on its board. The trust's chairman is adamant that BAT plays no role in shaping the strategies and goals of reducing butt litter. So why then is the trust equally adamant that it will limit its efforts to education and not join with other organisations to try and reduce the number of cigarettes being smoked, and then available to be discarded as litter?

All anti-litter campaigns openly embrace three broad strategies: reducing use, recycling and education to "do the right thing". Serious anti-litter organisations campaign to reduce packaging such as plastic bags, lobby for bottle deposit legislation and tougher fines for littering. The Butt Littering Trust deliberately limits itself to education. Imagine how seriously the community would regard a plastic bag manufacturer setting up a trust to educate shoppers not to discard bags, while lobbying hard to oppose any reduction in bag-use. This is exactly analogous to what BAT is doing through the trust. Grantees are warned that all communication with the public must adhere to the trust's key messages, with all public statements being vetted for "consistency in messages". Don't even think about urging smokers to quit.

But it gets worse. Along with long-time tobacco industry ally the Australian Hotels Association, the trust has recently opposed moves by

---

3   EPR Expert Reference Group 2015: 35.
4   EPR Expert Reference Group 2015: 5.

Newcastle City Council to ban smoking at outside al fresco restaurant and café tables where many non-smokers have complained that they must sit cheek-by-jowl with smokers who are not permitted to smoke indoors.[5] The trust argues that smoking bans have caused smokers to move outdoors, where many discard their butts.

The wider view is that reduced smoking opportunities means reduced smoking.[6] When smokers cannot smoke in particular settings, they smoke fewer cigarettes. When fewer cigarettes are smoked, fewer cigarettes are available to be dropped on the ground and less disease is caused as well. Reducing the prevalence of smoking would do more than any other strategy to reduce butt pollution. In the 1960s, nearly 70 percent of Australian men and around 30 percent of women smoked. Today, just over 17 percent smoke every day.[7] The only people who discard butts are smokers. Thirty percent of all Australian adults used to discard butts and now never do, because they are ex-smokers. Effective tobacco control reduces both the number of smokers in the community and the amount of cigarettes smoked per day by continuing smokers. It controls butt littering at source, because it reduces the number of "sources" who each have on average some 6,200 butts to dispose of each year.

Trying to persuade smokers to be more considerate, and law enforcement of anti-littering provisions, are two important components of litter-reduction efforts. But they are minor, band-aid contributors to the problem at large. BAT has a naked conflict of interest in addressing the litter question. The Butt Littering Trust directors are either willing or naively unwitting allies in this sham. Tobacco control advocates in Australia are now working with some success with local government authorities to alert them to the broader agenda of tobacco industry sponsored anti-litter campaigns.

---

5   Vallejo 2006.
6   Chapman, Borland, Brownson, Scollo, Dominello and Woodward 1999.
7   Australian Institute of Health and Welfare 2005.

53

Silver screen lights up with a deadly hidden message

At the end of every movie in the credits, we see businesses thanked for supplying products like designer clothing, cars and branded liquor. It should have surprised no one that the tobacco industry also did this for years, and even though they say today that they have stopped the practice, many would, quite reasonably, not believe them.

Today there is a movement in some areas of tobacco control to effectively censor smoking, either by banning it or by giving films that show smoking an adult classification. As the next few essays will show, I have always found this problematic and have lost friendships with some colleagues by saying so forcefully.

In the final scene of *Muriel's Wedding*, Muriel and Rhonda drive away for the last time from the bleak detritus of their past at Porpoise Spit. As they head triumphantly into their future and the tears of joy roll down our cheeks, Rhonda, in close-up, commandingly lights a cigarette.

No heavily identifying teenager watching could be left in any doubt that smoking is meant to fit as naturally with freedom, cutting the

Originally published as Chapman, Simon (1994). Silver screen lights up with a deadly hidden message. *Sydney Morning Herald*, 14 November.

parental chains and the Authentic Discovery of Self as tomato sauce on a meat pie. Yet the director always had a choice: smoking is no more or less natural to such endings than if the heroes had flashed an Amex card or shared a Kit-Kat. The power and hope of the ending could have been choreographed in a thousand different ways, with the cigarette option one that, even amid the concern about rising teenage smoking, is being taken by only one in five kids today.

But in many cases the crafted apposition of smoking with you-name-it is not a director's whim at all. For instance, in April 1983, Sylvester Stallone pledged himself to use Brown & Williamson's tobacco products "in no less than five feature films" in exchange for a fee of US$500,000.

The tobacco industry has long understood the value of product placement in movies. This year the US Federal Trade Commission released its annual report on cigarette advertising and promotional expenditures for 1992. After coupons and retail value-added promotions, "promotional allowances (paid to retailers and any other persons . . . to facilitate the sale of cigarettes)" was the second leading area of promotional expenditure, totalling US$1.5 billion (A$2 billion) – 29 percent of the second-largest advertising budget after cars in the USA. No breakdown was given for how much of this was paid to movie and television producers to ensure that cigarettes appeared in movies.

Throughout *Muriel's Wedding*, practically every character smokes. *Herald* letter writers have made the same comment about the ABC's *Janus*. In both *Janus* and *Muriel's Wedding* more unattractive, gormless, spivvy or violent characters smoke than do the heroes, so what is the balance of the message that comes across about smoking, particularly to the youth market – the future clients of both the tobacco industry and oncologists? Might not more directors be trying to make the point that it's losers who smoke?

There are murmurings in some health organisations about the possibility of film classifications based on whether or not a film portrays smoking in a positive light. In the same way that films depicting illicit drug use are now rated M or R, health groups are beginning to argue that tobacco – which kills more Australians every year than all other drugs, alcohol, road trauma, murder, AIDS and breast cancer combined – should not be seen as a trivial, ordinary behaviour. Whatever superficial appeal this argument may have, it will invite a very legitimate debate about censorship being the wolf in the sheep's clothing of healthism. By the same argument, should car chase scenes be kept from children? Shoot-outs? Gluttony? Plainly, that would be ridiculous. A director's judgement that smoking is important to a character or a film is one that could only be curtailed by the most totalitarian of governments.

So how should this debate proceed? Is the depressing answer one of open slather for the tobacco industry in films? Will the bad apples of advertising emerge as the innovators who pioneered the end of much stand-alone advertising, showing how product placement can work the same sales magic, immune from government control? Has the successful struggle during the 1970s and 1980s to ban tobacco advertising in Australia been a hollow victory?

If film and television producers are unashamed about assisting the tobacco industry in its ambitions by scripting positive smoking scenes in return for cash, then there should be no opposition to bold declarations to this effect in the credits. Being a willing sponge to tobacco dollars would become part of producers', directors' and actors' profiles in community debate, rather than allowing them to skulk behind noble virtues like freedom of artistic expression.

A central consideration must be whether or not the appearance of tobacco films has been commissioned. Commissioned product placement is obviously intended to be a form of tobacco advertising and is therefore almost certainly a breach of the *Tobacco Control Act (1992)* when such "advertisements" are "published" in Australia (imported films with tobacco product placement would be exempt, as is the case with magazines imported into Australia that contain tobacco advertising).

At the ninth World Conference on Tobacco and Health held last month in Paris, Professor Richard Peto of Oxford University reported that smoking now kills about two million people each year worldwide, half in middle age (35 to 69). This number is increasing rapidly as women's death rates reflect the historic increase in their smoking and as populations grow larger. Peto estimates that, in 2025, ten million people will die of diseases caused by smoking. Many will be the teenagers who are today watching films showcasing smoking.

Rupert Murdoch is very interested in movies. He's also very interested in selling lots of cigarettes – he's a member of the board of Philip Morris, the world's largest tobacco company. In the rush of excitement in the Australian film industry caused by Murdoch's Showground film studio initiative, it would be tragic if Australia turned a blind eye to what is a ballooning loophole in its internationally acclaimed tobacco advertising laws.

54

What should be done about smoking in movies?

Fourteen years after I wrote the last cautionary piece, the issue had begun to gain some momentum, so I returned to my concerns at greater length. This paper was quoted extensively by the High Court of Delhi when striking down the Indian government's ban on smoking in movies in a judgement on 23 January 2009.[1]

In 1997 Ron Davis (*Tobacco Control*'s inaugural editor) and I wrote an editorial titled "Smoking in movies: is it a problem?"[2] Since then, a growing body of research has examined the relationship between viewing of movies containing depictions of smoking, and subsequent smoking among youth. Reviewing this evidence, a 2008 National Cancer Institute monograph concluded:

The depiction of cigarette smoking is pervasive in movies, occurring in three-quarters or more of contemporary box-office hits.

---

1 *Mahesh Bhatt v Union of India & Anr.* See http://bit.ly/2cgMlyO.
2 Chapman and Davis 1997.

Originally published as Chapman, Simon (2008). What should be done about smoking in movies? *Tobacco Control* 17: 363–67.

Identifiable cigarette brands appear in about one-third of movies. The total weight of evidence from cross-sectional, longitudinal, and experimental studies indicates a causal relationship between exposure to depictions of smoking in movies and youth smoking initiation.[3]

The report's conclusion is consistent with commonsense and should give major impetus to what is a growing debate. If the highly choreographed imagery of tobacco advertising influences the uptake of smoking, then so will widespread positive depictions of smoking in movies, now arguably rivalling direct tobacco advertising as the world's largest vector for sustaining the appeal of smoking. Smoking in movies *is* a problem.

So what might be done about it? Many nations ban all tobacco advertising because of its influence on smoking. The idea that movies with smoking scenes should similarly be either banned or at least regulated through adult-only classification has gained traction in a small number of nations, particularly India, Thailand and the USA. The debate remains nascent elsewhere, with few signs of government interest.

In this commentary, I critically review three of the most prominent strategies proposed as ways of controlling smoking in movies. I caution that banning smoking from movies constitutes a fundamental threat to freedom of expression, inviting unavoidable ridicule for the inconsistencies and "airbrushing of reality" that its adoption would unleash. This is likely to alienate many ordinary and influential people who would otherwise be strongly supportive of comprehensive and tough tobacco control. I conclude that nations should pass or amend laws to require "no product placement" disclosures; global efforts should be increased to expose the extent and consequences of smoking in movies; and whistleblowers should be encouraged to expose instances of tobacco industry inducements to the movie industry so that prosecutions can arise where possible. Efforts should continue to persuade directors to be more judicious in their use of gratuitous smoking where this is unnecessary to the verisimilitude of their

---

3   National Cancer Institute 2008.

productions. And finally, smoking should become *one* element taken into account in film classification, but it should be considered in overall context on a case-by-case basis rather than triggering automatic upward classification, as occurs now with film classification in relation to other adult elements.

Is tobacco product placement still occurring?

Movies have long been prized vehicles for manufacturers to promote their products. When prominent actors smoke in box-office hits, powerful and indelible associations are added to smoking. Globally, hundreds of millions of young people view these movies every year, often regardless of their rating status. No one should therefore be surprised that the tobacco industry has a long history of promoting both smoking and particular brands by inducing producers to show products in the hands and between the lips of leading actors.[4] While the US-based tobacco industry has denied since 1990 that it continues product placement in movies, and the 1998 Master Settlement Agreement which the major companies have signed expressly outlaws the practice,[5] few experienced with the tobacco industry's track record trust these assurances. Orthodox tobacco promotional avenues are being closed through spreading national advertising bans and the tobacco industry actively exploits legislative loopholes in new media.[6] It would therefore be astonishing if tobacco interests were not still surreptitiously funding movie producers via third parties to have actors smoke in movies with major appeal to the industry's most important market segments, especially youth.

If this could be shown to be occurring in the USA, it would be simply another form of tobacco advertising, breaching undertakings in the Master Settlement Agreement.[7] If occurring in movie production in the increasing number of nations with laws incorporating comprehensive definitions of what constitutes tobacco advertising, it

---

4   Lum, Polansky, Jackler and Glantz 2008.
5   National Association of Attorneys General 1998.
6   Freeman and Chapman 2007b.
7   National Association of Attorneys General 1998.

would be prosecutable. Yet no such prosecutions have occurred. If paid product placement is indeed ongoing and as widespread as some tobacco control advocates imply, with myriads of directors insisting that actors smoke, it is also significant that no whistleblowers have emerged with examples of recent movies in which such inducements occurred. The movie industry contains many powerful individuals who would be appalled by such activity and who doubtless would like to expose such conduct if indeed it were happening.

Some tobacco control advocates see a movie cigarette and conclude "tobacco industry!" Sometimes it may well be, but often it is not, anymore than every time we see a car in a movie we should feel obliged to conclude "automobile industry!" People smoke, just as people drive, drink and eat. Filmmakers reflect this. An equally plausible explanation for smoking in movies, therefore, is that many movie directors are attuned to the richly signifying semiotics of smoking[8] and often judge that characters should smoke to convey particular associations. Here the options for control are far more complex. Three broad approaches have been proposed to reduce minors' exposure to smoking scenes in movies: banning all scenes of smoking (proposed, but now dormant after widespread opposition in India); *de facto* banning through pixelating the act of smoking and packs of cigarettes (Thailand); and one which appears to have the widest support: introducing an "R" classificatory rating either via movie industry voluntary codes or by law, preventing children under 17 years from admission to movies depicting smoking unless accompanied by an adult (this is the US guideline). Stan Glantz's US-based *Smoke Free Movies* website proposes an R rating thus:

> Any film that shows or implies tobacco should be rated "R." The only exceptions should be when the presentation of tobacco clearly and unambiguously reflects the dangers and consequences of tobacco use or is necessary to represent the smoking of a real historical figure.[9]

---

8   Klein, Richard 1993.
9   Smoke Free Movies 2008.

Banning all smoking in movies?

Film, the internet, magazines, literature and newspapers have a long history of being seen by various interest groups – political, moral/ religious and health – as vehicles that carry a diverse range of pernicious content said to be harmful to those exposed to it. Nations adopt a range of policies toward such content, ranging from massive state control of all content (for example, North Korea and Myanmar) through to large-scale active and passive censorship of material that offends political or religious sensibilities, as occurs routinely in many despotic, authoritarian and religiously fundamentalist nations.

At the opposite end of such policy are nations where freedom of speech and expression are enshrined as being of fundamental importance to the social and political fabric. In such nations, censorship – for whatever noble purpose – is met with principled resistance, with the onus being on those demanding censorship to demonstrate that the case for intervention is strong, and that the consequences of exposure are very serious. The few examples here are absolute prohibitions on promoting terrorism and producing or displaying child pornography, and on the overt incitement of violence and racial vilification.

Those who see movies as essentially vehicles for the transmission of authority-sanctioned health content meet opposition from those who argue that the role of film in open societies is far wider than being simply a means of mass communication of desirable or healthy role models to young people. Many movies depict social problems, people behaving badly and the seamy side of life. The role of cinema and literature is not simply to promote overtly pro-social or health "oughts", but to have people also reflect on what "is" in society or in screenwriters' imaginations. This includes a long list of disturbing, anti-social, dangerous and unhealthy realities. Numbered among these are domestic violence, animal cruelty, the exploitation of minorities, injustice, and neglect. Whether for educational purpose, entertainment or the broader purpose of artistic expression, filmmakers have often depicted highly socially undesirable activities such as racial hatred and vilification (e.g. *Schindler's List*, *Mississippi Burning*), genocide (*Hotel Rwanda*), gang violence (*Romper Stomper*, *A Clockwork Orange*) and crime (chose from literally thousands). It would be ridiculously simplistic to assume that by showing something most would regard as undesirable, a filmmaker's purpose was always to endorse such activity. People learn in ways far more complex than being fed a continuous diet of wholesome role models. Many would deeply resent a view of movies that saw them as the equivalent of religious or moral instruction, to be controlled by those inhabiting the same values.

Moreover, hundreds of millions of people around the world smoke. It would be unprecedented for cinema to have to "pretend" that this reality was not the case by never showing smoking in any movie, thereby implying that it was as heinous as (for example) child pornography, but less of a problem than the commonplace murder, mayhem and violence seen in countless films. It would invite ridicule from many people within and beyond the health sector who would see such a proscription on showing or mentioning smoking as an affront to freedom of speech. It is undoubtedly for this reason that the only nation which has sought to actually ban all smoking from movies (India) met with principled and successful resistance, including from many within the Indian civil society and arts communities.

Glantz's concession that exceptions should be allowed for "real historical figures" who smoked (such as Churchill or Mao Tse-Tung) in R-rating is notable here. It acknowledges that cinema should not "airbrush" historical reality. What is left unexplained here, though, is why it is permissible for children to see known historical smokers smoking, but not smokers set in a period such as the 1950s when the reality of social life was that smoking was widespread and unrestricted. Or indeed, why it would not be equally airbrushing of reality to show smoking in a movie set today depicting a group of people from a social or cultural group where smoking was the norm and therefore an accurate aspect of their lives?

Pixelating smoking in movies?

Thai law requires that any movie or program broadcast on television showing cigarettes or smoking must pixelate the cigarettes. The reasoning here would appear to be that as long as people do not actually see a cigarette, somehow the normative message will not get through to audiences. Bungon Ritthiphakdee, a Thai tobacco control expert, says that that local television movie and drama producers today seldom script scenes of people smoking since the law was introduced, because the required pixelation adds an extra production cost and more importantly, annoys viewers. Pixelation is therefore today largely confined to foreign produced, imported films.

Pixelation is common practice on television news crime reports: innocent until found guilty felons' faces are pixelated as they enter court before a trial. But is there anyone who doesn't think, "There's the felon!" – just as a pixelated cigarette would immediately tell viewers that here was someone smoking? It is difficult to imagine what Thai health authorities think not actually *seeing* the cigarette will achieve.

R-rate all smoking scenes?

In many liberal societies, sexual, violent and illicit drug scenes in movies invoke classification as unsuitable for very young children, although there is considerable variation between nations about what is permissible to screen to children. Parents do not have time to research the content of all movies and value movie classifications as a way of helping them avoid inappropriate, possibly disturbing content. This brings us to the widely supported proposal that smoking should not be banned in movies, but that all but manifestly anti-smoking scenes – even those where smoking is only "implied" – should cause a movie to be classified "R". Under the *Smoke Free Movies* policy,[10] this would mean that even *one* instance of smoking would see a movie classified as being equivalent to the Motion Picture Association of America's standard for those depicting "adult themes, adult activity, hard language, intense or persistent violence, sexually oriented nudity, drug abuse or other elements",[11] where such scenes are often sustained. Is this an equivalence that many in the community would find reasonable?

For example, the *Smoke Free Movies* currently rates the new Batman movie *The Dark Knight* as "promoting smoking" because, amid a cast of thousands, one minor character smokes a cigar.[12] While

---

10   Smoke Free Movies 2008.
11   Motion Picture Association of America 2007.

activists dedicated to eradicating smoking in children's movies engage in organised complaining about such closely monitored incidents, it seems improbable that many ordinary citizens would spontaneously rise up in community protest about such minor usage in the way they would about the sort of sustained adult content that currently sees movies classified as unsuitable for children, should those movies be not so classified. In this respect, arguments based on the unacceptability to the community of *any* smoking scenes are highly unlikely to find widespread support. Instead, they will likely be seen as overly extreme solutions proposed by single-minded interest groups.

Slippery slope problems?

In tobacco control, "slippery slope" or "thin edge of the wedge" arguments have a long and disreputable history. For many years the tobacco industry used such arguments to trivialise the health risks of smoking, arguing (for example) that if health warnings were to go on cigarette packs, then they should also go on a large range of other ordinary products that might be harmful too, despite these often being of incomparably lower risk (see for example a long list of "dangerous" products gathered by Brown and Williamson in 1984[13]). Such sophistry, however, does not mean that problems of inconsistency are not problematic to the determination of reasonable social policy. If even a single instance of smoking were to consign a movie to R status because of its potential to influence children to smoke, immediate parallel questions arise about a wide range of other potentially adverse role modelling cues in films.

Smoking causes massive health problems, but in that it is not unique. Globally, large-scale health and social problems flow from many activities that also often appear in movies. These include crime, physical inactivity, over-eating, excessive use of alcohol, unsafe sex, speeding and dangerous driving, gambling, risk taking such as extreme sport and adventure, motor cycle use and helmet-less cycling. For

---

12   Smoke Free Movies 2008.
13   Brown and Williamson 1984.

example, by the same reasoning that movies showing smoking might normalise or glamorise tobacco use, it could be argued that film should never show positive scenes of gluttony or actors enthusiastically eating fast food because of the obesity epidemic and millions of overweight and obese children struggle to control their weight. Countless comedy scripts would need to go back to the drawing board. Scenes of people drinking alcohol might be excised from children's movies – particularly if those drinking seemed to be enjoying it – because this might seed inappropriate ideas about alcohol in tender minds. All car chases and speeding scenes of course would be restricted to adult movies.

Smoking cartoon characters have been fingered as unacceptable[14] and a smoking Babar the elephant and a pipe-smoking Santa Claus have been condemned.[15] So by the same concerns, why not also R-rate the maniacal *Road Runner*, whose disrespect for the highway code might be taken literally by the same innocent children?

These examples are neither facetious nor hypothetical, but invite an "alphabet soup" of classificatory ratings, all respectful of the cases that could be mounted by other single issue health and social problem interest groups. For example, in August 2008, Dr Martin Schiff, a US weight-loss expert, called for movies promoting obesity to be classified "O" (for obesity): "Every day we see examples of overeating, gorging, food play and general disregard for health in movies and TV shows. No wonder millions of people are overweight." He nominated the family-oriented Abba musical *Mamma Mia!* for an "O" rating because it contained scenes of a lavish party and feast "where the participants seem to be eating anything and everything."[16]

Most will dismiss such calls as entirely unreasonable. But an illustration of how such inconsistency plays out in practice comes from scenesmoking.org, which rates the 2008 *What Happens in Vegas*, starring Cameron Diaz, as a "thumbs up/pink lung" because it contains no smoking. However, it does contain binge drinking, failure to wear seat belts, intoxication leading to possibly unprotected sex, gambling, and a parody of spousal abuse. With such a film receiving a ringing

---

14 Nakahara, Ichikawa and Wakai 2005.
15 Nakahara, Wakai and Ichikawa 2003.
16 Hiscock 2008.

endorsement from this youth-friendly organisation, ordinary people might be entitled to ask about consistency.

If R-rating proponents succeeded in having all smoking scenes restricted to R-rated movies, would this keep most children from seeing them? Hardly, as children's access to R and even X-rated movies is widespread.[17] A recent study showed that all 40 extremely violent movies were seen by a median of 12.5 percent of US adolescents aged 10 to 14 years. *Blade*, *Training Day* and *Scary Movie* were seen, respectively, by 37.4 percent, 27.3 percent and 48.1 percent of the overall sample and 82 percent, 81 percent and 80.8 percent of black male adolescents.[18] R-rating may deplete box-office takings, as R-rated movies are known to attract smaller audiences, but with rentals and downloaded movies easily accessible to children, it is doubtful whether fewer children in total would see them.

Do all scenes promote smoking?

Another problem with R-rating movies with any smoking scenes, other than those that openly proselytise against smoking in Surgeon General–warning style, lies with R-classification proponents' beliefs that all depictions of smoking are self-evidently alluring, which is why they need classifying for adults only. This is a simplistic notion which could result in some powerful anti-smoking messages being kept away from children.

Consider two examples. An ongoing story line from the immensely popular American TV series *Friends* (51 million people watched the final episode in the USA alone[19]) featured the character Chandler's attempts to quit smoking. Some scenes showed him smoking but the overall narrative was anti-smoking, despite scenes and lines often talking about the attractions of smoking. A rule that relegated any depiction of smoking to an R classification would see children deprived of the benefit of seeing such memorable indictments

17   Jackson, Brown and L'Engle 2007; Wingood, DiClemente, Harrington, Davies, Hook III and Oh 2001.
18   Worth, Chambers, Nassau, Rakhra and Sargent 2008.
19   http://fxn.ws/2dUHcQa.

of smoking. Those who want to banish such scenes from young eyes can thereby score some own goals.

In *In Her Shoes*, starring Cameron Diaz, Toni Collette and Shirley MacLaine, Diaz plays the insect-thin, dyslexic, rudderless younger sister of Collette's character. They have had an emotional rollercoaster of a childhood, and the film takes us through an emotional resolution as they become re-acquainted with their estranged grandmother (MacLaine). At one stage, Diaz reaches for a cigarette. The sagacious MacLaine says, "You shouldn't smoke. You have a history of lung cancer in your family." MacLaine takes the cigarette away, as a grandmother can.

If the movement to get all non-historical depictions of smoking R-certificated succeeds, then this powerful moment would relegate the film to R-rating (supposing that its other content had not already caused this). If that happened, then perhaps many thousands of young people around the world, lured by Diaz's box-office appeal, would be denied the richly contextualised and powerful message that the movie delivers: people who smoke are often very glamourous and cool, and drip with "attitude" but, like Diaz, they are often drifting, confused and, in the end, not particularly attractive characters. Why try to keep all this away from adolescents?

Such films present richly textured moral tales for young people to absorb and reflect on as they form their values and make decisions about matters like smoking. Only the crudest of early "hypodermic" media effects models[20] could posit that a single glimpse of smoking will, Pied Piper fashion, lure children ineluctably into a life of smoking. Film classification panels understand the importance of context in assigning their classifications, and are unlikely to be convinced that even one glimpse of smoking in any film is so self-evidently unacceptable that such an inflexible formulaic approach is justified.

The *Smoke Free Movies* project specifies an exemption for smoking scenes "when the presentation of tobacco clearly and unambiguously reflects the dangers and consequences of tobacco use". This also seems an overly narrow guideline. For example, a family movie that featured an ongoing narrative about a mother struggling to quit, whose smoking upset her family, who was exiled from friends by having to smoke in

---

20   Wartella and Reeves 1985.

alleyways outside restaurants, and who expressed regret about having commenced smoking, could send a powerful anti-smoking message that would fall well short of the prescribed "health consequences" message.

Alienating community support

For many years, tobacco control laboured to free itself from its early moralistic associations with dour temperance-based movements,[21] close brethren of movements which routinely protested at licentious literature and film, modern dancing and other devil's work. In the USA, there is some evidence that R ratings for smoking in the manner described have substantial community support.[22] But the USA is a nation with a broad rump of historical puritanism which is less evident in many nations. The mere popularity of a proposal should also not blind us to its shortcomings. Overly proscriptive, absolutist hostility to any sight of smoking in movies risks rekindling these historical associations which may alienate many otherwise strong supporters of tobacco control and stimulate bitingly sarcastic diversions[23] which could be avoided by more reasonable case-by-case policy.

What *should* be done

There are legally important differences between commercial speech (such as advertising) and free speech of the sort contained in cultural expression like movies and literature,[24] and any attempt to equate them as a basis for regulation, particularly on the basis of mere suspicion that the tobacco industry must be directing smoking scene traffic, will fail in most nations. But where product placement can be shown to be a direct result of tobacco industry promotional efforts, the matter crosses the line.

---

21 Tyrrell 1999.
22 McMillen, Tanski, Winickoff and Valentine 2007.
23 Queenan 2008.
24 Gostin 2002; Bayer, Gostin, Javitt and Brandt 2002.

Whistleblowers have made invaluable contributions to tobacco control. Potential informants should be actively fostered to speak out about product placement and legal action taken against any companies found to be engaging in it for having broken the Master Settlement Agreement ("No participating manufacturer may, beginning 30 days after the MSA execution date, make, or cause to be made, any payment or other consideration to any other person or entity to use, display, make reference to or use as a prop any tobacco product, tobacco product package, advertisement for a tobacco product, or any other item bearing a brand name in any motion picture, television show, theatrical production or other live performance, live or recorded performance of music, commercial film or video, or video game.")[25] Governments around the world should explicitly incorporate similar clauses in their tobacco advertising legislation.

The growing momentum of evidence so thoroughly summarised in the National Cancer Institute report should be publicised widely, with particular efforts to do this within the movie industry. This will accelerate critical discourse within the industry, which can only heighten awareness about its role in promoting smoking. *Smoke Free Movies'* efforts in this regard are exemplary, although as I have argued, likely to be generating unnecessary resistance from many because of their overly absolutist guidelines that all smoking, no matter how fleeting, should trigger an R rating.

Concerns that outright bans on smoking in movies "airbrush reality" raise the serious concerns I have outlined. But equally serious is the paucity of movies where the health consequences of smoking are even mentioned, let alone dramatised. This is airbrushing in the opposite direction. Here, tobacco control advocates should not insist that all movies with smoking be obliged to show its consequences, because such insistence erroneously assumes that movies are essentially health promotion vehicles requiring sign-off from health panels. Adolescents who smoke very rarely get sick and die in adolescence, so such an insistence would throw up the ridiculous spectre of all such films having to add an epilogue showing what happened to the smokers in later life. But the public health community could encourage writers

---

25   National Association of Attorneys General 1998.

and directors to engage with health consequence subplots more often than they do now. Many social movements have successfully partnered with the movie industry to increase exposure to their issues.

The discourse about the responsibility of directors has already had an impact within the industry. The Walt Disney Company's decision to no longer include any smoking in its family viewing fare will see the demise of the odd cigar-chomping pirate in such movies. Few could object to such gestures. But few sensible people see the problem as being much to do with the occasional sight of a cigarette or pipe in overtly "family entertainment". The main challenge comes with movies targeted at adolescents, where smoking can have a major presence. As I have argued, it is difficult to be categorical that *any* smoking in a movie means that the movie "promote" smoking. But it is undeniable that many such movies do, with the exact same consequences for the health of millions that were invoked as justification for controlling tobacco advertising. If the more reasonable proposition were promoted that smoking ought to considered as *one* element within movie rating panels' assessments of how a movie should be rated, I would predict that many within government and the movie industry would be more receptive, and more progress made.

55

Four arguments against the adult-rating of movies with smoking scenes

By 2011, the proposal that nearly all movies depicting smoking should be kept from the eyes of anyone under 18 years of age via an R-rating had got up a full head of steam in the USA. Matthew Farrelly and I went to town on it, setting out four arguments why it was a wrong-headed proposal. By July 2016, as I wrote this, no jurisdiction anywhere in the world has adopted this proposal.

A few years ago the Indian government tried unsuccessfully to ban all smoking scenes in movies.[1] Thailand pixelates cigarettes on television.[2] In the USA, over 20 public health agencies and the World Health Organization[3] are campaigning to require that most smoking scenes should trigger restricted (adult) film classification.[4] They believe that such ratings would significantly reduce the exposure of youth to

---

1 Kaul 2008.
2 Chapman 2008d.
3 World Health Organization 2009.
4 Smoke Free Movies 2010b.

Originally published as Chapman, Simon (2011). Four arguments against the adult-rating of movies with smoking scenes. *PLoS Medicine*, 23 August: e1001078.

smoking scenes in movies, which they argue directly causes the uptake of smoking.[5]

Should this policy be adopted, historical figures (such as King George VI in the 2011 Oscar winning *The King's Speech*) will still be able to smoke in films rated as acceptable for children. But nameless or fictional smokers would cause an adult rating, regardless of the historical or cultural accuracy of such casting, unless they were scripted to openly proselytise against smoking. Apparently it is unreasonable to airbrush the historical record of a well-known individual's smoking, but defensible for this to occur where whole populations or eras are concerned.

Efforts to expose and outlaw paid tobacco industry product placement in film[67] – which is unarguably a form of advertising – should be applauded, as should efforts to raise awareness within the film and television industries about the ways that gratuitous depiction of smoking can assist in normalising it. However, we have four concerns about the ratings classification proposal: two methodological, one practical, and one a matter of principle.

The first is the major problem in the evidence base of movie smoking scenes being inextricably entangled with a host of other variables in movies. The research bedrock of the restricted ratings proposal is a growing body of research said to satisfy criteria that exposure to smoking in movies causes smoking in youth,[8] including that there is a dose-response relationship between movie smoking exposure and likelihood of smoking uptake.[9] While the best of these studies control for several of potentially many subtle confounding factors associated with the dependent variable (youth who do and don't smoke) such as social, parental and psychological factors like self-assessed "rebelliousness" and risk-taking, clearly this can be only half the story. Some might also argue that, with rebelliousness being

---

5   National Cancer Institute 2008.
6   Lum, Polansky, Jackler and Glantz 2008.
7   Mekemson and Glantz 2002.
8   National Cancer Institute 2008.
9   Dalton, Sargent, Beach, Titus-Ernstoff, Gibson, Ahrens, Tickle and Heatherton 2003.

measured by items like "I like to do scary things" and "I like to listen to loud music",[10] the scales used to measure such constructs may be rather dated and of dubious validity. But, critically, potential important covariates of the independent variable (smoking in movies) are never considered. Smokers in movies never just smoke. And movies showing smoking have a lot more in them that might appeal to youth at risk of smoking than just smoking. Why is this "muddying" of the independent variable a critical consideration? Let us explain.

Teenagers select movies because of a wide range of anticipated attractions gleaned from friends, trailers and publicity about the cast, genre (action, sci-fi, teen romance, teen gross-out/black humour, survival, sports, super hero, fantasy and so on), action sequences, special effects, and soundtrack. It is likely that youth at risk for current or future smoking self-select to watch certain kinds of movies. These movies may well contain more scenes of smoking than the genres of movies they avoid (say, parental-approved "family friendly," wholesome fare like *The Chronicles of Narnia* or *Shrek*).

Teenagers at risk of smoking are also at higher risk for other risky behaviors[11] and comorbidities.[12] They thus are likely to be attracted to movies promising content that would concern their parents: rebelliousness, drinking, sexual activity or petty crime. Smoking will often be part of such movie tableaux, along with many other hard-to-quantify variables (character "attitude," irreverence, fashion sense) where the subtle and ever-changing semiotics involved present significant problems for questionnaire-based data gathering required for the calculation of attributable risk estimates (see below). Movie selection by those at risk of smoking is thus highly relevant to understanding what it might be that characterises the association between young smokers having seen many such movies and their subsequent smoking. Movie smoking may be largely artifactual to the wider attraction that those at risk of smoking have to certain genres of films. These studies rarely consider this rather obvious possibility, being preoccupied with counting incidents of smoking in the films.

---

10   Sargent, Beach, Adachi-Mejia, Gibson, Titus-Ernstoff et al. 2005.
11   Chen, Unger, Palmer, Weiner, Johnson, Wong and Austin 2002.
12   Hughes 1999.

By assuming that seeing smoking in movies is causal, rather than simply a marker of a preference for movies that have more smoking in them than the movie preferences of those less at risk, authors fail to consider problems of specificity in the independent variable (movies with "smoking"). It may be just as valid to argue that preferences for certain kinds of movies are predictive of smoking. The putative "dose response" relationships reported may be nothing more than reporting that youth who go on to smoke are those who see a lot of movies where smoking occurs, among many other unaccounted things.

If researchers also coded for potential covariates such as alcohol or recreational drug portrayal, violence, coarse language and sexual content, the depth of these very muddied waters might become apparent. One rare US study to have done this examined 71 top-grossing films over a four-year period and found that "the correlation between exposure to smoking in the movies and other adult content (nudity, violence, profanity) was so high [0.995] that it was impossible to disentangle their separate influence."[13] A challenge to the field would be to identify a subset of movies with much smoking, but no confounders like profanity, nudity, and violence, to examine variation in exposure to such movies and any relationship with subsequent smoking.

Our second concern is with the crude reductionism and questionable precision evident in the reasoning that allows conclusions like "390,000 [US] kids [are] recruited to smoke each year by the smoking they see on screen",[14] that introducing adult rating would prevent "probably 200,000 a year from starting to smoke",[15] and that smoking in movies claims "120,000 lives a year"[16] in just the USA. This epidemiological alchemy invites us to accept that these legions of children only smoke because of their exposure to movie smoking and that the resilience of this influence is so great that it retains a vice-like grip all the way through to the eventual deaths of these young smokers decades later, unmodified by other influences throughout these years.

---

13   Farrelly, Kamyab, Nonnemaker, Crankshaw and Allen 2011.
14   Smoke Free Movies (2010).
15   Smoke Free Movies (2006).
16   Smoke Free Movies (2006).

A lifetime of exposure to the sight of smoking in uncounted public, social and family situations; years of exposure to tobacco advertising and promotions still rampant in the USA and many other nations; exposure to smoking scenes often by the same influential movie and music stars in magazines,[17] music videos,[18] and on YouTube[19] - indeed "all the above" and more are ignored because of the impossibility of reliably quantifying such ubiquitous exposure over many years.

If the adult classification system for smoking was adopted, it would seem likely that the same youth at risk for smoking would still go to the same (then smoking-expurgated) kinds of films they now prefer: they don't select them only in anticipation of seeing smoking, the sight of which is commonplace. Meanwhile, they would still see copious amounts of on-screen smoking in the adult-rated films they already see with consummate ease, as well as all the other daily sightings of smoking that are conveniently not considered in these sorts of studies.

This leads to our third concern: the naivety of policy advocacy that assumes that film classification actually prevents young people from seeing "forbidden fruit." Glantz - a leading advocate for adult classification - has pilloried efforts to stop shopkeepers selling tobacco to minors because youth are street-smart enough to get older friends to buy cigarettes.[20] But similarly, youth very frequently access adult-rated movies via friends and download them legally and illegally by the millions from the web. In the USA in 2008, an estimated 10.397 million children aged 12 to 17 watched a movie on the internet, 5.6 times more than those who downloaded music. The average US teen saw 31.4 movies, of which only 10.8 (34 percent) were seen at a cinema.[21] Nearly all (98.9 percent) 15-year-old Swedish boys and 73.5 percent of girls have viewed pornography, often accessed through file-sharing sites.[22] Beliefs that restricting cinema viewing of smoking to adults is a

---

17   Chapman, Jones, Bauman and Palin 1995.
18   DuRant, Rome, Rich, Allred, Emans and Woods 1997.
19   Freeman and Chapman 2007a.
20   Ling, Landman and Glantz 2002.
21   Horovitz 2005.
22   Wallmyr and Welin 2006.

workable solution seem rapidly irrelevant with the exponential changes brought by the internet.

Fourth, and most fundamentally, we are concerned about the assumption that advocates for any cause should feel it reasonable that the state should regulate cultural products like movies, books, art and theatre in the service of their issue. We believe that many citizens and politicians who would otherwise give unequivocal support to important tobacco control policies would not wish to be associated with efforts to effectively censor movies other than to prevent commercial product placement by the tobacco industry.

The role of film in open societies involves far more than being simply a means to mass communicate healthy role models. Many movies depict social problems and people behaving badly and smoking in movies mirrors the prevalence of smoking in populations.[23] Except in authoritarian nations with state-controlled media, the role of cinema and literature is not only to promote overtly prosocial or health "oughts" but also to have people reflect on what "is" in society. This includes many disturbing, antisocial, dangerous, and unhealthy realities and possibilities. Filmmakers often depict highly socially undesirable activities such as racial hatred, injustice and vilification, violence and crime. It would be ridiculously simplistic to assume that by showing something most would regard as undesirable, a filmmaker's purpose was always to endorse such activity. Children's moral development and health decision making occur in ways far more complex than being fed a continuous diet of wholesome role models. Many would deeply resent a view of movies that assumed they were nothing more than the equivalent of religious or moral instruction, to be controlled by those inhabiting the same values. The reductio ad absurdum of arguments to prevent children ever seeing smoking in movies would be to stop children seeing smoking anywhere.

The call for movies with smoking to be adult-rated has been almost wholly conducted within the USA, where some 70 percent of Americans agree that smoking scenes should cause a movie to be thus rated.[24] Many Americans also believe in devil possession (58.6 percent),

---

23   Jamieson and Romer 2010.
24   McMillen, Tanski, Winickoff and Valentine 2007.

a biblical rather than evolutionary account of the origins of life (55.8 percent), UFOs (40.6 percent), and astrology (33.3 percent).[25] The popularity of beliefs is not always a reliable guide to their wisdom. In 2004, the "wardrobe malfunction" that exposed Janet Jackson's nipple on national TV for a second generated 540,000 complaints.[26] Such reactions perplex many outside the USA, who have long been used to far more relaxed regulation of film and television.

Proponents of the rating system for smoking argue that their proposal simply seeks to extend to smoking scenes the ratings system that now operates for sex and violence. Adult-rating advocates like to argue that smoking in movies should be treated identically to coarse language. However, non–adult-rated movies in many other nations frequently contain swearing, moderate violence and sex scenes, where panels appointed to judge the rating for the entire film have decided that these scenes do not overwhelm the overall suitability of the film to be screened to children. These panels are typically not constrained by prescribed formulae as would appear to be the case with swearing in the USA, but are asked to make a holistic judgement with reference to unspecified community standards.

The USA has First Amendment constitutional problems in banning above-the-line tobacco advertising[27] and largely because of this remains one of the few nations to have still not ratified the WHO's Framework Convention on Tobacco Control, which requires all tobacco advertising to be banned. Its public health community may therefore be drawn to advocacy for controls that they feel have some hope of progressing domestically, such as film classification. But other than in India and Thailand, we are aware of no significant momentum in governments or tobacco control circles for this to occur. This nascent momentum toward censorship and classification of smoking in movies deserves critical scrutiny from all who cherish open, civil society.

25 Rice 2003.
26 Freeman and Chapman 2007.
27 Bayer, Gostin, Javitt and Brandt 2002.

56

Factoids and legal bollocks in the war against plain packaging

In January 2014, Australia's Institute of Public Affairs (IPA) named me as one of Australia's all-time "dirty dozen opponents of freedom". It was an interesting selection in which I beat for a place Ivan Milat, the serial backpacker killer, former Queensland premier Joh Bjelke-Petersen, who banned all demonstrations in his state in 1977, and the Reverend Fred Nile, the Christian Democrats MP from New South Wales who is against abortion, homosexuality, nude beaches and lots more besides. In 2011 Tim Wilson, now a federal Liberal MP, was director of intellectual property and the Free Trade Unit at the IPA. He was an enthusiastic critic of the planned legislation for plain tobacco packaging. I noticed him throwing around a very large number ($30 billion) that he claimed the Australian government would be forced by the High Court to compensate tobacco companies every year over the savage impact that plain packs would have on their sales. I have rarely had so much fun unpacking a factoid. In 2012 the High Court rejected the tobacco industry's case.[1]

Originally published as Chapman, Simon (2011). Factoids and legal bollocks in the war against plain packaging. *Crikey*, 9 June.

With the passage of the government's bill on plain packaging now assured by the support of the opposition, the Greens and all but one of the independents, an ever-desperate tobacco industry is now concentrating on the legal apocalypse that they say will descend on Australia through the courts.

These arguments are all a paper-thin house of cards, starting with the central problem that plain packaging will not extinguish brand identities. All brands will still carry brand names allowing smokers to clearly exercise their freedom of choice to select between the much-vaunted but mostly non-existent differences in brands. This is critical, because in the highly unlikely event of a ruling by the High Court in favour of the industry, all calculations of compensation will need to take account that branding differences have only been diminished, not extinguished.

Given that some 30 to 40 nations now have appropriated massive sections of packs with graphic warnings and that not a cent has been claimed or awarded in brand damage anywhere in the world for this egregious assault on brand identity, the prospects of any claim for huge compensation even in the unlikely event of a favourable ruling are vanishingly small. The companies would need to demonstrate with precision that sales losses arose from losing colours, logos and different pack shapes, not brand names.

Given that consumption is falling every year, this task would be like unravelling gossamer while wearing boxing gloves.

Few of those megaphoning this legal Armageddon appear to have even read the draft bill itself. Section 11 makes it clear that plain packaging won't apply if it were to be determined (by a court) that its operation would result in an acquisition of property otherwise than on just terms. So in the unlikely event that the High Court says there is an acquisition of property (more on this below), the legislation would revert to a fallback position in the regulations under which "the trade mark may be used on the packaging of tobacco products, or on a tobacco product, in accordance with any requirements prescribed in the regulations".

---

1   My inclusion in the IPA's Dirty Dozen list is my most-prized award: http://bit.ly/2cREk7S.

In other words, the bill has been drafted with a get-out-of-jail-free card under which plain packaging will not proceed if the court said it was an unjust acquisition. So massive damages or compensation will simply not arise.

Moreover, Monash University's Professor Mark Davison has explained:

> As for the Constitutional argument that the legislation acquires property on other than just terms, Professor Craven, a noted Constitutional expert, has since observed on Radio National's *Background Briefing* that the tobacco industry's prospects of success are about the same as a three-legged horse has of winning the Melbourne Cup. The reason for his view is simply explained. The extinction of rights or the reduction of rights is not relevant. The government or a third party must acquire property as a consequence of the legislation.
>
> The government does not wish to use the tobacco trademarks. Nor does it want third parties to do so. It does not desire to or intend to acquire any property. The proposition that prohibitions on the use of property do not constitute an acquisition of property was confirmed by the High Court as recently as 2009. In that case, the High Court held that the government was entitled to extinguish property rights in licences of farmers to take bore water.[2]

But the industry and its errand boys, such as those at the Institute of Public Affairs, nonetheless know that the threat of a massive legal penalty will get them headlines. A big number is required and the number that has been selected is $3 billion . . . per year. So where did this satisfyingly large number come from? It started circulating in May 2010 and has been repeated countless times since by frothing shock-jocks and some who should have known better.

Step forward Tim Wilson, the director of intellectual property and the Free Trade Unit at the IPA. Wilson sent a submission[3] to Senator

---

2 Davison 2011.
3 http://bit.ly/2gjnDkO.

Steve Fielding's inquiry into plain packaging where we can examine his prowess with the numbers.

At page four in his executive summary he says plain packs would lead to a court order to award the tobacco industry between $378 million and $3,027 million per year. Table 2 (page 13) in his submission shows two lines of numbers for the total value of tobacco sales in Australia in 2006: one for the value including excise tax (which goes to the government) and one for the sales value ex-tax (in other words the returns to manufacturers and retailers combined). By taking the trouble to differentiate the two, Wilson must know that no court would order the return of the tobacco tax component to the companies: it's the ex-tax value that fuels such a pipe-dream.

Wilson then calculates the ex-tax value on two assumptions: a 10 percent and a 30 percent fall in sales each year that might follow the introduction of plain packs. He calculates these two figures at $378 million and $1.135 billion. So where does the $3 billion factoid come from? Are you ready for this? The tax-included sales value of a 30 percent fall is $3.027 billion.

So how reasonable are Wilson's assumptions that plain packs will cause a fall of a minimum 10 percent through to 30 percent a year? Between 1999 and 2003 the average annual fall in total dutied cigarettes was just 2.6 percent. The most sales have *ever* fallen in one year was just shy of 10 percent in 1999 after the combined impact of a change in the way cigarettes were taxed (from weight to per stick) and a big boost to the national quit campaign by federal health minister Michael Wooldridge.

Most analysts of the likely impact of plain packaging believe that its main impact will be on children over the next generations. Just as no Australian aged under 19 today has ever seen a local tobacco ad or tobacco sponsored sporting event, no child growing up after 2010 will ever see carcinogenic tobacco products packaged in carefully market-researched attractive boxes. Smoking rates by kids today are the lowest ever recorded. Plain packs are expected to continue that downward momentum, starving the industry of new generations of new smokers as older smokers quit and die early. Plain packs will probably not influence long-term, older smokers much.

Wilson's $3 billion number is thus based on a projected decline that is so far off the planet of declines ever recorded, it is dreamland stuff. Worse, it appears to be a willful selection of the tax-included biggest number he could sight in his own table. To the delight of the industry, it has now become a virulent factoid, with Google showing more than 7,000 hits for "plain packs cigarettes" and "$3 billion". Tim, you are a true contributor to informed public debate.

57

The slow-burn, devastating impact of tobacco plain packaging

Plain tobacco packaging was unquestionably the biggest policy fight to which I have ever contributed. In the years between 2008, when I wrote (with Becky Freeman and Matthew Rimmer) a "case" for the proposal, right through to the implementation in December 2012, I spent uncounted hours writing 19 opinion page articles on the issue, giving many dozens of media interviews, assisting journalists with background information, and talking daily to close colleagues on strategy for defending the policy and promoting it to other nations. Some 20 countries have now or are in the process of adopting plain packaging. In this piece, I wrote about the early data on its impact in Australia.

It is three years since Australia fully implemented its historic tobacco plain packaging law.[1] From 1 December 2012 all tobacco products have been required to be sold in the mandated standardised packs, which with their large disturbing graphic health warnings, are anything but "plain".

---

1   Chapman and Freeman 2014.

Originally published as Chapman, Simon (2016). The slow-burn, devastating impact of tobacco plain packaging. *Conversation*, 3 December.

Ever since, there have been frenzied efforts by the tobacco industry and its ideologically baggage carriers to discredit the policy as a failure. The obvious sub-text of this effort has been to megaphone a message to other governments that they should not contemplate introducing plain packaging because it has "failed": smoking, it is claimed, has not fallen any faster in Australia after plain packaging that it was before. All that has occurred is that illicit trade has increased, they argue.

The supreme irony here is of course that if such criticism were correct, then to paraphrase Hamlet's mother Gertrude, "The tobacco industry doth protest too much, methinks." Why would the industry and its astro-turfed bloggers waste so much money and effort denigrating a policy which was having little or no impact? Why take the Australian government to the High Court (and fail 6 to 1) to try and block the law? Why invest in supporting minnow tobacco growing states like the Dominican Republic, Honduras and Cuba in their efforts to have the World Trade Organization rule against plain packaging? Why not just ignore an ineffective policy instead of making it only too obvious to all by such actions that it is in fact a grave threat to your industry?

Two key assumptions have underscored efforts to discredit the impact of plain packaging. First, critics assume that the impacts of the law should have been evident immediately it was implemented: as one colleague put it recently, "within ten seconds of the law passing". Second, they assume (but never actually state) that the impact of plain packaging on smoking by children (the principal target) and adults was supposedly going to be greater than anything we have previously observed in the entire history of tobacco control.

In 1999, the late Tony McMichael, professor of epidemiology at the Australian National University, published a classic paper called Prisoners of the Proximate,[2] where he wrote about the need to understand the determinants of population health in terms that extend beyond proximate single risk factors and influences. In tobacco control, both proximal (discrete, recent and quick-acting) and distal (ongoing, slow-burn) effects of policies and campaigns can occur. Price rises (and falls through discounting) can have both immediate and lasting effects,

---

2   McMichael 1999.

jolting smokers into sometimes unplanned quitting and also slowly percolating an unease about the costs of smoking that translate into quitting down the track.

Tobacco advertising bans are a good example of a policy that has such slow-burn effects across many years. Few if any quit smoking in direct response to tobacco advertising bans. They work instead by causing the next generations of kids to grow up in an environment devoid of massive promotional campaigns depicting smoking in positive ways.

I have often heard smokers say, "Plain packaging won't make me quit smoking". This is akin to the myopic self-awareness of those who swear "Advertising (for any product) never influences me" while noting that it only influences the more impressionable.

Plain packs were unlikely to act suddenly in the way tax rises do, although the unavoidably huge graphic health warnings may well have acted like straws that broke the Camel's back of worry about smoking. Their impact was far more likely to be of the slow-burn sort, where the constant reminder that tobacco, unique among all products, is the only consumer good treated this way by the law. It is exceptionally dangerous, with a recent estimate[3] being that two in every three long-term smokers will die from tobacco use.

In 1993 I wrote a now highly cited paper[4] in the *British Medical Journal* which talked about the impossibility of "unravelling gossamer with boxing gloves" when it came to being certain about precisely why smokers quit. I took a day in the life of a smoker who quit, and pointed to the myriad of influences both distal and proximal that coalesce to finally stimulate a person to stop smoking. While a smoker might nominate a particular policy, conversation with a doctor or anti-smoking campaign as being "the reason" they quit, much of what went on before provides the broad shoulders of concern that carry the final attribution. There are synergies between all these factors and the demand to separate them all is like the demand to unscramble an omlette.

---

3   Chapman 2015b.
4   Chapman 1993.

So what has happened to smoking in Australia since plain packs? Data released this month from a national schools survey[5] involving more than 23,000 high school children found smoking rates were the lowest ever recorded since the studies first commenced in 1984. This momentum is starving the tobacco industry of new smokers which is one important reason why all tobacco companies are now busily acquitting e-cigarette brands.

With adults, National Accounts data[6] just released show that for the 11 quarter-year periods since March 2013, consumption of tobacco products in aggregate fell an unprecedented 20.8 percent, while the previous 11 quarters it fell 15.7 percent and in the 11 before that only 2.2 percent.

The last available data on adult smoking prevalence we have is from 2013 and shows that just 12.8 percent of Australians over 14 smoked on a daily basis, again the lowest on record and again, the biggest percentage falls experienced since the surveys commenced.

Meanwhile, the tobacco industry plods along funding heavily lambasted[7] studies which purport to show that none of this is happening.

The argument that plain packaging would cause illicit trade to boom was made with monotonous regularity by Big Tobacco between April 2010, when plain packaging was announced, and its December 2012 implementation. When the industry lost its case in the High Court, the argument was quietly dropped. Today the industry explains illicit trade entirely by the heinous government tobacco tax rises cloaked in a sanctimonious rhetoric of speaking up for poor smokers and corporate citizen concern about tax avoidance bleeding Treasury. In all this it fails to mention that it has long used tax rises as air cover to quietly raise its own profit margins.

As I wrote recently in *The Conversation*,[8] "From August 2011 to February 2013, while excise duty rose 24 cents for a pack of 25, the tobacco companies' portion of the cigarette price (which excludes

---

5   White and Williams 2015.
6   http://bit.ly/2d0zxOw.
7   See http://bit.ly/2cbp4BH.
8   Chapman 2015b.

excise and GST), jumped A$1.75 to A$7.10. While excise had risen 2.8 percent over the period, the average net price had risen 27 percent. Philip Morris' budget brand Choice 25s rose A$1.80 in this period, with only 41 cents of this being from excise and GST."

Ireland, England and France have already passed laws that will introduce plain packs. Norway and Canada will soon, and New Zealand, Chile, Turkey, South Africa and Brazil have also made high level noises about joining in too.

58
Pleased as Punch: interview with the tobacco industry

I mostly refuse to engage with the tobacco industry because, as the High Court judge in the UK's 2016 plain-packaging judgement put it, values and objectives "collide in the most irreconcilable ways". But when the leading tobacco industry magazine, *Tobacco Reporter*, invited me to give uninhibited responses to nine questions about plain packaging in 2015, I couldn't resist.

Q. Professor Chapman, you were one of the strongest supporters of the introduction of plain packaging legislation in Australia. The objectives of the legislation were to reduce the attractiveness and appeal of tobacco products to consumers, particularly young people, increase the noticeability and effectiveness of graphic health warnings, reduce the ability of the retail packaging of tobacco products to mislead consumers about the harms of smoking, and, in the long term, contribute to the reduction of smoking rates. Two years after the law has been enforced, are you happy with its impact? Assuming you are, could you please explain why?

Originally published as Rossel, Stefanie (2015). Pleased as Punch. *Tobacco Reporter*, February.

A. Very happy. A highly chemically engineered, addictive product which is forecast to kill 1 billion people this century on average ten years early is now being packaged in a way commensurate with its unparalleled status as the most deadly consumer product ever marketed. My only regret is that the gangrene pictorial warning does not yet incorporate a scratch-and-sniff tab impregnated with putrescence or cadavarine which would allow smokers additionally unforgettable insight into the world of smoking that will await many of them.

Q. There has been much debate about the lack of hard data on the development of the tobacco market and smoking in Australia since plain packaging became mandatory. On which evidence do you base your findings?

A. Tobacco companies of course know *exactly* the impact it is causing in Australia and likely to cause when it spreads internationally. They know this impact day by day, suburb by suburb, shop by shop and brand by brand because they have instant sales data and can map this to both proximal and distal factors intended to both promote and reduce smoking. The industry's apoplexy about plain packs is all we need to know about whether plain packaging is biting. In a nearly 40-year career, I have never seen the industry attack any policy – including tax – with the venom and aggression that we are seeing with plain packs.

Q. Even two years after its implementation, the relevance of the introduction of plain packaging is difficult to evaluate. Judging from the hype that emerged around its introduction and the great expectations about the potential impact of this unprecedented, drastic measure by the tobacco control community, as well as the fierce opposition from the tobacco industry, one would have expected an immediate, obvious effect of the legislation. Today, in the absence of reliable, unequivocal data, it appears that the public health community, not unlike the tobacco industry, rejoices at every set of data that seems to prove their point, while at the same time they excuse any other findings claiming plain packaging legislation was merely part of a comprehensive package of tobacco control activities and that it was still too early to look at its effectiveness. Could you please comment on this discrepancy? What do you think, is plain packaging already a success in its own right or just an "experiment", as the then health minister Nicola Roxon termed it when it was implemented? When *would be* the right time to assess the effectiveness of the legislation in your opinion?

A. I am unaware of anyone with any experience or credibility in tobacco control who forecast "an immediate, obvious effect" from plain packaging. This is so obviously and deliberately an industry straw-man game. No Australian born after 1 July 1993 (so now aged up to 21) has ever seen a local tobacco advertisement or sponsored event. They have grown up understanding that, unique among all consumer products, tobacco is the only product subject to a total advertising ban. Similarly, those born after December 2012 will now grow up never seeing a product with 60-plus carcinogens packaged in beguiling livery, reflecting the best efforts of your industry to keep smokers' minds off that reality. Measures like advertising bans, graphic health warnings, smoke-free policies, plain packaging and all other elements of comprehensive tobacco control have worked synergistically to get both adult and children's smoking prevalence to today's record lows. Australia today has the world's lowest smoking prevalence, with only 12.8 percent smoking daily. It is a template that if replicated will save hundreds of millions of lives this century.

Q. Asked about the effectiveness of plain packaging, the tobacco industry, as would have been expected, basically said it had no effect whatsoever and argued that it was rather the series of significant tax hikes that impacted on cigarette sales. What is your opinion on that? Was the introduction of plain packaging a necessary measure or would tax hikes alone have done the trick?

A. On the same day that the Australian government announced plain packaging, it introduced an overnight 25 percent hike in tobacco tax (1 May 2010). Treasury modellers predicted a 6 percent fall in consumption, but an 11 percent fall occurred. In August 2011, we witnessed BATA's David Crow acknowledging this decimating impact to a Senate committee but almost begging the government to continue it rather than progress plain packaging. What should that tell us?

Q. Recent population health surveys from several Australian states indicate that smoking prevalence among adults has gone up. A New

South Wales population health survey showed that in 2013 16.4 percent of adults smoked, up from 14.7 percent in 2011. The latest figures from Queensland reveal that for 25- to 34-year-olds, 28 percent of men smoke, compared with 19.8 percent in 2012, and for women it has risen 4 percent to 17 percent. In South Australia smoking rates were up from 16.7 percent to 19.4 percent. The New South Wales *Health of Young People Report* reveals an upward trend since 2011 for smokers aged between 16 and 24. Apparently, plain packaging has not deterred these people from taking up smoking. Could you please comment on these figures?

A. Your question conspicuously avoids the rhino in the living room: national data from a 24,000-strong national sample which shows the lowest ever smoking prevalence post-plain packs (12.8 percent daily), that younger people are delaying the take-up of smoking – the age at which 14- to 24-year-olds smoked their first full cigarette increased from 14.2 in 1995 to 15.9 years in 2013 – and that smokers reduced the average number of cigarettes smoked per week by 13.5 percent, from 111 cigarettes in 2010 to 96 in 2013.

The New South Wales and South Australian state data you cite are not statistically significant, and if they were in the opposite direction we would not be able to claim that rates were decreasing. The website for the New South Wales data states clearly that 2010 and 2012 data are not comparable ("In 2012 mobile phones were included in the survey methods for the first time and this increased the number of younger people and males in the survey sample. Both of these groups have relatively higher smoking rates, leading to a higher overall reported rate of current smoking. The 2012 prevalence estimate reflects an improvement in the representativeness of the survey sample. The rate for 2013 has stabilised.") If the tobacco industry really believed these cherry-picked figures signified an increase in smoking in Australia, it would be voluntarily introducing plain packs as fast as it could.

Your industry is so amusing in the way that it regularly flip-flops between strenuously arguing plain packs have no effect on prevalence or sales and then megaphoning factoids like the infamous one circulated by the industry-sponsored Institute of Public Affairs that plain packs would work so well that $3 billion a year would be ordered by the courts for compensation. When we drilled down into this, the factoid was based on an assumption of a 30 percent fall *each year* in consumption. Would it be too much to ask you to make up your mind? Is it a policy that won't work, or the most damaging policy ever introduced anywhere?

Q. As it looks, it is the lack of reliable, hard data that makes it so difficult to assess the impact of plain packaging. What would be a suitable solution to this problem? In a contribution to abc.net.au in July 2013, you call for publicly available data on tobacco-tax receipts and projections in Australia – would this be a good way out of the dilemma? And would this also be a solution favoured by the public health community?

A. Since I wrote that, the Australian Bureau of Statistics has released data showing a decrease in chain volume of tobacco sales of 6.3 percent from the March 2013 to the September 2014 quarters.

Q. Australia's plain packaging legislation is currently facing a landmark challenge at the World Trade Organization (WTO) that was filed by five countries, among them cigar-producing nations Cuba, the Dominican Republic and Honduras, which say that brandless packaging is an assault to their trading rights, threatening their trademarks and local economies. In your book you are quite confident that it is highly unlikely Australia will lose the case – why?

A. "Landmark" is your word. A sad collection of minnow nations all with pathetic tobacco control, high smoking rates and high corruption indeces are leading this tawdry exercise. There has been a massive amount of legal scholarship published by extremely senior people on the prospects of the WTO challenge succeeding. All give its success about the same probability as a three-legged horse winning the Grand National or Kentucky Derby. Five tobacco transnationals were humiliated 6–1 in the Australian High Court, another result that all but industry consultants predicted.

Q. Several countries in the world, among them European Union member states, have already made efforts to follow Australia's example (see *Tobacco Reporter* December 2014). Under EU law, restricting the use of brands is problematic, since it infringes intellectual property rights, and national and international trademark law, as well as articles contained in the Charter of Fundamental Rights of the European Union and even the European Convention on Human Rights. The outcome of the WTO case left aside, what makes you so sure that the domino effect we have seen with other tobacco control measures will occur in this case, too?

A. Some 77 nations have "infringed the intellectual property rights" of your industry by requiring graphic health warnings and thereby appropriating large areas of this "intellectual property". Not a cent has been paid in compensation anywhere. There is not one component of comprehensive tobacco control that has been first adopted by one country and which has not then rapidly dominoed globally.

Q. Tobacco (and plain packaging) has also been a hot topic in the Trans-Pacific Partnership (TPP) talks. TPP is a proposed regional free-trade agreement. As of 2014 12 countries throughout the Asia-Pacific region, among them the United States, have participated in negotiations on the TPP. The trade agreement also contains investor-state dispute settlements (ISDS) clauses which enable foreign corporations to sue a host country for laws or policies, or even court decisions, they find inconvenient and objectionable. In how far could TPP put an end to Australia's plain pack "experience" and prevent the "global plain-pack domino spectacle", as you put it?

A. Australia's Trade Minister Andrew Robb has now twice taken the trouble to state publicly that Australia will not allow the TPP to jeopardise plain packaging. There are many products on which different governments impose strong restrictions or even outright bans for health or cultural reasons. Examples include Islamic nations (with severe restrictions on alcohol sales), firearms, asbestos, exotic and endangered fauna, and pornography. I somehow don't like the prospects of transnational liquor companies deciding that they could force Saudi Arabia to allow liquor, or publishers to sell *Penthouse* openly from cafés and newsstands in Mecca. No firearms company has taken Australia to any court or tribunal for its heinous action in 1996 of banning civilian ownership of semi-automatic rifles and pump-action shotguns, weapons favoured by gunmen who almost weekly wreak havoc in the USA.

59

The case for a smoker's licence

In August 2011, after the High Court of Australia cleared the way for the Australian government to implement plain packaging, I was often asked by journalists and interviewers, "So what's next in tobacco control?" In 2005 I'd published a paper in which I briefly canvassed the idea of a "licence" to smoke premised on the idea of smokers passing knowledge test of the risks they faced if they decided to smoke.

I decided to fully develop the proposal in the article below, which has now been opened by 24,000 readers. All big ideas that have been implemented in tobacco control have at first been seen as radical and from some fantasy land inhabited only by public health ideologues. But advertising bans, smoke-free public areas and transport, graphic health warnings on packs and plain packaging have all become realities and together have been associated with smoking rates tumbling in many nations. Those who ridiculed these policies are today busy wiping egg off their collected visage.

Smoker licensing seems similarly "out there" today, but may well seem a normal policy in years to come.[1]

Originally published as Chapman, Simon (2012). The case for a smoker's licence. *PLoS Medicine*, 14 November: 1001342.

The prolonged use of tobacco causes the death of about half its users,[2] with a billion people this century predicted to die from tobacco caused disease.[3] In particular, the cigarette is an exceptionally dangerous product: no other commodity or human activity causes a remotely comparable number of annual deaths.

The history of tobacco control has seen policies introduced that were initially considered radical, but which rapidly came to be considered normal[4] and essential to the goals of reducing use and the burden of disease caused. No other consumer product is subject to total advertising bans nor required to be sold in plain packaging, as will occur in Australia from December 2012.[5] Again uniquely, 47 nations now require large graphic warnings on tobacco packaging.[6] Smoke-free public transport, workplaces, restaurants, bars and stadiums are common in an increasingly large number of nations. The World Health Organization's Framework Convention on Tobacco Control, which requires such measures, has been ratified by 174 nations.[7]

Despite these developments, tobacco sale is subject to trivial controls compared with other dangerous products that threaten both public or personal safety. This paper describes a proposal for a major development with further potential to reduce tobacco use: the tobacco user's license, and considers several anticipated objections.

Tobacco vs pharmaceuticals access

Access to firearms, fireworks, explosives and dangerous chemicals is often heavily restricted for both personal and public safety reasons. However the most instructive comparison with how tobacco products are sold is with the way governments regulate the sale of other drugs:

---

1 An 18-minute video explaining the concept can be found here: http://bit.ly/2c66LL9.
2 Doll, Peto, Boreham and Sutherland 2004.
3 Proctor 2001.
4 Chapman and Freeman 2008.
5 Chapman and Freeman 2010.
6 Physicians for a Smoke-Free Canada 2012.
7 Framework Convention Alliance. Home page 2012.

pharmaceuticals. Those known to be benign with little potential for harm, or which are unlikely to create dependency, tend to be freely available as over-the-counter products in pharmacies, and increasingly in supermarkets and convenience stores. Mild analgesics, cough and cold remedies and bronchodilators are good examples.

However, pharmaceuticals likely to cause health problems if used incorrectly or for too long, or which require users to be monitored so the drug or dosage can be modified, are sold by pharmacists to those with prescriptions issued by medical practitioners and, increasingly, nurses.[8]

Prescriptions are "temporary licences"

While prescriptions are strictly speaking a prescriber's note of authority to a pharmacist to dispense restricted drugs to a named individual, the prescription system is in effect a system of temporary licensing to use restricted substances. Travellers carrying restricted drugs across borders can be required to show that they have a "licence" to be in possession of some drugs. It is a criminal offence to supply prescription drugs to those without a prescription and those doing so can face pharmacy or medical deregistration, fines and possibly imprisonment in serious cases.

To obtain their drugs, users must attend a doctor, pay a sometimes significant consultation fee, and, if assessed as needing a drug, then visit a pharmacist. There, they will pay again to receive a limited supply of the drug, sometimes with provision for several repeats. After this, users are required to return to a doctor should they need more drugs.

This is how nearly all nations regulate drugs designed to ease pain, reduce symptoms, prevent disease and prolong life. It is seen as a sensible, established system designed to prevent misuse of drugs and to better ensure that access to such drugs is supervised in the interest of patient health.

By contrast, tobacco products can be sold by any retailer. Mixed businesses, supermarkets, petrol stations, kiosks, barbers, bars and

---

8   Kroezen, Francke, Groenewegen and van Dijk 2012.

vending machines are examples of the nearly ubiquitous tobacco retailing environment.[9] Unlike prescribed pharmaceuticals, smokers can buy unlimited quantities of tobacco. Many nations outlaw sales to minors, but prosecutions are rare and sales to children common. In contrast to the highly regulated way we allow access to life-saving and health-enhancing pharmaceuticals, this is how we regulate access to a product that kills half its long-term users. *Prima facie*, there would seem to be a case for redressing this bizarre but historically based inconsistency.

The tobacco user's licence

The proposed smoker's license described below merits serious consideration as a major platform in the tobacco control endgame now being considered in nations with advanced records of reducing smoking. Earlier, less elaborated accounts have been described in 2005,[10] and by LeGrande et al. in 2007[11] and 2009.[12]

Smart-card technology

All smokers would be required to obtain a smart swipecard licence[13] to transact any purchase from a licensed tobacco retailer. Retailers could not sell to anyone without a card, because there would need to be perfect reconciliation between tobacco stock supplied by wholesalers to retailers and that sold to licensed smokers. Penalties for unreconciled sales to unlicensed persons would be severe, with threat of loss of retail licence, as now applies with pharmacists supplying restricted drugs anyone without a prescription.

Licence application could be made online or at authorised tobacconists, with supported data-linkable, proof-of-age cross-referencing (passport, driver's licence, birth certificate) required to

---

9   Chapman and Freeman 2009.
10   Chapman and Liberman 2005.
11   Laurance 2007.
12   LeGrande, Titmus and Srivastva 2009.
13   Chien, Jan and Tseng 2002

validate identity. The government licensing authority would validate these identities via data linkage, then mail the licence.

A database of all smokers

With rapidly increasing internet access, most smokers would probably elect to transact their licensing online, thereby providing an email address. This could be used by governments as a way of efficiently communicating new and potentially cessation-motivating information to all smokers, with tailored messages for different age groups. Every time a sale was transacted, data of exquisite specificity would be added to the national database. This would enable both immediate and longitudinal national, regional and local monitoring of tobacco sales in ways that could provide invaluable information about smoker responsiveness to tobacco control initiatives as well as industry price discounting and new brand launches. Such information would be of great assistance to policy and program planners wanting to maximise cessation.

Pre-commitment to a maximum daily consumption

The smartcard licence would be encoded with a maximum purchase limit chosen by the licensee at the time of application. There could be three grades of licence: one to ten cigarettes per day (max. 70 per week), 11 to 20 (max. 140 per week), and 21 to 50 (max. 350 per week. Loose tobacco equivalents could be calculated. A smoker wanting to purchase a pack would request their brand and swipe their licence in the smartcard terminal. With the speed that credit card and EFTPOS terminals now approve or deny a transaction, the terminal would instantly confirm that the licensee was either able to purchase a new supply or that the chosen limit had been reached, in which case the terminal would display the earliest date when a new supply could be purchased. Limits would be calculated over a 14-day period. Licensed smokers could purchase their chosen quota as infrequently as once every two weeks, to avoid the imposition of any need to visit retailers more often.

The more cigarettes a licensee opted for, the higher the fee. Some 90 percent of smokers regret having started smoking[14] and 40 percent make a quit attempt each year,[15] most failing. Many smokers are known to support tobacco control policies like tax rises and smoking restrictions because they believe such measures will assist them to quit or reduce their consumption.[16] It is likely that some smokers may use the opportunity to set a lower daily limit via a licensing scheme than they might normally smoke in an effort to reduce their usual consumption. Cutting down before quitting is a common approach to eventual cessation.[17]

The pre-set daily limit would preclude smokers consuming more than planned unless they borrowed cigarettes from other licensed smokers. As these would be valued by other smokers, such borrowing would be marginal. The limit would also act as a barrier to unplanned "binge" smoking that occurs now, particularly when alcohol is involved.[18]

Smokers could also adjust their consumption limit upwards by going online and paying the extra licensing fee, in the way consumers are used to doing with changing their internet download limits. At annual licence renewal time they could also elect to change their limit.

Maximum daily limit

There would be an upper limit of 50 cigarettes per day, averaged across 14 days. Very few smokers consume more than this. Allowing purchasers to buy more than 50 may encourage some to obtain a license with the intent of on-selling tobacco to unlicensed smokers. A limit of 50 cigarettes is unlikely to attract such enterprise as it would not provide the on-seller with substantial profit.

Failure to purchase one's pre-committed allocation (for example, when travelling overseas or temporarily quitting) would not allow smokers to purchase the backlog of unpurchased supplies at a future date.

---

14   Fong, Hammond, Laux, Zanna, Cummings, Borland and Ross 2004.
15   Hyland, Borland, Li, Yong, McNeill, Fong, O'Connor, Cummings 2006.
16   Wilson, Weerasekera, Edwards, Thomson, Devlin and Gifford 2010; Borland, Yong, Siahpush, Hyland, Campbell, Hastings, Cummings and Fong 2006.
17   Hughes and Carpenter 2006.
18   Hoek, Maubach, Stevenson, Gendall and Edwards 2011.

Cost of licence fee

The licence fee would be neither trivial nor astronomical. It would be set at a sufficient level to give smokers some pause in deciding whether to obtain or renew their licence. Market research could be used to determine the appropriate level. For the sake of illustration, assume that the lowest level (up to ten cigarettes per day) would be $100 a year (27 cents a day) and the highest $200 (54 cents a day). This could be paid in quarterly installments or in full.

Periodic renewal

The licence would need to be renewed each year. As with initial application, this could be done online, as are many annual or periodic payments, or at authorised tobacconists. The status of the renewal would be recognised by smart-card terminals in every retail outlet, as would any change in the smoker-determined weekly limit.

Incentive to surrender licence

There is some evidence that financial reward can stimulate cessation.[19] The incentive to surrender one's license and obtain a cumulative refund of all licence fees paid may promote cessation. As a quit incentive, all licence fees paid during a smoker's licensed smoking history would be fully refundable, with compound interest. Licence surrender would be permanent and reapplication not permitted. If a licence fee was $100 for up to ten cigarettes per day, someone commencing at 18 could collect $1,000 plus interest if deciding to quit a decade later. Smokers could be reminded of this via email each year. Consideration should be given to ending this provision in middle age (say 40 years) as a major incentive to encourage quitting. The 50-year follow-up of the British doctor's cohort study showed that "those who stopped before middle age . . . had a pattern of survival similar to that of men who had never smoked".[20] This information could be heavily publicised to promote permanent license surrender at the start of middle age. Those who at the start of the

---

19   Cahill and Perera 2011.
20   Doll, Peto, Boreham and Sutherland 2004.

scheme had obtained their first licence when aged over 40 could have this extended to 50; 50 to 60 and so on.

Cooling-off period

Application for licence surrender would incorporate a mandatory six-month "cooling-off" period where smokers could change their mind and cancel their revocation application if they relapsed. Some smokers relapse far beyond six months but it may be that ready access to unlimited supplies of cigarettes is an important contributory factor here, and that inability to purchase legally would reduce later relapse. Those who did relapse after licence expiry could be encouraged to use nicotine replacement therapy.

Poor smokers

As smoking prevalence diminishes, an increasing proportion of smokers are on low incomes and unemployment or disability support. Some in this group may find it hard to pay for a licence. This argument has often been used by the tobacco industry to oppose tobacco-tax rises. Those advocating keeping tobacco tax low perversely seek to "help" poor smokers by keeping tobacco affordable, which encourages use. Poor smokers, as a group, are known to be more responsive to price than those on higher incomes, in terms of both quitting and reducing use,[21] so the additional licence cost should add to this effect.

Tourists and temporary visitors

Tourists and other temporary visitors wanting to purchase tobacco could apply for a licence abroad prior to travel, or on arrival, in the same way that local cell phones are hired by travellers during their stay. Provision would exist for licences of shorter duration, to accommodate short trips. Short-term licence fees would not be refundable.

Existing adult smokers

The government would announce the scheme a year in advance of its implementation and encourage early application with "early bird" discounts. Consumers are used to this with, for example, the

---

21   Siahpush, Wakefield, Spittal, Durkin and Scollo 2009.

introduction of mandatory highway toll windscreen transponders. Anyone already aged 18 or over who wanted a smoker's licence could be thus "grandfathered" and allowed to buy a licence if they chose.

New smokers to pass a test of risk knowledge

A person turning 18 who wished to henceforth legally purchase tobacco could apply for a licence. However, unlike the commencing cohort of adult smokers at the start of the scheme, newly licensed smokers would have to pass a knowledge-of-risk test (see examples in the box). Applicants for their first driving licence must pass knowledge tests. Sometimes these are elementary, but they can also involve learning detailed information about breaking distances at different speeds and the meaning of a large variety of road signage. To better ensure that new smokers were making an informed choice, something the tobacco industry has long declared that it believes applies to smokers' decisions ("The tobacco industry believes that people who smoke do so fully informed of the reported health risks of smoking"),[22] new applicants would be required to demonstrate a satisfactory level of knowledge that might encompass issues like:

* probabilities of various diseases in smokers vs non-smokers
* the impact on day-to-day functioning of diseases like emphysema and heart disease
* average number of years lost by continuing smokers
* financial cost of smoking to an individual across increasing durations of smoking
* chemical additives used in cigarette manufacture.

Applicants would be given online educational material of direct relevance to the test, and a large, growing question bank would be developed based on this material, with random on-screen questions being given to each applicant. Such a test would disadvantage applicants who had intellectual impairment (see below). However, the same concerns apply to any knowledge test, such as for a driving license or requirement to demonstrate understanding of a contract, lease or other legal transaction.

---

22   Tobacco Institute of Australia 1994.

Examples of multiple-choice questions that could be asked of licence applicants:

- If 100 people were diagnosed with lung cancer, how many would we expect to be alive in five years' time?
- What fraction of smokers do you believe will die early because of their smoking?
- On average, how much longer do non-smokers live than people who have smoked for a long time?
- A long-term smoker who dies from a disease caused by his or her smoking can expect to lose how many years off normal life expectancy?
- If a person smokes an average of fewer than ten cigarettes a day during their lifetime, what are their chances of dying from a smoking caused disease compared to a 20-a-day smoker?
- How many times would a typical 20-a-day smoker inhale smoke deep into their lungs between the ages of 20 and 40?
- If 100 people try to stop smoking, regardless of which method they use, on average how many do you think will not be smoking 12 months later?
- How many known carcinogens (chemicals which are known to cause cancer) are there in cigarette smoke?

The tobacco industry might well find the legal implications of such "informed consent to smoke" attractive. Any smoker seeking legal redress later from a tobacco company for having been misled, would have passed the test, making such a line of argument difficult to sustain.

Dysfunctional smokers

Some young smokers with profound mental health or intellectual disabilities would be unable to pass the licensing test. Such people would be likely to be under care or on a disability pension. Special provision could be made for another adult, carer or institutional representative to obtain a license on their behalf, after consideration of their circumstances.

Gradual increase in the minimum age for purchase.

A Singaporean group has proposed that commencing with the birth cohort born in 2000, from the year 2018, anyone turning 18 would be unable to buy tobacco thereafter.[23] The idea here is that current smokers born before 2000 should be the last generation of smokers. However, libertarian objections that adults should be free to take informed risks, as with smoking, may render such a plan politically unacceptable.

However, a possibly less objectionable variation on this idea is that from a given year, the legal age for smoking would be raised each year by one year. As very few smokers commence experimenting with smoking after 23 years, the expectation is that the incremental, progressive rise in the legal smoking commencement age would effectively see very few people take up smoking when the minimum legal age reached around 23 years. Some would object that those aged 18 and over are adults who can vote, be conscripted for wars and so on, and increasing the minimum age for smoking beyond 18 is therefore unreasonable. However, precedents exist for varying age-limit restrictions (e.g. a legal drinking age of 21 in parts of the USA; legal refusal of car hire to young and very old drivers; and age-related insurance premium differences).

Potential objections to the scheme

1. We should regulate the industry, not smokers

Some may argue that a regulatory strategy focused on smokers rather than on the tobacco industry is inappropriate, and that regulation should be directed "upstream" at the industry and its products. This is a false dichotomy because user licensing is not being proposed as an alternative to industry or product regulation but as complementary to these. A core argument for the licensing of tobacco retailers has always been that removal of the licence (and so the right to sell) could be used as a strong deterrent to selling to minors. This has always been a

---

23   Khoo, Chiam, Ng, Berrick and Koong 2010.

very poorly rated tobacco control strategy because it relies on the direct observation of sales to minors by regulatory agents, and this is often difficult and time-consuming. Licence cancellations and prosecutions are therefore rare and a so a very weak disincentive to selling to minors. The instant swipecard licence verification ensures that retailers *only* sell to licensed adult smokers. Also, many platforms of industry and product regulation directly affect smokers (price, packaging, pack warnings, duty-free bans, ingredient regulation), so the criticism that an explicitly user-focused form of regulation is somehow problematic seems misplaced.

2. Cost of administration

The costs of the scheme would include administrative staff costs to process licence applications, renewals and license surrender refunds; publicity costs to inform smokers about the scheme; and retail swipecard terminals. The cost of the scheme would be drawn from the licensing fees, with retailers paying all costs associated with the swipecard terminals. Lost cards would incur a replacement charge.

As explained, the accumulated licence fees would in theory all be (eventually) refundable to smokers wishing to surrender their licences. However, not all smokers would surrender their licence by the final age limit specified for surrender and refund (40 years). This would leave a large pool of funds that could be used to administer the scheme.

3. Further stigmatisation of smokers?

Every current smoker's experience has been that tobacco products have always been sold alongside other unrestricted commodities. This will have powerfully conditioned the view that cigarettes are "ordinary" commodities and that a proposal like this is self-evidently draconian. Some smokers may feel that they are being treated like registered addicts, and that the licence epitomises their stigmatisation.[24]

Such understandable reactions reflect many decades of smoking being considered "normal". Open sale of tobacco is consonant with the lack of understanding of tobacco's harmfulness when cigarettes became a mass distributed and advertised commodity at the start of the

---

24 Bell 2011; Carter and Chapman 2006.

20th century. However, today's smokers have all experienced a range of profound changes in the way that smoking and cigarettes are socially perceived and regulated. Having to go outside to smoke in now virtually any indoor public setting, having disturbing graphic warnings on packs, and regular exposure to public awareness campaigns resting on negative subtexts about the undesirability of smoking have all coalesced to drive smoking lower and to make most smokers make quit attempts and regret having started. It would be almost unimaginable for a smoker today to express the hope that their own children would grow up to smoke as well.

The requirement to have a prescription (a temporary licence) to legally obtain pharmaceuticals is never decried as stigmatising or insulting. Those responsible for planning the introduction of smokers' licences could try to amplify this analogy.

4. Licensing is unprecedented and would "sanction" smoking

Many nations register methadone users and some allow registered heroin-dependent people access to heroin (Switzerland, the Netherlands). In California, Canada and the Netherlands, licenses are issued for the medicinal use of cannabis. The Northern Territory government in Australia has introduced a photo-ID system integrated with limits on the purchasing of bulk, cheap wine and large single purchase amounts of alcohol.[25] In Australia, the over-the-counter purchase of cold-relief medicines containing pseudoephedrine involves one's identification and address being recorded in a national database, as a means to limit supply to reduce diversion into illicit methamphetamine manufacture.[26] In all of these examples, different forms and levels of drug user licensing have been introduced as a means of allowing limited access to different drugs while controlling wider use. Tobacco, which harms far more people than all those drugs combined, currently has no form of user regulation. (In Japan, where cigarette sales are dominated by vending machines, smokers wanting to use the machines must have licences, but the system is incomparable to the current proposal in every other respect).[27]

---

25 Northern Territory Government. Department of Justice 2008.
26 South Australian Consolidated Regulations 2011.

5. A slippery slope?

Opponents of the idea would be quick to suggest that Orwellian social engineers would soon be calling for licences to drink alcohol and to eat junk food or engage in any "risky" activity. This argument rests on poor public understanding of the magnitude of the risks of smoking relative to other cumulative everyday risks to health. Other than religious-based restrictions on alcohol sales in some Islamic nations, no other product is subject to the restrictions routinely applied to tobacco marketing and packaging in many nations today. In Australia, the first restrictions on tobacco advertising commenced in 1976 – 36 years ago. Since then, similar restrictions have not been implemented for any other consumer good. Any slope would appear to be decidedly unslippery.

6. Black market concerns

Might licensing cause a growth in black-market tobacco? As obtaining a licence would not be onerous nor very expensive (relative to the cost of smoking itself), there would be few reasons why most current smokers intending to continue would not obtain one. A licence would enable easy access to tobacco purchasing, whereas those without a licence would need to take trouble to find illicit sources of supply. Here, some would argue that illicit drug trade flourishes in some nations in spite of such drugs needing to be sourced illegally from criminals. The implication here is that many smokers would be similarly willing to transact with criminals. However, this analogy is badly flawed because while illicit drugs can *only* be sourced illegally, tobacco would still be readily obtainable legally. It is therefore difficult to foresee why significant proportions of smokers would elect to source their tobacco "underground", dealing with criminals simply because of an easily obtained licensing requirement.

The main explanations for high demand for illicit tobacco are the cheaper price at which illicit tobacco sells, the ease of cross-border traffic in some nations, and the high levels of corruption in which illicit trade

---

27   Keferl 2009.

can flourish.[28] None of these factors would in any way be influenced by a user licensing system and so are not arguments against licensing.

Conclusion

The current suite of comprehensive tobacco control policies, embodied in the Framework Convention on Tobacco Control, were developed during decades when sometimes large majorities of populations smoked, (particularly males).[29] Today, nations which have taken tobacco control seriously have smoking prevalence near or below 20 percent and are setting medium-term prevalence targets of 10 percent. Discussions about "endgame" strategy are becoming more common in tobacco control circles and have begun to be articulated by governments and the public.[30] New Zealand has announced a goal of being smoke-free by 2025.[31] In England, 45 percent of the population and one-third of smokers support a total ban on the sale of tobacco products.[32]

In the past 30 years, many nations have introduced legislation for tobacco control that previously seemed unimaginable: total and sponsorship advertising bans, widespread smoke-free policies, large graphic warnings and now, plain packaging. A smoker's licence may today seem a radical step toward ending the epidemic of tobacco cause disease, but it is far less radical than prohibiting the sale of tobacco, which is not a strategy that has yet been supported by any international expert report or political forum. The New Zealand government, in setting its 2025 "smoke-free" goal, did not say it would actually prohibit the sale of tobacco. A smoker's licence allows smokers the choice to continue smoking within a regulatory framework that promises new disincentives to smoke and a major financial incentive to quit.

This proposal is unlikely to gain traction in impoverished nations with poor electronic retailing infrastructure, extensive networks of

28 Joossens and Raw 2008.
29 Framework Convention Alliance 2012.
30 Thomson, Edwards, Wilson and Blakely 2012.
31 New Zealand Government 2012.
32 Shahab and West 2010.

unlicensed tobacco retailers, high corruption indexes and extensive illicit retailing, and where low priority is given to tobacco control. It will be of most interest to high-income nations which are actively pursuing tobacco control goals.

The requirement for a licence would send a powerful symbolic message to all smokers and potential smokers that tobacco was no ordinary commodity, akin to grocery items, confectionary or any product on unrestricted sale. It would mark tobacco as a product uniquely deserving of such regulation and thereby invite reflection among smokers on why this exceptional policy had been introduced. This may diminish self-exempting views that smoking is just another unexceptional risk in "life's jungle."[33]

---

33   Oakes, Chapman, Balmford, Borland and Trotter 2004.

60

E-cigarettes: the best and the worst case scenarios for public health

When it became obvious that e-cigarettes were not a nine-day wonder but potentially a major player in tobacco control – for better or for worse – I decided to try and scope those better and worse scenarios in this essay for the *British Medical Journal*.

The World Health Organization's recent report on electronic nicotine delivery systems repeatedly notes the poverty of evidence to guide policy. It recommends that governments regulate the products, their promotion, and where they can be used in public as well as supporting research into their safety and efficacy in smoking cessation.[1,2] The report is due for consideration at the sixth conference of the parties to the WHO Framework Convention on Tobacco Control, which will be held on 13–18 October 2014 in Moscow.

In this essay, I consider the best and worst case scenarios for e-cigarettes; claims that they assist in smoking cessation and their value if

---

1   World Health Organization 2014.
2   Iacobucci 2014.

Originally published as Chapman, Simon (2014). E-cigarettes: the best and the worst case scenarios for public health. *British Medical Journal* 349: g5512.

users continue to smoke; and, finally, the tobacco industry's interests in these products.

Best-case scenario

The best outcome with e-cigarettes would be a massive, rapid migration of smokers into vaping, akin to the magnitude of the replacement of film by digital cameras. Unparalleled declines in diseases caused by smoking would occur, starting with cardiovascular and respiratory diseases and followed years later by cancers caused by smoking. Overwhelmingly, vapers would be smokers whose principal motivation was smoking cessation. Although some might vape and smoke ("dual users") temporarily, nearly all would completely quit smoking.

Uptake of vaping among former smokers and never-smoking children would be extremely low, and longitudinal studies of children who started vaping would show negligible transition to smoking. Like adults, children would use e-cigarettes as a gateway out of smoking, not into it.

Continuing research would affirm that direct and secondhand vape was inconsequential to any health outcome, despite the particle sizes of vape being comparable with those in cigarette smoke.[3] Public awareness of this would reduce antipathy to vaping in enclosed areas, and vapers would feel less antisocial and welcomed into areas from which smoking is exiled.

The tobacco industry, seeing its tobacco sales in free fall, would divest itself of smoked tobacco products and drop all global opposition to effective tobacco control, such as standardised packs and tax rises.

As rates of smoking disease plummet, the inventors of e-cigarettes would share the Nobel Prize for medicine. The history of tobacco control would have a final chapter on the triumph of harm reduction and the role of innovation. E-cigarettes would have made smoking history.

---

3   Grando 2014.

Worst case scenario

The story could, however, be very different. Under the worst-case scenario, global uptake of e-cigarettes would be on the scale of cell phones. Most smokers would switch, but many who would never have smoked – including children – would start vaping, attracted by its coolness and "no risk" hype and then maintained by nicotine dependency.

However, to the delight of the tobacco industry, the long decline in the number of smokers would stall because most vapers would also keep smoking. Many smokers would prevaricate, convinced that reducing rather than quitting was good enough. The number quitting would be eclipsed by those taking up vaping who had never smoked. Substantial proportions of non-smoking vapers, particularly young people, would drift into smoking. They might find the rigmarole of buying and refilling capsules inconvenient, or simply be curious about how smoking compared. Many would find the nicotine jolt from cigarettes more satisfying than e-cigarettes.[4] The net impact would be an increase in smoking prevalence or a slowing of its decline.

Following emerging evidence about angiogenesis and apoptosis,[56] the International Agency for Research in Cancer's recent decision to give priority to examining the role of nicotine in cancer[7] would produce consensus that it is far from being "as safe as coffee," as e-cigarette advocates had been advising.

Longitudinal studies would show that daily lung basting with the nicotine and fine particles[8] in vapour – averaging 150 puffs a day (around 5,000 a year)[9] – over many years is far from benign, but by then the imagined benevolent harm-reducing genie would be well out of the bottle, strongly resisting being returned.

---

4 Martínez-Sánchez, Ballbè, Fu, Martín-Sánchez, Saltó, Gottlieb, Daynard, Connolly and Fernández 2014.
5 Grando 2014.
6 Cardinale, Nastrucci, Cesario and Russo 2012.
7 Straif, Loomis, Guyton, Grosse, Lauby-Secretan, El Ghissassi et al. 2014.
8 Fuoco, Buonanno, Stabile and Vigo 2014.
9 Etter and Bullen 2014.

Governments would have allowed e-cigarette advertising, reprising the same themes used to promote cigarettes. The public smoking "performance" would be fully resocialised, signifying all that smoking did 50 years ago: elegance, sexuality, modernity, freedom. A teenager without a highly personalised e-cigarette would be semiotically naked.

All smoke-free areas would allow vaping, but emerging evidence about harms[10] would meet the decades-long resistance and "smokers'/vapers' rights" arguments fought over cigarette smoke.[11]

Public health experts who threw all caution to the wind, and vilified those who wanted good evidence to lead policy, would be written into public health history as overly excitable, amnesic or myopic quislings, willingly or unwittingly orchestrated by commercial interests.

Cessation

So where do we stand today? The central platforms of the promise of e-cigarettes are smoking cessation and harm reduction via the seemingly undeniable logic of "every cigarette forgone to vaping is harm reducing".

Vapers' chat rooms brim with jubilant testimony about permanent quitting. That is undeniably good news for those who have quit. But claims about stratospheric rates of smoking cessation from such communities[12] are valueless in estimating potential population cessation impacts across all e-cigarette users, for the same reason we would never use data from whisky appreciation societies to generalise about national Scotch consumption.

The most important data on outcomes from "real-world" population cessation are from England.[13] Twenty percent of those attempting to quit with e-cigarettes in the past year were not smoking on the day they were questioned, compared with 15.4 percent of those who attempted to quit unassisted and 10.1 percent of those who used

---

10 Schobera, Szendreia, Matzena, Osiander-Fuchsb, Heitmannc, Schettgend, Jörrese and Fromme 2014.
11 Champion and Chapman 2005.
12 Farsalinos, Romagna, Tsiapras, Kyrzopoulos and Voudris 2014.
13 Brown, Beard, Kotz, Michie and West 2014.

over-the-counter nicotine replacement therapy. Substantial relapse would be expected from all of these groups. An 80 percent failure rate, with relapse to follow, is a long way from the miracle cure currently being hyped.

Reduced use

There is strong evidence for a causal association between disease and early uptake, amount smoked and duration of smoking, but the evidence on "reverse engineering" harm by continuing to smoke while cutting back is far from strong. A 2007 systematic review[14] examining the health effects of reducing smoking by more than half found only a "small health benefit." Since then, four cohorts[15] of a total of 535,620 people followed for up to 25 years have reported findings such as "no evidence that smokers who cut down their daily cigarette consumption by > 50 percent reduce their risk of premature death significantly".[16] The largest, from Korea,[17] found no association between smoking reduction and all cancer risk but a significant decrease in risk of lung cancer, with the size of risk reduction "disproportionately smaller than expected".

The impact of any smoking cessation policy or strategy is a function of its effectiveness multiplied by its reach. So here, there is cause for some optimism. The rapid growth in e-cigarette use in some nations, despite the modest early results on quitting, may nonetheless translate into a large number of ex-smokers across the population who attribute their quitting to e-cigarettes. But that would be only part of the story. What proportion of these quitters would have stopped anyway had e-cigarettes been unavailable? Would we just be seeing substitution of cessation methods? Would the overall cessation volume rise? How many vapers who did not quit and became dual users might have prevaricated and kept smoking because they vaped?

---

14 Pisinger and Godtfredsen 2007.
15 Song, Sung, and Cho 2008; Hart, Gruer and Bauld 2013; Tverdal and Bjartveit 2006.
16 Tverdal and Bjartveit 2006.
17 Song, Sung, and Cho 2008.

Why are tobacco companies investing in e-cigarettes?

All tobacco transnationals have now acquired e-cigarettes lines. Tellingly, no company has stated that it is actively working to decrease cigarette sales or desisted from aggressively opposing effective tobacco control policy.

Only the most naive or captured advocates for vaping could fail to acknowledge that the tobacco industry wants people who vape to smoke and vape, not vape instead of smoking. To the credit of some advocates, nascent policy proposals to accelerate the decline of smoking and calls for governments to set dates for combustible tobacco to be "phased out" have been made. But to date, no government has even gestured serious intent about this.

Big Tobacco is already buying out e-cigarette minnows and shutting out competition through patent-law actions. Here it is following its global playbook in buying up almost all small national tobacco companies. Many e-cigarette start-ups may be salivating at the prospect of getting rich quickly, but what will be the public health outcome of this entirely predictable momentum?

Big Tobacco thinks all its Christmases have come at once. E-cigarettes will allow companies to profit from nicotine addiction around the clock: in places where you cannot smoke, you may be able to vape if the WHO's recommendations are ignored. E-cigarettes can also offer a cornucopia of childfriendly flavours familiar at preschoolers' birthday parties. With e-cigarette advertising awash across all media, those arguing that there will be no major collateral benefits for tobacco companies via smoking are myopic.

E-cigarettes also promise hope of new respectability to tobacco companies. The same tobacco company staff who scheme to attack effective tobacco control and bust open low income, high illiteracy markets[18] with cigarette promotions suddenly have opportunities to present themselves as the harm-reducing solution to the "terrible" health problems that arise because of their work.

Disturbingly, some experienced in tobacco control are now aggressively advocating the importance of freely advertising e-

---

18   Agaku and Filippidis 2014.

cigarettes to promote wider uptake. For decades the tobacco industry maintained the public farce that they had no interest in children smoking and that their advertising was crafted to attract only smokers, with some magic barrier preventing it from attracting the attention of non-smokers and especially children. Privately, they of course understood completely that, "The base of our business is the high school student"[19] and that voluntary controls were a "phony way to show sincerity, as we all well know."[20]

Yet today, some public health advocates of e-cigarettes blindly insist that the deluge of advertising will have zero effect on non-smoking teenagers and is not "intended" to catch their interest. Big tobacco must find it hard to believe its luck that it has such people on tap to make these arguments for them. In Utah, the state with the lowest tobacco use in the USA, the department of health reports that use of e-cigarettes in high school students has tripled since 2011. Seven percent of grade ten students were current users. Nearly one-third of these reported that they had never smoked cigarettes.[21]

Nations with advanced tobacco control programs have achieved all-time lows in youth smoking. In Australia today only 3.4 percent of 12- to 17-year-olds smoke daily.[22] This reduction is slowly starving the tobacco industry. But in the name of accommodating the pleas of often-exaggerated claims about the size of the smoking population who "cannot" quit, some policy approaches to e-cigarettes risk placing these invaluable, hard-won gains at risk.

Smokers desperate to quit should be able to access e-cigarettes at pharmacies, perhaps with a permit or prescription. Nearly every nation has such a system of controlled access to drugs with abuse or dependency potential. Only two countries, the USA and New Zealand, allow direct-to-consumer advertising of prescribed or restricted drugs. Only people with commercial interests and extremist advocates argue that it is a sensible idea to attract children into addiction.

---

19   Achey 1978.
20   Knight and Chapman 2004.
21   Utah Department of Health 2013.
22   Australian Institute of Health and Welfare 2014b.

Scheduling e-cigarettes would allow them to be overseen for quality and safety, carefully monitored through research, with their availability relaxed or tightened on the basis of evidence or benefits or harm. Every imaginable mistake was made with the way tobacco was sold and marketed. Early caution is critical if we are not to repeat those mistakes with a product that so far has an unimpressive record in doing what its advocates claim for it and which threatens to renormalise the smoking performance and possibly hold many smokers longer in their addiction. The WHO is to be commended for its caution.

61

Spotless leopards? Decoding hype on e-cigarettes

The e-cigarette issue is a fascinating development in tobacco control. My view at present is one conditioned by a strong concern not to repeat the disastrous mistakes of earlier false harm-reduction promises that were made for filters and during the "lights and milds" labelling fiasco. Both of these saw millions of smokers falsely reassured that they could keep smoking rather than quit. Most smokers who use e-cigarettes continue to smoke and there is as yet insufficient evidence both about the longer-term trajectory of vaping, dual use and smoking cessation, and about the possibility that e-cigarettes may cause as yet unseen significant health problems. Few smokers know about the health consequences of their smoking for many years longer than e-cigarettes have so far been in use.

I presented the talk below, which was an attempt to summarise these concerns, to the Oceania Tobacco Control Conference in Perth on 21 October 2015 and then published it in my Smoke Signals column in the *Conversation*.

Originally published as Chapman, Simon (2015). Spotless leopards? Decoding hype on e-cigarettes. *The Conversation*, 22 October.

E-cigarettes are the latest innovation in nicotine delivery products to fly the harm-reduction flag. They follow the massive failures of cigarette filters.[1] Over decades, filters falsely reassured millions of smokers that they were reducing their exposure to harm and so could keep smoking. We also had the lights and milds fiasco[2] – which saw 80 percent of Australian smokers select those misleadingly labelled brands, which were outlawed by the ACCC[3] from 2005 as a consumer fraud. Along the way we saw reduced-carcinogen brands and even asbestos-filtered cigarettes.[4]

There was massive publicity about harm reduction from filters and low tar, and massive consumer uptake, but not a blip in the incidence of tobacco caused disease in those who still smoked. Thanks to harm-reduction arguments, countless smokers continued smoking who might otherwise have quit. The tobacco industry drove these arguments and was supported by many in public health who thought they were no-brainers. Nigel Gray, a giant of global tobacco control, admitted that the decades-long, well-intentioned low-tar harm-reduction policy was a disaster.[5]

Meanwhile, we continued with the core policies of trying to prevent uptake, encourage quit attempts and denormalise smoking via smoke-free policies to protect non-smokers. Together, these objectives have delivered Australia the lowest smoking prevalence in the world.[6] For 35 years since the early 1980s, we have seen continually falling incidence rates of tobacco-caused disease. Female lung cancer seems likely never to reach even half the peak we saw in males. Awkwardly for some, Australia has become world leader in reducing smoking without any mass cessation clinic network or major embrace of e-cigarettes.

---

1   Centers for Disease Control and Prevention, National Center for Chronic Disease Prevention and Health Promotion, and Office on Smoking and Health 2010.
2   Borland, Yong, King, Cummings, Fong, Elton-Marshall, Hammond and McNeill 2004.
3   http://bit.ly/2cAVDZy.
4   Levin 2013.
5   Gray 2000.
6   http://bit.ly/2d0ysGy.

Today, demands are being made to rush in soft-touch regulation to allow e-cigarettes to be manufactured, flavoured, promoted and used virtually without restriction. This is all being done on the shoulders of an argument that insists that after 50 years of tobacco control, there remain many smokers who can't or don't want to give up their nicotine dependence, and that in just a few years, sufficient evidence has already accumulated to show that e-cigarettes are both benign and great for cessation.

But the "can't quit" argument has received remarkably little critical interrogation. We know that hundreds of millions[7] of heavily dependent smokers have quit since the early 1960s, most without any assistance at all. We know that today's smokers smoke fewer cigarettes per day than at any time in the past, exactly the opposite of what the hardening hypothesis would predict.[8]

The demands of the "We don't want to quit, we love nicotine" vaping activists to access e-cigs and use them without restrictions must be balanced against the risks of what these demands might mean for population-wide progress toward the goal of keeping smoking heading south. Comprehensive tobacco control is not just about the preferences of vapers. It is most importantly about continuing to starve the tobacco industry of new recruits and ensure that smoking is made history.

If we think of e-cigarettes as a transformative genie in a bottle, we need to think very carefully before letting it out, because putting genies back in their bottles is much more difficult than impulsively letting them out. If they prove to be benevolent, all's good. But if they bring false hopes and keep many people smoking, we may be looking at the early days of a third major false god of tobacco harm reduction.

That genie is well out of the bottle in England and the USA, and other countries need to watch what is happening there very closely. Today, I want to examine four cornerstones of the public health case being megaphoned for e-cigarettes.

---

7   Smith and Chapman 2014.
8   Chapman 2015a.

1. E-cigarettes are benign and nicotine risks "like drinking coffee or something".[9]

No one sensible makes the argument that e-cigarettes are likely be even remotely as harmful as smoking.

The 2015 annual report of Public Health England[10] endorsed the "95 percent less harmful" than smoking estimate. They took this from a consensus report authored by 12 people.[11] Six of these were subsequent signatories to the 53-signature letter to the Dr Margaret Chan at the WHO calling for minimal regulation.[12] Six had no research track record or experience in tobacco control whatsoever. Two had financial ties to the tobacco or e-cigarette industries. There is no transparency about how this group was selected. But this was plainly not a group which was ever likely produce a consensus that was anything but glowing about e-cigarettes.

But let's assume they may have been in the risk comparison ballpark. If e-cigarettes are 95 percent less harmful, then we would *only* see 300,000 deaths a year globally from e-cigarettes, instead of 6 million[13] if every smoker switched.

On present trends (England's Robert West suggests that e-cigarette growth may have already plateaued in England), that scenario is as likely as pigs flying. A far more likely scenario – as I will argue – is one that sees a continuing stream of smokers quitting mostly unaided as they always have; significant numbers attributing their quitting to e-cigs; but a slowing in overall quit attempts as many dual using vaping smokers keep smoking at reduced rates, in the erroneous belief that they are reducing harm.

Robert West group's Smoking Toolkit study has been monitoring tobacco use in England every month since 2007, including e-cigarettes since 2011.[14] Significantly, the latest data from August show the lowest percentage of English smokers trying to quit since 2007 (31.6 percent

---

9   Kremer 2013.
10 McNeill, Brose, Calder and Hitchman 2015.
11 Nutt, Phillips, Balfour, Curran, Dockrell et al 2014.
12 Abrams, Axell, Bartsch, Bauld, Bordland et al 2014.
13 http://bit.ly/1hIyq1l.
14 http://bit.ly/OSS8yt.

down from a high of 42.5 percent in 2007).[15] If the net impact of e-cigarettes is that quit attempts fall and more stay smoking than who quit with e-cigarettes, we may see a repeat of the major harm-reduction follies of the past.

The quality of evidence we have for declaring e-cigarettes to be benign has been described in another review as very poor. A 2014 review[16] concluded:

Due to many methodological problems, severe conflicts of interest, the relatively few and often small studies, the inconsistencies and contradictions in results, and the lack of long-term follow-up, no firm conclusions can be drawn on the safety of ECs. However, they can hardly be considered harmless.

This review was not even referenced in the Public Health England review.

The health problems caused by tobacco develop over decades. Every year will bring us more and more information about what the consequences of the typical daily vaper inhaling nicotine, propylene glycol, and an unregulated cocktail of fine and ultra-fine particles[17] like flavouring agents approved for ingestion in foods but not for inhalation[18] an average 120 times a day[19] (43,800 times a year). We will also see what the International Agency for Research in Cancer[20] has to say about whether nicotine is carcinogenic, having declared its assessment to be one of its priorities in 2014.

---

15 West, Beard and Brown 2016.
16 Pisinger and Døssing 2014.
17 Schobera, Wolfgang, Katalin Szendreia, Wolfgang Matzena, Helga Osiander-Fuchsb, Dieter Heitmannc, Thomas Schettgend, Rudolf A. Jörrese and Hermann Fromme 2014.
18 The Flavor and Extract Manufacturers Association of the United States 2012.
19 Etter and Bullen 2011.
20 World Health Organization International Agency for Research on Cancer 2014.

2. How good are e-cigarettes for smoking cessation?

Earlier this year, a paper co-authored by five of England's best tobacco control researchers, including Robert West and Ann McNeill, reported the world's first prospective cohort data on the question of quitting via vaping versus other methods.[21] Their data are of great importance because by distinguishing daily from non-daily vapers, they allow the differentiation of casual and experimental users from daily users. Their study also provides data on outcomes 12 months later.

The paper commenced by noting that:

> Smoking prevalence in England has been declining from 20 percent in 2012 to 18.4 percent in 2014, and in 2014 smoking cessation rates were the highest since at least 2008. This simultaneous increase in e-cigarette use and cessation *may be coincidental*, and it is therefore vitally important for longitudinal studies to be conducted to assess the impact of e-cigarette usage on quitting behaviour.

So what did the study find? "Daily use of e-cigarettes while smoking appears to be associated with subsequent increases in rates of attempting to stop smoking and reducing smoking, but not with smoking cessation. Non-daily use of e-cigarettes while smoking does not appear to be associated with cessation attempts, cessation or reduced smoking."

A companion paper broke down the data further by type of e-cigarette product.[22] Daily tank system users were the only group that showed a significant improvement in smoking cessation. But of 1,643 smokers followed up at 12 months, only 69 – just 4.2 percent – were daily tank vapers at 12 months, and just over one in four of these – only 19, or 1.2 percent of the total sample – had quit. This is hardly the stuff of revolutionary dreams for population-wide cessation!

In August, the English Smoking Toolkit study reported that the large majority (over 80 percent) of e-cigarette users are dual users who also continue to smoke.[23]

---

21 Brose, Hitchman, Brown, West and McNeill 2015.
22 Hitchman, Brose, Brown, Robson and McNeill 2015.

61 Spotless leopards? Decoding hype on e-cigarettes

The recent Public Health England annual report downplayed this elephant in the room in its fingers-crossed optimism that dual use should be seen as just a transitory phase that smokers go through before they quit smoking. As I will argue soon, the tobacco industry has other ideas about this.

So putting these studies together for England – "e-cigarette central" – where, in plain language, are we today?

- Non-daily vaping has no impact on cutting down or quitting.
- Daily vapers make more quit attempts than non-vaping smokers, but they don't succeed any better than those who don't vape.
- Daily *tank* vapers do better at quitting, but the numbers involved are very small.
- 80 to 90 percent of vapers are dual users.
- While this has been happening, quit attempts among English smokers at large are at the lowest level since 2007.

3. Do vaping smokers cut back more than non-vaping smokers?

The Brose et al. paper from England reported that at 12 months, 13.9 percent of daily e-cigarette users *reduced* cigarette smoking substantially.[24]

But let's turn the last figure around. Even among those smokers who vaped daily, 86.1 percent did not even cut back smoking substantially. That's how good e-cigarettes are at just *reducing* smoking. They are far less successful, for example, than workplace smoking bans, where we see 20 percent reductions from reduced smoking opportunities.

I'm sure you'll agree that all the Big Tobacco companies now selling both cigarettes and e-cigarettes must be simply mortified by this news.

---

23   http://bit.ly/2cIN2Df.
24   Brose, Hitchman, Brown, West and McNeill 2015.

4. But does reducing daily smoking substantially reduce deaths from smoking caused disease?

Let's suppose that most daily, sustained vapers *did* cut back substantially (by more than 50 percent; which they don't), would this be harm reducing? We've known for decades that three synergistic variables (age of smoking onset, amount smoked and duration of smoking) are critical in predicting mortality from smoking. There is a dose-response relationship that no one disputes here: those who smoke more are more likely to die from their smoking than those who smoke less.

From this, it's understandable that many smokers believe that, just as they know water to be wet, cutting down the number of cigarettes they smoke will reduce their harm. But this is quite a different claim. The epidemiological data on lifetime risk is about total pack years and does not consider the question of whether the cumulative risks of smoking can be "reverse engineered" by reducing.

But there is large-scale research on this and it is not good news for the "cutting down obviously reduces risk" dogma. Four cohort studies published since 2006 have reported on whether reducing smoking, as opposed to stopping smoking altogether, confers any mortality benefit.

A Norwegian cohort of 51,210 people followed from the 1970s until 2003 found "no evidence that smokers who cut down their daily cigarette consumption by > 50 percent reduce their risk of premature death significantly."[25]

A Scottish study of two cohorts followed from the 1970s to 2010 also found no evidence of reduced mortality in reducers, but clear evidence in quitters. It concluded "that reducing cigarette consumption should not be promoted as a means of reducing mortality."[26]

The largest study, from Korea involving nearly half a million men followed for 11 years, found no association between smoking reduction and all cancer risk but a significant decrease in risk of lung cancer, but with the size of risk reduction being "disproportionately smaller than expected".[27]

---

25 Tverdal and Bjartveit 2006.
26 Hart, Gruer and Bauld 2013.

Vapers who keep on smoking – which is most of them – are fooling themselves if they think they are seriously reducing risk.

I now turn to the future of vaping. "Think of the children!" is a common sarcastic slur made daily by vaping activists across social media. These self-absorbed misanthropes, today's W.C. Fields clones in their disdain for children, could not care less about the implications of e-cigarettes for teenagers. All they care about is their unhindered access to unregulated vape gear and their rights to vape anywhere: in workplaces, next to you on planes, and presumably while driving the school bus, inside childcare centres and hospitals. They want access to flavours like Gummy Bear and Bubble Gum that would cause a riot at a three-year-old's birthday party. Vape is apparently so close to pure air that any restrictions are totally unwarranted.

In England, vaping by non-smoking kids is very uncommon. Nearly everyone thinks that is self-evidently a good thing. But the same cannot be said about the USA, where data from the US National Youth Tobacco Survey show that while cigarette smoking continues to fall in American teenagers, e-cigarette use has been dramatically increasing[28] since 2011 and is now way ahead of cigarette smoking: there are now some 67 percent more[29] middle and high school kids vaping than are smoking.

Apologists for teenage vaping actually try to argue that this is a good development! You see, all those teenage vapers would have been smoking were it not for e-cigs. The small problem here is that this rise was not associated with a rise in dual or multiple tobacco or nicotine product use, and the decline in cigarette smoking had been falling before e-cigarettes arrived.

Some argue there is no problem in having tobacco and nicotine naive youth taking up e-cigarettes and becoming addicted to nicotine. Others would prefer authorities like the US Surgeon-General and the International Agency for Research in Cancer, not vape shop owners and industry spin merchants, to assure us there's nothing to worry about with such uptake. But as yet they have not.

---

27 Song, Sung, and Cho 2008.
28 Neff, Arrazola, Caraballo, Corey, Cox, King, Choiniere and Husten 2015.
29 http://bit.ly/2cREnAv.

Nearly all businesses survive and flourish by retaining existing customers and critically, stimulating new customers to start. If you sell tractors or sheep-dip chemicals, you will have little expectation of finding new customers who don't own sheep or land where a tractor might be needed. But if you are selling products which have potential to be used by more than those already using them, you are vitally interested in non-users. Cigarette and e-cigarettes fit that description perfectly.

Leopards don't change their spots. For decades the tobacco industry told us – and still does – that it is not the least bit interested in teenage smoking. If British American Tabacco succeeds on getting its hands on the Cancer Council Victoria's teen smoking data, we all can be assured that it will keep the contents strictly within its opposition to plain packs division and never show the data to its salivating "capturing new smokers and vapers" divisions.[30]

The global e-cigarette market today is a mixture[31] of Big-Tobacco-owned brands and those owned by start-up incumbents. The tobacco industry is rapidly acquiring those minnows it regards as likely to be most profitable and strategic. Wide-eyed vaping advocates would have us seriously believe that the tobacco industry, with its billions of dollars in assets and long history of acquisitions, will not somehow soon swallow up most of these just as it did small tobacco companies all over the world.

No tobacco company currently acquiring e-cigarette brands is desisting in any way from attacking effective tobacco control. Plain packs are being attacked. Every day BAT bleats on Twitter about how high tobacco tax – the most important plank in comprehensive tobacco control – is causing more illicit trade. The message is clear: taxes should be lowered, to make smoking more affordable and to arrest brutal falls in smoking.

Quite obviously, this is not an industry that wants smokers to stop smoking. It's an industry with a business plan to have smokers keep smoking and also to vape when they can't smoke. It is an industry that understands how to erode the nicotine "downtime" from smoke-free

---

30 McKenzie and Baker 2015.
31 Kendell 2014.

policies that have badly reduced sales. And guess what? This is exactly what most smokers who vape are doing.

The concept of e-cigarettes being a "gateway" into smoking has been rightly criticised as being imprecise and vague, often being little more than crude "after, therefore because of" reasoning. But glib dismissals of the rapid rise of teenage use with "kids just try stuff" throw-away lines ignore the many appeals of vaping to teenagers and the fact that youth smoking is the lowest on record. Increasingly, most kids don't "just try" smoking.

A very useful model of how e-cigarettes may work as a catalyst for smoking has recently been published. The authors provide a causal hypotheses for the initiation of e-cigarette use and for the potential transition to tobacco smoking that highlights the combined factors of:

• perceived negligible risk
• attractive taste options
• lower price
• inconspicuous use
• higher level of peer acceptance.

This model could stimulate important research into understanding e-cigarette uptake and any apparent transition to smoking.

We are well on track to see the end of the tobacco epidemic in this country. E-cigarettes may have a role in that. Time will tell. But there are major concerns about the core claims being made for e-cigarettes. Australia should consider any policy changes in harm reduction very carefully. We should all be open to quality evidence that might suggest that this time we have something different. But equally, we do not want to repeat mistakes of the past.

62

Ten myths about smoking that will not die

In March 2016, a lightbulb turned on in my head that I could write something for my column in *The Conversation* that knocked the stuffing out of common myths I hear often about smoking. Ten immediately came to mind and then another ten followed (see next chapter). *The Conversation* has a creative commons licence, meaning that others can republish any material originally published there.

The I Fucking Love Science (IFLS) website republished the two columns, as did three other online publications. As I write this in September 2016, the two columns have had 1,782,660 views, of which 84 percent were via IFLS. This was far more than all 60-odd of my *Conversation* columns combined. So it was hard to leave it out of this selection.

Across 40 years I've come to recognise many factoid-driven myths about smoking that just won't die. If I asked for a dollar each time I had to patiently refute these statements, I'd have accumulated a small fortune.

Originally published as Chapman, Simon (2016). Ten myths about smoking that will not die. *The Conversation*, 10 March.

Their persistence owes much to their being a vehicle for those who utter them to express unvoiced but clear subtexts that reflect deeply held beliefs about women, the disadvantaged, mental illness, government health campaigns and the "natural".

Let's drive a stake through the heart of ten of the most common myths.

"Women and girls smoke more than men and boys"

Women have never smoked more than men. Occasionally, a survey will show one age band where it's the other way around, but from the earliest mass uptake of smoking in the first decades of last century, men streaked out way ahead of women. In 1945 in Australia, 72 percent of men and 26 percent of women smoked.[1] By 1976, men had fallen to 43 percent and women had risen to 33 percent. As a result men's tobacco-caused death rates have always been much higher than those of women. Women's lung cancer rates, for example, seem unlikely to reach even half the peak rates that we saw in men in the 1970s. Currently in Australia, 15 percent of men and 12 percent of women smoke daily.[2]

But what about all the "young girls" you can see smoking, I'm always being told. In 2014, 13 percent of 17-year-old male high school students and 11 percent of female students smoked.[3] In two younger age bands, girls smoked more (by a single percentage point). Those who keep on insisting girls that smoke more are probably just letting their sexist outrage show about noticing girls' smoking than their ignorance about the data.

"Quit campaigns don't work on low socio-economic smokers"

In Australia, 11 percent of those in the highest quintile of economic advantage smoke, compared with 27.6 percent in the lowest quintile.[4]

---

1   Greenhalgh, Bayly and Winstanley 2015, 1.3.
2   Greenhalgh, Bayly and Winstanley 2015, 1.3.
3   Greenhalgh, Bayly and Winstanley 2015, 1.6.
4   Greenhalgh, Bayly and Winstanley 2015, 9.1.

More than double. So does this mean that our quit campaigns "don't work" on the least well-off? Smoking prevalence data reflect two things: the proportion of people who ever smoked, and the proportion who quit. If we look at the most disadvantaged groups, we find that a far higher proportion take up smoking than in their more well-to-do counterparts (60.5 percent vs 49.6 percent have ever smoked[5]) while when it comes to quitting 66.6 percent of the most disadvantaged have quit compared to 47.7 percent of the least disadvantaged[6]).

There are more disadvantaged smokers mainly because more take it up, not because disadvantaged smokers can't or won't quit. With 27.6 percent of the most disadvantaged smoking today, the good news is that nearly three-quarters don't. Smoking and disadvantage are hardly inseparable.

"Scare campaigns don't work"

Countless studies have asked ex-smokers why they stopped and current smokers about why they are trying to stop. I have never seen such a study when there was not daylight between the first reason cited (worry about health consequences) and the second most nominated reason (usually cost). For example, a national US study covering 13 years showed that "concern for your own current or future health" was nominated by 91.6 percent of ex-smokers as the main reason they quit, compared with 58.7 percent naming expense and 55.7 percent being concerned about the impact of their smoking on others.[7]

If information and warnings about the dire consequences of smoking "don't work", then from where do all these ex-smokers ever get these top-of-mind concerns? They don't pop into their heads by magic. They encounter them via anti-smoking campaigns, pack warnings, news stories about research, and personal experiences with dying family and friends. The scare campaigns work.

---

5   Greenhalgh, Bayly and Winstanley 2015, 9.2.
6   Greenhalgh, Bayly and Winstanley 2015, 9.2.
7   Hyland, Li, Bauer, Giovino, Steger and Cummings 2004.

"Roll-your-own tobacco is more 'natural' than factory-made"

People who smoke rollies often look you in the eye and tell you that factory-made cigarettes are full of chemical additives, while roll-your-own tobacco is "natural" – it's just tobacco. The reasoning here is that we are supposed to understand that it's these chemicals that are the problem, while the tobacco, being "natural", is somehow OK.

This myth was first turned very unceremoniously on its head when New Zealand authorities ordered the tobacco companies to provide them with data on the total weight of additives in factory-made cigarettes, roll-your-own and pipe tobacco. For example, data from 1991 supplied by W.D. & H.O. Wills showed that in 879,219 kilograms of cigarettes, there was 1,803 kilograms of additives (0.2 percent) while in 366,036 kilograms of roll-your-own tobacco, there was 82,456 kilograms of additives (22.5 percent)![8] Roll your own tobacco is pickled in flavouring and humectant chemicals, the latter being used to keep the tobacco from drying out when smokers expose the tobacco to the air 20 or more times a day when they remove tobacco to roll up a cigarette.

"Nearly all people with schizophrenia smoke"

It's true that people with mental health problems are much more likely to smoke than those without diagnosed mental health problems. A meta-analysis of 42 studies on tobacco smoking by those with schizophrenia found an average 62 percent smoking prevalence (with a range from 14 to 88 percent). But guess which study in these 42 gets cited and quoted far more than any of the others?

If you said the one reporting 88 percent smoking prevalence you'd be correct. This small 1986 US study of just 277 outpatients with schizophrenia has today been cited a remarkable 1,135 times. With colleagues I investigated this flagrant example of citation bias[9] (where startling but atypical results stand out in literature searches and get high citations – "wow! This ones got a high number, let's quote that

---

8   Tobacco Control 1994.
9   Chapman, Ragg and McGeechan 2009.

one!"). By googling "How many schizophrenics smoke" we showed how this percolates into the community via media reports where figures are rounded up in statements like "As many as 90 percent of schizophrenic patients smoke".

Endlessly repeating that "90 percent" of those with schizophrenia smoke does these people a real disservice. We would not tolerate such inaccuracy about any other group.

"Everyone knows the risks of smoking"

Knowledge about the risks of smoking can exist at four levels.[10] Level 1: having heard that smoking increases health risks. Level 2: being aware that specific diseases are caused by smoking. Level 3: accurately appreciating the meaning, severity, and probabilities of developing tobacco related diseases, and Level 4: personally accepting that the risks inherent in levels 1–3 apply to one's own risk of contracting such diseases.

Level 1 knowledge is very high, but as you move up the levels, knowledge and understanding greatly diminish. Very few people for example, are likely to know that two in three long-term smokers[11] will die of a smoking caused disease, nor the average number of years that smokers lose off normal life expectancy.

"You can reduce the health risks of smoking by just cutting down"

It's true that if you smoke five cigarettes a day rather than 20 your lifetime risk of early death is less (although check the risks for one to four cigarettes a day here[12]). But trying to "reverse engineer" the risk by just cutting down rather than quitting has been shown in at least

---

10   Chapman and Liberman 2005.
11   Chapman 2015c.
12   Bjartveit and Tverdal 2005.

four large cohort studies to confer no harm reduction.[13] If you want to reduce risk, quitting altogether is the goal.

"Air pollution is the real cause of lung cancer"

Air pollution is unequivocally a major health risk. By "pollution" those who make this argument don't mean natural particulate matter like pollen and soil dusts, they mean nasty industrial and vehicle pollution. The most polluted areas of Australia are cities, where pollution from industry and motor vehicle emissions are most concentrated. Remote regions of the country are the least polluted, so if we wanted to consider the relative contributions of air pollution and smoking to smoking-caused diseases, an obvious question to ask would be "does the incidence of lung cancer differ between heavily polluted cities and very unpolluted remote areas?" Yes it does. Lung cancer incidence is highest in Australia in (wait for this . . .) the least polluted very remote regions of the country, where smoking prevalence happens also to be highest.[14]

"Smokers should not try to quit without professional help or drugs"

If you ask 100 ex-smokers how they quit, between two-thirds and three-quarters will tell you they quit unaided: on their final successful quit attempt, they did not use nicotine replacement therapy (NRT), prescribed drugs, or go to some dedicated smoking-cessation clinic or experience the laying on of hands from some alternative medicine therapist. They quit unaided.[15] So if you ask the question "What method is used by most successful quitters when they quit?" the answer is cold turkey.

Fine print on an English National Health Service poster states a bald-faced lie by saying that "There are some people who can go cold turkey and stop. But there aren't many of them." In the years before[16]

---

13 For example, Tverdal and Bjartveit 2006.
14 http://bit.ly/2ebdiHa.
15 Chapman and MacKenzie 2010.

311

NRT and other drugs were available many millions – including heavy smokers – quit smoking without any assistance. That's a message that the pharmaceutical industry would rather not megaphone.

"Many smokers live into very old age, so it can't be that harmful"

People who use this argument should probably just wear a badge saying "I'm not very bright" to save us the trouble of having to listen to their interesting theories on disease. In just the way that five out of six participants in a round of deadly Russian roulette might proclaim that putting a loaded gun to their head and pulling the trigger caused no harm, those who use this argument are just ignorant of risks and probability. Many probably buy lottery tickets with the same deep knowing that they have a good chance of winning.

---

16   Smith and Chapman 2014.

63

Ten *more* myths about smoking that will not die

As Oliver Twist said, "Please sir, can I have some more?" With the readership of the first piece going berserk, I could hardly avoid writing a second set of ten myths.

Last week I wrote about factoid-driven myths that just refuse to die. In less than a week over 1.145 million people have clicked on the piece. The median number of readers across 59 of my *Conversation* columns until now has been 4,550, with the previously most-read piece attracting 55,285 readers.

There's plainly a big appetite for smoking myth-busting, so here are ten more.

"Today's smokers are all hardcore, addicted smokers who can't or won't give up"

This claim is the essence of what is known as the "hardening hypothesis"[1]: the idea that decades of effort to motivate smokers to quit has seen all the low hanging fruit fall from the tree, leaving only deeply addicted, heavy smokers today.

Originally published as Chapman, Simon (2016). Ten *more* myths about smoking that will not die. *The Conversation*, 16 March.

The key index of addicted smoking is number of cigarettes per day. This creates a small problem for the hardening hypothesis: in nations and states where smoking has reduced most, average daily cigarettes smoked by continuing smokers has gone down, not up. This is exactly the opposite of what the hardening hypothesis would predict if remaining smokers were mostly hardcore.

"Smoking is pleasurable"

Repeated studies have found that around 90 percent of smokers regret having started, and some 40 percent make an attempt to quit each year. There's no other product with even a fraction of such customer disloyalty.

But I'm always amused at some die-hard smokers' efforts explain that they smoke for pleasure and so efforts to persuade them to stop are essentially anti-hedonistic tirades. Many studies[2] have documented that the "pleasure" of smoking centres around the relief and pleasure smokers get when they have not smoked for a while and the next nicotine hit takes away the discomfort and craving they have been experiencing. This argument is a bit like saying that being beaten up every day is something you want to continue with, because hey, it feels so good when the beating stops for a while.

"Light and mild cigarettes deliver far less tar and nicotine to the smoker than standard brands"

Several nations have outlawed cigarette descriptors like "light" and "mild" because of evidence that such products do not deliver lower amounts of tar and nicotine to smokers, and so are deceptive. The allegedly lower yields from cigarettes labelled this way resulted from a massive consumer fraud. Cigarette manufacturers obtained these low readings by laboratory smoking machine protocols which took a standardized number of puffs, at a standardized puff velocity. The

---

1   Chapman 2015a.
2   Tiffany 2009.

smoke inhaled by the machine was then collected in glass "lungs" behind the machine and the tar and nicotine weighed to give the readings per cigarette.

But the companies didn't tell smokers two things. So-called light or mild cigarettes had tiny, near-invisible pin-prick perforations just on the filter (see picture). These holes are not covered by the "lips" or "fingers" of the laboratory smoking machine, allowing extra air to be inhaled and thus diluting the dose of tar and nicotine being collected.

But when smokers use these products, two things happen. Their lips and fingers partially occlude the tiny ventilation holes, thus allowing more smoke to be inhaled, and smokers unconsciously "titrate" their smoking to obtain the dose of nicotine that their brain's addiction centres demand: they can take more puffs, inhale more deeply, leave shorter butt lengths or smoke more cigarettes.

Today, where use of these descriptors has been stopped, the consumer deception[3] continues with the companies using pack colours to loudly hint to smokers about which varieties are "safer".

"Filters on cigarettes remove most of the nasty stuff from cigarettes"

We've all seen the brown stain in a discarded cigarette butt. But what few have seen is how much of that same muck enters the lungs and how much stays there. This utterly compelling video[4] demonstration shows how ineffective filters are in removing this deadly sludge. A smoker demonstrates holding the smoke in his mouth and then exhales it through a tissue paper, leaving a tell-tale brown stain. He then inhales a drag deep into his lungs, and exhales it into a tissue. The residue is still there, but in a much reduced amount. So where has the remainder gone? It's still in the lungs!

---

3 Connolly and Alpert 2013.
4 http://bit.ly/2d4Gkva.

"Governments don't want smoking to fall because they are addicted to tobacco tax and don't want to kill a goose that lays golden eggs"

This is perhaps the silliest and fiscally most illiterate argument we hear regularly about smoking. If it was true that governments really wanted to maximise smoking and tax receipts, they are doing a shockingly bad job. Smoking in Australia has fallen almost continuously since the early 1960s. In six of the ten years 2001–2011, the Australian government received less tobacco tax receipts than it did the year before.[5]

Plainly, as smoking continues to decline, diminishing tax returns will occur although this will be cushioned by rising population, which will include some smokers. In the meantime, tobacco tax is a win-win for governments and the community. It reduces smoking[6] like nothing else, and it provides substantial transfer of funds from smokers to government for public expenditure. Those of us who don't smoke do not squirrel away what we would have otherwise spent on smoking in a jam jar under the bed. We spend it on other goods and services, benefitting the economy too.

"Most smokers die from smoking-caused diseases late in life, and we've all got to die from something"

Smoking increases the risk of many different diseases, and collectively these take about ten years[7] off normal life expectancy from those who get them. Smoking is by far the greatest risk factor for lung cancer. In Australia, average age of death for lung cancer is 71.4,[8] while life expectancy is currently 80.1 for men and 84.3 for women,[9] meaning that on average men diagnosed with lung cancer lose 8.7 years and women 12.9 years (mean 10.8 years). Of course, some lose many more (Beatle George Harrison died at just 58, Nat King Cole at 45).

---

5 Greenhalgh, Bayly, and Winstanley 2015, 13.6.
6 Chapman 2015b.
7 Doll, Peto, Boreham and Sutherland 2004.
8 Australian Institute of Health and Welfare 2011.
9 Australian Institute of Health and Welfare 2016.

If a 20 a day smoker starts at 17 and dies at 71, 54 years of smoking would see 394,470 cigarettes smoked. At ten puffs per cigarette, that's some 3.94 million point-blank lung bastings. It takes about six minutes to smoke a cigarette. So at 20 a day, smokers smoke for two hours each day. Across 54 years, that's a cumulative 1,644 days of smoking (4.5 years of continual smoking if you put it all together). So by losing ten years off life expectancy, each cigarette smoked takes about 2.2 times the time it takes to smoke it off the life expectancy that might otherwise have been enjoyed.

"Smokers cost the health system far more than the government receives from tobacco tax."

In June 2015, a senior staff member of Australian libertarian senator David Leyonhjlem, Helen Dale, tweeted: "Evidence is unhealthy choices are cheaper for the state – the person dies instead of staying on life support."[10] In Australia, a now old report looking at 2004/05 data estimated the gross healthcare costs attributable to smoking "before adjustment for savings due to premature death" were $1.836 billion.[11] In that financial year, the government received $7,816.35 billion in customs and excise duty and GST.

Someone who thought that the fiscal ledger was all that mattered in good government might conclude from this that smokers easily pay their way and perhaps we should even encourage smoking as a citizen's patriotic duty. With smokers being considerate enough to die early, these noble citizens lay down their lives early and thus contribute "savings due to premature death" like failing to draw a state pension or needing aged care services late in life. Philip Morris notoriously gave this advice to the new Czech government in 1999.[12]

---

10 http://bit.ly/2cIN8uE.
11 Greenhalgh, Bayly, and Winstanley 2015, 17.2.
12 Fairclough 2001b.

Other assessments though, might well point to the values inherent in such advice. History's worst regimes have often seen the economically non-productive as human detritus deserving death. Primo Levi's unforgettable witnessing of this mentality in Auschwitz comes to mind.

"Big Tobacco is starting to invade low-income nations, now that smoking is on the wane in the wealthiest nations."

Sorry, but US and British manufacturers have been aggressively marketing cigarettes in places like China since the early years of last century. These collectible posters[13] show many featuring Chinese women. But the large populations, the often lax tobacco control policies and the higher corruption indexes of many low- and middle-income nations make many of these nirvanas for Big Tobacco. There are fewer more nauseating experiences than reading the oleaginous corporate social responsibility reports of tobacco transnationals and then seeing how they operate in smokers' paradises like Indonesia. This documentary says it all.[14]

"Millions of cigarette butts on the world's beaches leach lots of toxic chemicals into oceans"

Cigarette butts are the most discarded items in all litter. Every year uncounted millions if not billions are washed down gutters in storm water and find their way into rivers, harbours and oceans. Cigarette filters and butts contain toxic residue and experiments have shown that when laboratory fish are placed in containers with leachate extracted from used cigarette butts for for 48 hours, 50 percent of the fish die.[15] From this, we sometimes hear people exclaim that cigarette butts are not just unsightly, but they "poison the oceans".

But a confined laboratory container does not remotely mirror real life exposures in oceans or rivers. There are some 1,338,000,000 cubic

---

13 http://bit.ly/2cAVCEL.
14 Thompson 2009.
15 Slaughter, Gersberg, Watanabe, Rudolph, Stransky and Novotny 2011.

kilometres of water in the world oceans, so the contribution of cigarette butts to the toxification of all this could only excite a homeopath.

If we want to reduce tobacco litter, we need not wander into such dubious justifications. The best way by far is to keep reducing smoking. Industry attempts at portraying themselves as corporately responsible by running dinky little clean-up campaigns or distributing personal butt disposal canisters distracts from their efforts to keep as many smoking as possible.

"Tobacco companies care deeply about their best customers dying early"

Naturally, all businesses would rather their customers lived as long as possible so that the cash registers can keep ringing out long and loud. Tobacco companies wish their products didn't kill so many, but worship the god nicotine for its iron grip on so many.

Visit any tobacco transnational's website and you will find lots of earnest and caring talk about the companies' dedication to doing all they can to reduce the terrible harm caused by their products. All the major companies have now invested heavily in electronic cigarettes, so isn't this a sign that they taking harm reduction seriously?

It might be if the same companies were showing any sign of taking their feet off the turbo-drive accelerator of opposing effective tobacco control policies. But they are doing nothing of the sort. All continue to aggressively attack and delay any policy like tax hikes, graphic health warnings, plain packaging and advertising bans, wherever in the world these are planned for introduction.

For all their unctuous hand-wringing about their mission to reduce harm, they are all utterly determined to keep as many smoking as possible. Big Tobacco's business plan is not smoking *or* e-cigarettes. It's smoking *and* e-cigarettes. Smoke when you are able to, vape when you can't. It's called dual use and some 70 percent of vapers are doing just that. The tragedy now playing out in some nations is that some gormless tobacco control experts are blind to this big picture.

64
Letters to editors

I've written hundreds of letters to newspapers over the years, and always invited the letters editor of the *Sydney Morning Herald* to come and talk to my public health advocacy students each year. The letters page of newspapers is one of the most read. I didn't keep most of those I wrote, but here are a few I did and which I'm pleased were published.

Community armouries, *Sydney Morning Herald*, 9 November 1992

M.J. Kay's concerns about community gun armouries in urban areas are baseless (Letters, 5 November). If governments can ban the importation of firecrackers and radar detectors, they can certainly restrict the importation and manufacture of guns to those that can be easily disarmed by removal of the firing mechanism. Most guns already come apart. This way, community armouries would store only the firing mechanisms, thus saving space, reducing costs and negating concern about thefts (stealing a piece of a gun would be pointless). It would also allow shooters to retain their precious guns in their homes for purposes of cleaning, fondling and full dress rehearsals of their paranoid fantasies about dispelling the invading hordes from the north. When the invasion is announced or when they want to kill a few bunnies or shoot at human silhouettes down at the gun club, they can slip down to their local police station and check out their missing bit. This proposal will not stop all gun deaths, but it will put a critical pause between the rage of a domestic violence episode, or the despair of a potential suicide, and the final, bloody consequence that happens some 700 times year in Australia when guns are in the next room.

Tobacco sponsorship of sport, *Sydney Morning Herald*, 6 February 1993

At the cricket on Saturday the camera lingered on a shirtless, hatless couple, both smoking. Richie Benaud commented, "While it's their own business I know, they would be much more sensible if they wore hats" and then went on to talk about the preventability of melanoma.

With lung cancer killing many more Australians annually than skin cancer, Benaud's very pardonable excursion into other people's business might well have mentioned the couple's smoking as well. But then, the sun doesn't sponsor the cricket.

The economics of smoking, *Financial Review*, 26 May 1994

It is getting more and more amusing to follow the antics of the tobacco industry and its "independent" economic advisers (20 May). Professor Robert Tollison, a long-time friend to the international industry and apparently their intellectual "big gun", has come all the way from Kentucky to give us the following beauties. First, tobacco taxation is regressive. Ummm, well . . . yes . . . *all* sales taxes are regressive when all people don't earn the same. The corollary of his argument is presumably that the price of cigarettes should be lowered. What a perverse way to help the poor. Next, smokers don't get sick from smoking (sound familiar?) and even if they did, according to Tollison, would "be penalised by labour markets for excessive absenteeism with lower wages." Oh, really? Perhaps while he's here, he should stop by and tell all those duffers in the life insurance industry that their own figures on smokers dying younger and having higher health costs are all wrong. And finally, $9.1 billion out of the estimated $12.5 billion annual benefits of smoking are accounted for by . . . ready?. . . the $9.1 billion that smokers spend on their addiction. And I suppose this means that if they didn't smoke, it would all be put in jam tins forever with not a cent spent elsewhere in the economy!

The truth about the economics of smoking that the industry dares not mention is that the 60 percent of lung cancer deaths that occur before age 70 assist in pruning what some economists refer to as the "unproductive sector" of the population. This is the same sort of thinking that the Nazis used in their death camps, where human life was valued only while it could contribute to the German war effort. The frail, the aged and the sick were simply killed. Tobacco serves the same purpose but the industry can't bring itself to point out this benefit because it involves admitting that smoking kills.

Nick Greiner, *Sydney Morning Herald*, 24 June 1996

So Nick Greiner is "relaxed" about chairing W.D. & H.O. Wills (22 June), rationalising that tobacco is a legal product. The same base expediency of course was used by those in Victorian England who sent children down mines and up chimneys, and by those who profited from the entirely legal slave trade before the bleeding hearts ended those nice little earners. No matter that smoking kills 19,000 Australians a year, with about 55 percent of these dying before age 70. If it's legal, there's little more to be said it seems.

Greiner says that smokers have "full information" about the risks of smoking. This is from the chairman of a company that has always refused to tell consumers which chemical additives it uses In cigarettes and has spent a public relations fortune over the years trying to muddy public awareness that smoking doesn't cause lung cancer – it's only a "statistical association".

Nick Greiner does not smoke himself – a phenomenon not uncommon among tobacco barons. Doubtless he would argue that he chooses not to smoke. While the male head of a lingerie company would not be expected to "choose" to wear women's underwear, smoking is a choice open to all. It is scarcely imaginable that the chairman of Ford would drive a Toyota or the head of the Meat Marketing Board would be a vegetarian. Such lack of personal confidence in their products would probably see them not long in their jobs. The tobacco industry does not seem to mind such an irony.

Gun deaths, *Sydney Morning Herald*, 28 March 1996

Your correspondent John Harvey (22 March) uses an argument that is depressingly common among the gun lobby. It runs, "There are far larger causes of death than guns . . . why don't people arguing about gun control turn their attention (for example) to road carnage? This is about as sensible as saying to a heart specialist, "Why don't you try to cure cancer?" or to an environmentalist, "What are you doing about unemployment?"

He argues that gun deaths are as rare as shark attack deaths. In 1994, 522 Australians were killed by guns. No one died from shark attack that year. And he caps it all by calling gun registration "discredited". Why is it, then, that we have maintained such a discredited system for handguns in this state since 1927? And why is it, Mr Harvey, that the UK, which has three times Australia's population and crime rate to match, had only 72 gun deaths in 1993? The UK has some of the world's toughest gun laws, and yet I can just hear Mr Harvey saying, "And that didn't stop Dunblane." This is like saying, "If you can't fix every problem, don't try to fix any of them." Tougher gun laws, including registration, will not eliminate gun violence, but there is plenty of evidence that they will reduce it.

Killing with kindness, *Financial Review*, 18 September 1996

The IPA's Alan Moran's views on "sin taxes" like those on tobacco (13 September) will have earned him a pat on the back if not the wallet from one of his board, Nick Greiner, down at W.D. & H.O. Wills. Moran's gripe is tobacco tax is regressive, therefore making low-income smokers spend a higher proportion of their income on tobacco than the wealthy. He thinks it "remarkable" that voices preoccupied with equity have not gone into bat for this heinous burden on the poor.

What is truly "remarkable" is the extent to which Moran and his ideological ilk have the gall to appropriate concern for the poor in full knowledge that international evidence has repeatedly shown that the lowest socioeconomic groups have the highest responsiveness (both cessation and reduction in number of cigarettes smoked) to cigarette price increases.

Because these groups have the highest smoking rates and the highest rates of smoking-caused diseases, price policy is of enormous importance in any efforts to narrow these socioeconomic differentials and reduce diseases like lung cancer. This is of course why the tobacco industry and its apologists have become born-again social welfare advocates. They want the poor and the other main price sensitive group, children, to smoke more.

The corollary of Moran's position is presumably that the price of cigarettes should be lowered. What a perverse way to help the poor. Killing with kindness comes to mind.

Cigarette lighter recall, *Sydney Morning Herald,* 20 December 1996

Philip Morris' decision to recall cigarette lighters because they posed "a potential risk" is like White Star line recalling the *Titanic* because it had splinters in the handrails.

Boxing reform, *Sydney Morning Herald*, circa 1997

Several weeks ago the National Health and Medical Research Council called for professional boxing to be banned because of the brain damage it causes nearly all participants. This well-motivated but unrealistic proposal seems to have disappeared without trace. Might I suggest instead that the NH&MRC, in a spirit of compromise, lobbies for the rules of boxing to be reversed? The main objective under the present rules is to hit your opponent's head so hard that his brain sloshes with such force against the skull that unconsciousness occurs. By contrast, a foul stroke is recorded when the boxer hits his opponent in the testicles. This can be very painful, occasionally dangerous, but never life-threatening. Under the reversed rules, a foul stroke would become one that strikes the head and the crowd-pleaser redefined as a lusty blow flush to the orchestra stalls. Think of the new impetus to the development of evasive footwork. Think of new generations of young men with bruised egos but intact brains. With the search on for new demonstration sports for the 2000 Olympics, "cod-walloping" could be Australia's responsible entry.

Support for tobacco executive, Sydney Morning Herald, 23 August 2003

Kathryn Greiner's analogy suggesting the University of Sydney may as well refuse tobacconists' children places because the Senate voted against endorsing her BAT chairman husband is quite facile. Unlike Nick Greiner, tobacconists' children have no fiduciary responsibility to promote transnational tobacco company policy that if successful results in the early and painful deaths of thousands of Australians. Mrs Greiner's moral support for her beleaguered husband is touching but please, spare us such nonsense.

65

Bertrand Russell's *Why I am not a Christian*: a book that changed me

In my early 20s, I read all of Orwell, Koestler and Dostoyevsky but an invitation to nominate just one book that changed me was easy to name. After this was published, a retired Christian couple from Yorkshire wrote a nice letter inviting me to come and stay with them for a few days. I couldn't make it.

In 1969 at the age of 17, after eight schooners of lager and a night of murderous vomiting following my final matriculation exam, I left my home in the New South Wales country and moved to a university hall of residence in the parental Gomorrah of Sydney. In the room opposite was an earnest man from Hong Kong, ten years my senior, who late at night would tap on my door to invite me to play chess and drink jasmine tea. He was doing a PhD on the mathematical philosopher Gottfried Leibniz and his room was full of books with titles that both frightened and excited me at the prospect of all I would need to know, now that overnight I was no longer a child. On the first night I entered his room the spine of one burnt into my head: Bertrand Russell's *Why I am not a Christian*.

Originally published as Chapman, Simon (2000). *Why I am not a Christian*: a book that changed me. *British Medical Journal* 320: 1152.

Such profanity promised to fit well with other unwritten books that swirled in my callow head: *Why I no longer live with my parents*; *Things to do with naked girls*; *Mind-altering drugs for beginners*. I asked if I could read it, and recall switching off my light at 3.30 am, drunk with excitement at the eloquent defilement that I'd just consumed. Not since I'd wolfed down *Lady Chatterley's lover* in an afternoon at 13, after being handed it by a conspiratorial librarian with pearls and hair in a bun, had I had such joy from a book.

I'd been brought up in the high Anglican church and God had been a problem for me ever since I'd asked my parents at around ten, "If God made the world, who made God?" – something Russell now informed me was the naif's way of phrasing the argument from first cause. The imperious Canon from our cathedral had been invited home for afternoon tea to plug the dyke of the boy's worrying scepticism. Staring at me with that look, he'd said there was simply no need to keep on asking the question. It all just started with God. Sure . . . right, I thought. How puerile. Church for me had been the pageantry, the lusty singing on cold Sunday mornings, the scented mothers fussing with scones and jam after the service, but particularly the chance to pash choirgirls after practice on Thursday nights. I'd had little truck with the theology and the stuff about heaven seemed patent anthropocentric wish-fulfilment, clasped to the bosoms of the mostly aged parishioners who seemed determined to believe in it all.

The shackles of the afterworld fell off that night, and in rode the exhilarating awareness that gut-level scepticism with all sorts of comfort zones were likely to have whole tribes of authors out there brilliantly dashing the sacrosanct crockery onto the concrete of no-prisoners argument. Russell's book was soon followed by Joachim Kahl's *The misery of Christianity: or a plea for a humanity without God*. This was a catalogue of horrors wrought in the world in the name of religion, while championing the values that many religions wanted to claim as their own. Jean Paul Sartre's essay *Existentialism and humanism* consolidated the rift while securing the importance of taking responsibility for your beliefs and values. As an undergraduate, it also gave me a French philosophical badge I could wear along with my pretentious Gitanes cigarettes and taste in excruciating films by Bresson, Renoir, Resnais and Truffaut.

Looking back, Russell's book and much of what I learnt about his life embodied two of the most important things in my life today: passion for justice and intellectual scepticism. It'll be in my own 17-year-old's Christmas stocking this year.

66

Why do researchers donate their time and money to help private conference organisers make big bucks?

Every day without fail I delete invitations to fake conferences, to pay for the privilege of publishing my research on any topic to a predatory junk science "journal" (I get invitations to send my work in metallurgy, neurological surgery and accountancy among many others) or to join their editorial boards (presumably so they can exploit my reviewing skills for research areas I know less than nothing about). But I also get asked to donate my time and money to help commercial conference companies make lots of cash. Here's why I refuse.

Research conferences are part of every academic's calendar. They provide opportunities to interact with global and national stars in your field, and present early opportunities for new research to be released to an audience of peers. The typical conference is run by learned societies or research associations, who contract professional conference organisers to handle the grunt work and take their cut. Plenary program speakers are selected by scientific program committees of experienced researchers and the speakers often given free registration

Originally published as Chapman, Simon (2011). Why do researchers donate their time and money to help private conference organisers make big bucks? *Crikey*, 15 November.

and travel support in recognition that their names will be magnets to those attending, boosting attendance.

Another model is the entirely commercial conference business, where conference companies select topics that they judge will attract interest and run conferences independent of any scientific body.

IIR Conferences[1] (aka Informa) is Australia and New Zealand's leading commercial provider of conferences, seminars and portentous sounding "summits". In December the 7th Australian Wind Energy Conference[2] will be held in Melbourne. I was invited to speak on the claims of anti-wind-farm groups who claim that wind turbines can make people sick. Except for two other Melbourne locals, most of the other listed speakers are senior wind energy company people, government officials and politicians.

Registration is $2,995 plus GST – $3,294.50 all up. And if you really want to spray your money around, you can purchase the PowerPoints for the two days of plenaries – a snip at $764.50. I'm used to giving my PowerPoints away at conferences.

When I was invited, I asked for my expenses to be paid and they offered to reimburse airfares and taxis and graciously to waive the registration fee. Terrific. I wouldn't have to pay to hear myself speak! But they would not pay for two nights in a hotel (I live in Sydney) – maybe $400 to 600 – because they had "a limited budget". I said I would not charge a speakers' fee.

The idea here apparently, is that I and other speakers should effectively put our hands in our pockets to assist the company in their efforts to make lots of money. If they were to get just 100 payers through the door, they would pull $299,000 before selling a single PowerPoint set.

So when they refused to pay my hotel, I withdrew.

As I wrote last year,[3] I've received IIR brochures over the years and routinely binned them, wondering about how connected and important an audience would be who would shell out such sums to hear from people you can readily hear at many public sector conferences at a

---

1 http://www.informa.com.au/.
2 http://bit.ly/2cURSxv.
3 Chapman 2010.

fraction of the price. I'm going to a four-day international conference in Singapore in March where the registration is $620 and the PowerPoints are free.

Last year, when invited to speak at one of their meetings, I called three other participants asking the terms on which they were participating. One, when asking for travel, was told, "As a speaker, you will receive full complimentary access to both days of the conference including all speaker papers, luncheons and networking functions. Speakers are normally asked to cover their own travel expenses," but that they would make an exception with him. However, none I spoke with were getting fees. Some but not all public-sector workers are unable to accept fees, making this a nice little honey pot to exploit.

So why do public-sector experts give up their valuable time to effectively donate their time and expertise to for-profit companies like IIR? And why do they give away their PowerPoints to be sold at such an extravagant cost, seeing that such companies play no role in their content?

67
Why I block trolls on Twitter

Many people who use Twitter experience being trolled, often by anonymous accounts. I got a steady stream from the outset, and soon discovered the block and later the mute functions, which to me are the equivalents of the spam filter with email, the call screening and blocking functions on phones that save you from sales agents or people you just don't want to speak with, or a sign near your doorbell saying you won't buy from door-to-door sales people.

Most of my trolling comes from vaping obsessives because I've been sceptical of core claims that have been made. Most of these tweeps have nothing else in their feeds. I have often awoken to dozens of tweets from the same person, and opening gambits strewn with abuse, typically from a dedicated vaper with a handful of other vaping followers.

My first column[1] last week was quickly trolled by a small group of mostly UK-based vaping activists. Of 49 comments posted, 17 were

---

1 Chapman 2015d.

Originally published as Chapman, Simon (2015). Why I block trolls on Twitter. *The Conversation*, 12 January.

Reason blocked	*n*	%	Reason blocked	*n*	%
Vaping/e-cigs	227	67.8	Climate-change denial	5	1.5
Mixed abuse	26	7.7	Israel/Palestine extremism	4	1.2
Pro-smoking	23	6.9	Anti-cycle helmets	3	0.9
Racist	18	5.3	Pro-gun	2	0.6
Anti-wind farm	13	3.9	Religious fundamentalism	2	0.6
Extreme libertarian	12	3.6			

Table 67.1 (*n* = 335)

removed by *The Conversation*'s moderator before the comments were closed off after two days. I saw some of these before they were removed. They were mostly from one-track trolls I have long blocked from my Twitter account.

Using this app,[2] I can see I've blocked 335 accounts since November 2011 (see Table 67.1). By far the biggest category here is a well-connected network of electronic cigarette advocates, most of whom have small followings of mainly fellow vapers. In many cases their feeds show they have apparently no other interests other than talking about their love for nicotine and hammering anyone who expresses any scepticism about any of the glowing claims being made. One troll actually went to the trouble of opening 16 different accounts, populating them with random followings and then firing off venom to me in his or her first tweet each time, hoping I wouldn't guess it was the same person.

I'm targeted because, along with many others in public health, I support regulation[3] of e-cigarettes and have written "hasten slowly" commentaries[4] trying to temper some of the often commercially driven hype in circulation about these products. Anything less than doctrinaire enthusiasm for almost complete lack of regulatory oversight will not be tolerated, apparently.

---

2 http://blockedby.me.
3 Stanton 2014.
4 http://bit.ly/2cnMjIH.

Keyword	n	%
Tobacco or smoking	2,513	19.8
Wind*	1,208	9.5
Plain†	1,176	9.2
Vaping/e-cigs	373	2.9
Solar‡	116	0.9
All others	7,334	57.7
Total	12,720	

Table 67.2 *tweets about wind farms and turbines †tweets about plain tobacco packaging ‡tweets about solar energy or solariums

A month ago, I downloaded my Twitter feed and did keyword counts of all the times I have ever tweeted anything with the words ecig, e-cig, vape or vaping, and compared this with the frequency of other issues I often tweet about (see Table 67.2).

So there is a giant disconnect between what I tweet about and the preoccupations of those whom I choose to stop clogging up my Twitter feed and thereby distorting for my followers the extent of my interest in e-cigarettes. Blocking is a bit like putting a sticker on your mailbox saying "No junk mail accepted", except that unlike with junk mail, it works!

The concept of an internet troll is unavoidably subjective: what one person regards as hostile or inflammatory can be genuinely intended by the sender as an attempt to engage in debate. But having a Twitter account is not an obligation to engage with anyone seeking to do this, no matter what adamant trolls might want to insist. I take a similar attitude to hostile, ignorant, obscene or simply tediously persistent tweeters hitting my Twitter feed that I often give to such attempts at interaction communicated through other means. Like millions of others, I block such people on email using junk filters. I don't engage with uninvited door-to-door or telephone proselytisers and promoters either.

Obsessed vapers, like golf, dope or wine bores, apparently cannot understand why anyone would not want to share their preoccupation and not engage in the endless back-and-forth's evident in their feeds with each other.

Trolling often comes in waves and a little searching of new followers' feeds which look suspicious often quickly reveals networks of those I have blocked. There's a good deal of mutual goading to troll the recalcitrant. So I sometimes block such people pre-emptively before they have tweeted.

In Australia, there is a highly civil dialogue about e-cigarettes that is well advanced between colleagues in research and public health who might be described as either highly optimistic or sceptical and cautious about the potential key benefits and risks. There is much common ground. There is also zero tolerance of the sort of infantile name-calling that infests much social media advocacy on vaping. Twitter is a terrific vehicle for disseminating new research and data but the block and mute functions are a godsend to denying trolls the attention they crave.

68
Publishing horror stories: time to euthanase paper-based journals?

I was deputy editor, then editor, of *Tobacco Control*, the *British Medical Journal*'s specialist journal from its foundation in 1992 until 2008. During that time online publication of research journals began and the open access movement built early momentum. I have always been an enthusiastic supporter of both. In 2010 I experienced a publishing saga for a research paper that was eventually published late in 2013. This was the worst publishing experience of my career, but most colleagues have similar horror stories. Those wanting to read the paper at the centre of the saga today cannot unless they pay an extortionate US$41 to liberate it from behind a paywall. I put a preprint of it on my university's eScholarship repository.[1]

Paper journals other than those subsidised by society membership, and a handful with very large circulations, are surely on their last legs. Here are a few reasons why.

---

1   Chapman, Haynes, Derrick, Sturk, Hall and St George 2014.

Originally published as Chapman, Simon (2013). Publishing horror stories: time to euthanase paper-based journals? *British Medical Journal Blogs*, 27 September.

Every researcher has exasperating stories of the glacial pace of research publication. But as a former research journal editor of 17 years, I know that researchers' ideas on what constitutes "glacial" varies enormously. I've received "hurry up" letters from authors a week or so after submission, and have often played a game with other editors about the record number of review requests that have needed to be sent out before the required number of usable reviews were returned. Mine was 16.

While every researcher wants their paper peer-reviewed expeditiously by the best people, the noblesse oblige to reciprocate reviewing to others is often sadly lacking. Unresponsive and delayed reviewing and, less commonly, tardy revisions from authors are two factors over which editors have little control. If peer reviewed publications are to continue as a core academic currency, universities and research institutes should require their research staff to show evidence of at least as much reviewing as papers published. This data should be audited and published.

But in my experience, by far the biggest delay factor in publication times is the limitations imposed by the old model of paper-based publication, where publishers give editors a set number of issues and pages to fill each year, and publishing backlogs begin to form despite the best efforts of editors to match their rejection rate with the space available.

All these problems have combined to see many journals now offer online publication shortly after acceptance. It is not uncommon today to see subscriber or pay-per-view journals with vast numbers of "online first" publications available. One journal I know, which publishes about 75 original articles a year in its paper edition, is currently showing a paper-edition backlog of nearly 130 online-first papers, the most recent of which will not be published "properly" in print for nearly two years.

This is fast becoming a farcical situation. In my field, it has been a long time since I first read research in a paper journal or walked into a library to browse new paper copies of serials. To read a paper first in a printed journal would mean that I was up to two years out of date, reading material that was first published online. Why do publishers and a (surely) diminishing number of readers persist with the fiction that "real" publication means final publication in the paper version of a journal? Paper journals are fast becoming a kind of belated souvenir of online publishing that often happens many months or even years earlier.

If research matters, then we'd all assume that the importance of its findings ought to be somehow aligned with mechanisms to get those findings into the public domain as fast as possible after peer review.

In 2010, I submitted a co-authored paper on the research dissemination behaviours of a peer-voted list of 36 of Australia's top public health researchers in six fields. I chose the *American Journal of Public Health*, considered one of the leading journals in that field. I'd published seven papers with them before, which have had 794 combined citations. I've thought of it as a journal where I send some of my best work. Below is a timeline of the saga of trying to get that paper published, first in the *American Journal of Public Health* and then in the *Journal of Health Communication* (ranked fifth out of 72 for impact factor by *Journal Citation Reports* in the Communication category).

1. American Journal of Public Health

5 Dec 2010	Paper submitted online.	
23 Dec 2010	Electronic acknowledgement of receipt.	[18 days]
15 May 2011	I enquire about progress, as their submission system is still saying the paper is "under review".	[148 days]
21 May 2011	Assigned editor apologises, saying he was not made aware of the paper's submission until 8 April 2011. ("communication unfortunately seemed to be obstructed")	[6 days]
6 June 2011	Editor rejects paper after review, but invites major revision.	[16 days]
11 July 2011	Major revision submitted, but problems seeing it in the online system.	[1 day]
22 July 2011	Major revision successfully submitted online.	[10 days]
27 July 2011	A co-author of the paper receives an invitation to review it!	[5 days]

11 Nov 2011	Revised paper rejected after two perfunctory reviews which stressed lack of interest for US readership because Australia is "different".	[103 days]

Time from first submission to final rejection: 341 days

2. Journal of Health Communication

15 Nov 2011	Paper submitted online.	
15 Feb 2012	Reviews received and revision offered.	
21 May 2012	Paper accepted.	[97 days]
2 May 2013	I email the journal and query the paper's progress. I note that the journal has an "ifirst" facility to publish pre-paper editions.	[1 day]
3 May 2013	Editor apologises about the backlog and says, "Your paper is in the next batch to go to the publisher. You will see proofs in the next month."	[346 days]
18 Sept 2013	Proofs arrive.	[138 days]
20 Sept 2013	Corrected proofs returned.	[2 days]

Time from first submission to proofs arrival: 673 days

iFirst publication: Anyone's guess!!

Paper publication: Probably long after the retirement of at least two authors.

This has been by far my worst experience in a 35-year publishing career, but like most colleagues I've had many papers published many, many months after acceptance. This time it was a saga of online submission failure, staff changes, dropped balls and incomprehensible, outrageous delays. The differences between the original submission and the accepted version were mostly – as often happens – insubstantial matters of presentational preference (move this here, that there; reference this paper; and the profoundly naive "delete extra spaces between words"). The material in the paper is now nearly three years old. As authors, we are presumably meant to be happy and grateful that that our work will grace a journal. But the old model of paper publishing needs be euthanased fast and replaced with online open access publishing featuring open-reviewing (moderated for trolls) and smart reader-rating metrics that don't allow gaming by authors.

69
My mother's death

In 1995 the Northern Territory's Assembly became the first legislature anywhere in the world to pass legislation allowing voluntary enthanasia. This was effectively nullified by the passage of federal legislation in 1997 introduced by the Christian fundamentalist Liberal MP Kevin Andrews. I led a project in 1994 to publish a book of prominent Australians' views on "the last right" – the right to assisted suicide for the terminally ill. This was my own contribution to the book.

On 10 February 1984, my mother Margaret died in bed at her home. About a year before she had been diagnosed as having breast cancer. She had a mastectomy soon after, followed by radiotherapy. For the next nine months she seemed mostly her usual optimistic self. She looked forward to coming to Sydney every three months to see her oncologist. At her November 1983 visit, it was discovered that the cancer had metastasised into her lungs. She came from the hospital straight to my office, where, looking at my face for the slightest sign of hope, she told me that she had made up her mind to fight it.

Originally published as Chapman, Simon (1995). My mother's death. In Simon Chapman and Stephen Leeder (eds), *The last right: Australians take sides on the right to die*. Port Melbourne, Vic.: Mandarin Books.

After I started university in 1970, Mum would sometimes come and have dinner with me and my student friends. She threw herself into every conversation about politics, sex and all the big topics. Then, as at home, I recall her many times saying things like, "Heavens, when my time's up, I don't want to linger around in pain and misery . . . I'd like to just go off at a time of my own choosing." If someone had knocked on the door with a survey about voluntary euthanasia, she would have told them the same.

But from the moment she was told the news about her lungs, all this changed. There was not a moment when even a crack appeared in her resolve to "fight it". She dredged up all that fighting spirit stuff – the sort that had been with her during the London Blitz, which had allowed her to live in the drab back room of her first business after migrating to Australia, knowing she would work her way out of it. From that morning on, her life became focused on how she was going to beat this thing.

Two days later she went back into hospital and was knocked sideways with chemo- and radiotherapy. I visited her every day in a huge barn of a public ward and sat with her as she lay almost motionless, screened off by a thin white curtain. I had never seen anyone looking so sick. Still through this, she would cling to the smallest fragment of hope passed to her by the doctors and nursing staff trying to give her comfort. "The doctor said it had all gone well . . . he said I'd be feeling much better in a week or two, and then it will be wait and see." "The way I see it, if I don't give it a go, then I'd never give myself a chance, would I?"

After two weeks she came home and was so exhausted she could barely bother to walk a few yards into the back garden to get some sun. She insisted on cooking us what would be her last Christmas dinner.

As the cancer grew, her breathing became increasingly shallow and rapid. Three weeks before she died an oxygen cylinder was brought in beside her bed. When you can't breathe properly, every moment of your life becomes preoccupied with getting the next breath. Lack of oxygen – hypoxia – causes disorientation and confusion. My sister and I had been taking it in turns to go down to her house in a small town and help. In the evenings we would sit with her and feed her junket through a straw. When we left the room, we left a bell near her hand so she could ring it if she needed anything.

I was sleeping on the floor in the next room the night she died. Dad woke me at 4 am and asked me to come and see if Mum was alright. I could see straight away that she was dead. The bell had fallen to the floor. Her body was still warm. Dad felt it right that the local doctor should be phoned right away so she could come down and tell us what was obvious. I pretended to phone and then sat with Dad drinking scotch, every now and then going back in with him to hold Mum. The last thing she said to me was about how the next day she was going to tell the doctor that she wanted to go back into hospital for another try with "the treatment".

When the news about her lungs came through, we knew Mum was going to die. We didn't know when, but we knew it could be soon. All we wanted to do was comfort her, give our love and hope that it would happen with minimal suffering. Both my sister and I stifled the impulse to talk with her as we would have normally. We said to each other, "She's going to die. The only thing she has to look forward to is this crazy hope she clings to. Who are we to try to take that away from her?" Dad has always been frightened and appalled by talk of death, regarding it as profane and unseemly. This made us keep him away from our often angry discussions about the way medicine conspired with the fear of death to build these optimistic artifices that were deceitfully called "treatment". So the option that she take no further therapy was never really discussed.

I fell upon the phrase that the treatment she received after her November lung cancer diagnosis was in fact a form of medically sanctified torture. I said this to everyone I met when they asked how things were going. I did literature searches in oncology journals, confirming my understanding that the probability of the treatment she was getting giving any decent remission was practically zero.

The last weeks of her life were appallingly wretched. She existed in total exhaustion between the kingdoms of fear and anger, whipped along by what we sensed was an unflagging burden of virtuous stoicism. There seemed no respite from this tyranny of false hope. Our temptation to ease the subject into the open with her retreated beneath the force of the plea behind her often terrified eyes that we didn't. One night as I stroked her arm, she angrily brushed my hand away.

Where does this false hope, this "Break my bones, but don't dare take away even the tiny chance I have" thing come from? Partly it must come from our culture's denial and sanitisation of all things to do with death. Expressions like "brave", "battle with cancer" and "never stopped trying" say much about the way we spurn any resignation about imminent death.

Yet how needless much of her suffering all seemed. I tried to put myself in her consultant's shoes. Here was a warm, articulate woman only 64 years old, begging for hope . . . pleading with them to do something, jumping at any nuance of a chance, stoically prepared to weather any misery involved. Was it fair of me to expect him to deny her any chance, no matter how remote or at what suffering? If her two children, with a lifetime of talking with her, were not prepared to raise the subject of putting up the white flag and accepting death, why should I expect him to do it on the basis of having known her for a cumulative total of perhaps a few hours?

It seems to me that above everything else, many in medicine feel the need to do *something* in the face of threatened death. It is almost as if it is sacrilegious to do nothing, particularly in circumstances when death may be still months away. If it can muck in with techno-chemical heroics which signify the defiance of all odds, there will be plenty of people there to cheer it along, and very few who will feel it reasonable to be angry if these attempts fail as they almost invariably do in cases like my mother's. Culturally, medical heroics dovetail with the arrogance of our collective belief in our earthly immortality. They represent the institutional expression of the cultural denial of death. For doctors trained and expected to rescue, revive and restore, the open recognition of the limits to medicine can come close to an admission of failure.

And if the decision to be frank about doing nothing is difficult, what of hurrying things along – what of the attitude that says, "If I am honest with this person, I will not seek to hide that it is nearly certain they will die within weeks. These weeks are likely to become progressively miserable and will become more devoid of hope for any reprieve. Is part of my duty of care at such times to offer to end this suffering if it is requested?" In my mother's case this misery did not mean pain that could be relieved with drugs, giving the doctor a valued and sanctioned palliative care role. It meant instead that she would slowly suffocate to death over several weeks while becoming increasingly disoriented. She would have never wanted that. Who in their right mind would? And what sort of medical ethics says that she should just have to put up with it?

If her doctor had not tempted her with treatment, she would have developed hypoxia but avoided the weeks of nausea and misery brought on by the treatment. The local GP who attended her in her last weeks did not offer and Mum did not ask if her life might end with a sedative injection or drink. Each day she visited I would ask as Mum lay gasping in the next room, "How much longer do you think she has?" The answer was always indeterminate. Medicine devoid of any vocation to actively assist in the right to die has no answer to such pointless suffering.

There are those who argue that there *is* some point to such suffering. I say let them feel free to exercise that option with their own deaths if it brings them a higher comfort. But I have only contempt for ethics that insist such degrading suffering should be compulsory for those whose fates select such paths. Any laws or codes of conduct which institutionalise a denial of the dying's right to determine their time of death do not reflect a civilised view of the end of life. The hastening of death in such circumstances, when the dying who have requested it are often incapable of taking action themselves, will require assistance. It follows for me that doctors and others should be able to assist such deaths with impunity where it is beyond any doubt that the dying person has consented.

Would my mother's experience have been any different if she had lived her life knowing that as well as tending you all through your life when you are sick, doctors could be there, like priests, to come at your call and give you the medical equivalent of the last rites? To supply you with a way of choosing your own time to go? If she had grown up in a culture when it might be as natural as day and night to say, "My time is near, let's have the doctor help me avoid the worst of the suffering", would she have felt impelled to put herself through so much wretchedness for what was really no chance at all?

And how different might her death have been if her doctor had decades of a medical tradition behind him which better enabled him to be frank rather than surreptitious about what lay ahead; about the futility of aggressive chemicals and radiation in prolonging her life; and who could instead offer options of assisted, painless death at a time of her choosing.

So yes – to both questions.

70

Dying with dignity with dementia

My father died in 1999, 17 years after my mother. Unlike Mum, he died peacefully, and at an advanced age. But he'd lived with increasingly advancing dementia for many of those years he lived alone. Many who support voluntary euthanasia will have dementia to some degree during the period that they may also be suffering from illnesses that make their life seem unbearable to them. Dementia poses huge challenges to so many who would hope to die with dignity. For all his deterioration, I feel my father still enjoyed much in his life until his death.

My father Alec, who died peacefully at 89 in his sleep, had dementia and lived in a nursing home for the last seven years of his life. After Mum died, he lived alone in their Mittagong home for about a decade, but as he moved into his 80s, we noticed that many ordinary tasks were getting beyond him. He could no longer operate the television, stabbing away randomly at the keys on the remote and unable to follow the simple large print step-by-step instructions we'd left for him.

Other than making tea and toast, cooking was too challenging so he ate most meals at a local truck-stop hamburger joint around the

Originally published as Chapman, Simon (2016). Dying with dignity with dementia. *The Conversation*, 28 January.

corner from his house. My sister and I in Sydney would get occasional confused phone calls where his frustration was obvious but the precipitating incident forgotten as he called to ask for help about something he then couldn't recall. Finally, a local widow he had been seeing for a few years ("We deny each other nothing," she told us more than once) apologetically told us that his confusion was getting too much for her.

Both my sister and I worked full time and we had no spare rooms in our homes, so we very reluctantly began the search for a suitable nursing home. We found one about five minutes away from my sister's house, where he had a pleasant self-contained two-roomed flat with a garden view. From the day he moved in, Dad complained that the place was full of old people, even though he was among the oldest. He was a private man and kept mostly to himself.

My sister and I would have a ritual call to each other every Friday to see who'd have him home Saturday, and who would take Sunday. He'd go with us to shops and cafés, but mostly liked just sitting on the lounge, where he would try to read the newspaper. We often saw that he was holding it upside down. If friends came around to our place, they found him always well dressed, congenial and up for a chat.

We started to get increasingly bizarre and panicked phone calls from him at the nursing home. He was English and moved to Australia in 1949. "Where are you?" he'd demand. "I'm here with my bag packed and the plane to England will leave soon. The house has been taken over by people who are not looking after it, and I've got to get over and sort it out."

We'd call him back after 20 minutes and he would have no recollection of his earlier panic. I would sometimes purposefully make the same comment to him to try and understand the size of the mental prison in which he lived. Five to ten minutes after remarking to Dad that we'd soon need to put a brick on the heads of our two teenage sons to stop them getting too tall, I'd say it again. He never once remarked that I'd already said that.

One night at 1 am the Bowral police called me. They had found him wandering in the backstreets of the town, confused after getting himself to Central and catching the train. I drove the 90 minutes down from Sydney and found him contentedly drinking tea with the night-duty police. I gently asked him what he was doing there, but it soon became obvious he didn't understand the question.

At Bondi Beach one day, I went to the kiosk to get him an ice cream. When I returned he'd gone from the bench where we'd been sitting. He had hailed a taxi, but couldn't say where he'd wanted to go and was taken to a police station, where they traced him from his wallet.

We twice bought his last living sister, Rose, out from the Isle of Wight to stay. They would talk for hours in remarkable detail about their life together in Portsmouth before he left England.

On one occasion when I was alone with him, he said to me tearfully that his life was awful, that he couldn't get anything straight in his mind and that he had nothing in common with the other residents. When he melted a plastic electric jug by placing it on the cooktop, he was moved to a heart-breaking tiny, bleak room in a secure section of the nursing home.

But in all this, across his gradual decline, he rarely seemed sad. My sister often made the same observation. He took great pleasure in food, dancing with my wife to country music like Hank Williams in our living room, watching the passing parade of people in public places and visual video feasts like *Baraka* and *Powaqqatsi*, drinking in the ambiance of family dinners, and most especially, in his beloved whiskey.

On his arrival from the nursing home around 10 am, we'd offer him tea or coffee. He would pause and then ask a little hesitatingly if he might not have a small tincture. We'd oblige and then notice him topping up several times before he dozed off for a midday nap. One day the matron at the nursing home took me aside and told me earnestly that she wondered if I knew that Dad had a drinking problem.

I said I knew he liked a drink, but what was the problem? Was he endangering others, rowdy, abusive? She looked at me hard and explained patiently that (at 88) he might become addicted. I told her that he could have as much whiskey as he wanted.

On his last day, my brother-in-law Paul drove him to Picton, where they had a counter lunch and Dad drank a schooner. He went to bed that night and was found dead in bed the next morning.

Dad's dementia was not profound. He knew who we were, although was often confused about our children. He dressed himself impeccably in a coat, collar and tie every day regardless of the weather, was never incontinent and right to the end could hold a conversation about banalities. He was always moved by television news of tragedy. One evening when he stayed overnight, he silently wandered in the dark into our bedroom, where, *in flagrante delicto*, we failed to notice him until he asked, just inches away, "Is that you, Si?" There was no recollection in the morning.

I've long been an advocate for voluntary euthanasia and am an ambassador for Dying with Dignity. I edited a book on the views on it of 63 prominent Australians in 1995,[1] when the Northern Territory's chief minister, Marshall Perron, had just introduced his bill for the brief period that it became law before being overturned by Commonwealth legislation in 1997 that effectively removed the rights of Commonwealth territories to legislate. The recent film *Last cab to Darwin* dramatised the case of one man who thought he wanted to be helped to end his life.

Choosing when to go is a common conversation for baby boomers as we move into our final decades. I'm always quick to say that I never want to move to a nursing home, and will take steps to end my life at a time of my choosing should I ever find it not worth living. Such decisions seem relatively uncomplicated when I contemplate being given a terminal diagnosis late in life or being told that I have a disease like motor neurone disease.

But many of us will not be given such a diagnosis. Dad slipped into increasingly obvious dementia over ten or so years. It's hard to know what he perceived about his decline. He never talked about ending his life. He had many long hours of joy in the years he lived with his deterioration. He certainly died with dignity, but it could have easily been different.

The gradual but very unpredictable realities of cognitive decline are one of the most challenging that anyone open to ending their own life will face.

---

1   Chapman 1995.

Alzheimers Australia lists the following facts about dementia in Australia today:

- There are more than 342,800 Australians living with dementia.
- This number is expected to increase by one third to 400,000 in less than ten years.
- Without a medical breakthrough, the number of people with dementia is expected to be almost 900,000 by 2050.
- Each week, there are 1,700 new cases of dementia in Australia; approximately one person every six minutes. This is expected to grow to 7,400 new cases each week by 2050.
- There are 24,700 people in Australia with younger onset dementia (a diagnosis of dementia under the age of 65, including people as young as 30).
- Three in ten people over the age of 85 have dementia.
- An estimated 1.2 million Australians are caring for someone with dementia.
- Dementia is the second leading cause of death (the second leading cause in women) in Australia and there is no cure.
- On average symptoms of dementia are noticed by families three years before a firm diagnosis is made.[2]

---

2 http://bit.ly/2d0zUJ5.

71

Can academics ever retire?

I wrote this piece a few months into my "retirement" from the University of Sydney. Seventeen months on, I've had not a nanosecond of regret. I'm writing a book, am moving toward my 70th column for *The Conversation*, teaching short courses in exotic locations, and researching and publishing some of the most important work I've ever done. Retirement of course allows more time for many pleasures that were limited by work demands. But writing has always been in the very front line of those pleasures. I've been very blessed to have a lifetime job where such pleasure could be taken nearly every day.

When your local butcher or grocer retires, it's perfectly clear what this means. They are no longer there in the shop when you next go in. Someone else has taken over, or the shop has changed to another business. If you see them in the street it would be bizarre to ask them about what's good value this week. Their retirement is unambiguous. They don't cut up meat or select fruit from the city markets anymore. They go on big trips, play more golf, take things easy.

Originally published as Chapman, Simon (2015). Can academics ever retire? *The Conversation*, 30 April.

But when academics retire it's far from clear what this means. Some things are obvious. They stop taking on the supervision of new postgraduate research students, although often agree to keep assisting those who have not yet graduated. They greatly reduce their teaching, now reserved for guest lectures and making appearances in seminars where a reflective voice of experience is called for.

They are excused from committees and interminable reporting duties, and from losing two months of their life every year applying for research grants, in the knowledge that 85 percent of applications will be rejected. I will never forget my sheer joy as I finished writing comments on the last masters student assignment I knew I would ever mark. Marking is universally experienced as the most spirit-dulling duty of academic work. It helped that the last one was, like so many, as good as they can get.

But having now been effectively retired for seven months (I'm currently eating up a career's worth of untaken long service leave prior to formal retirement), there are many things that are never-ending. Some of these present challenges in how to respond without appearing rude and unhelpful. Others force reflection on just how much academic life is a vocation, not just a job. And others are a joyous apotheosis of what you've always wanted to do, but could rarely find time for.

I started my public health career in 1974 and loved almost every minute of the next 40 years. I never recall a day when I resented going into work, usually before 7 am, and often working 70 to 80 hours a week.

Academic work becomes rapidly vocational. You quickly realise that you live to work, far more than you are working to live. When you publish work that you find out has been very useful in policy debates, precipitated change or altered the way that something is talked about, it's simply gratifying.

The heart of academic life is having research questions eating away at you like musical earworms. For pure scientists, these questions can often be highly theoretical and arcane. But for me, the starting point was always wanting to pursue strategically useful research questions where I knew there was an appetite for change that could make important differences in people's lives.

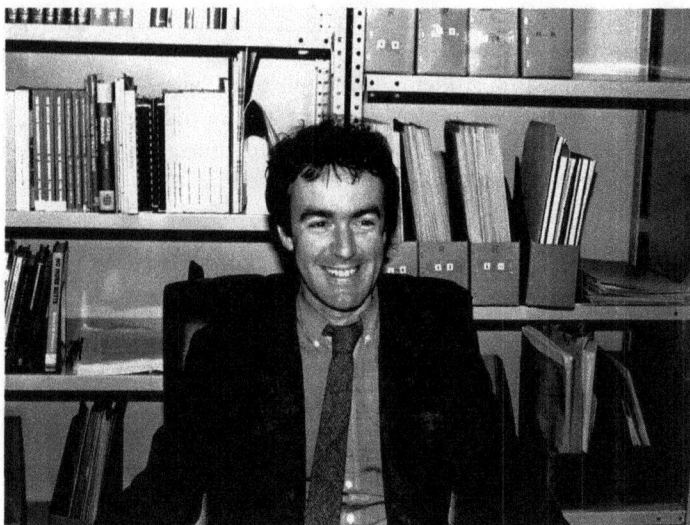

The author at 30.

When you stop drawing a salary, your curiosity about those questions does not suddenly switch off. You don't suddenly have an epiphany, as you might if you had worked in the Venetian blinds industry, that you just no longer have any interest in what you did every day for the last 40 years. But your appetite for setting out to answer these questions reduces, and so you focus only on those in which you are passionately interested and which can be researched without a team of funded colleagues. Here free data obtainable from the internet open up many possibilities.

My profile has long caused me to get many daily requests from all over the world. The most common are for reviewing others' papers, grants and book proposals. I have always subscribed to the *noblesse oblige* of reviewing others' work, just as I expect others will review mine. Regrettably, as a long-time journal editor, I know how far from universal that value is.[1]

---

1   Chapman and Hayen 2011.

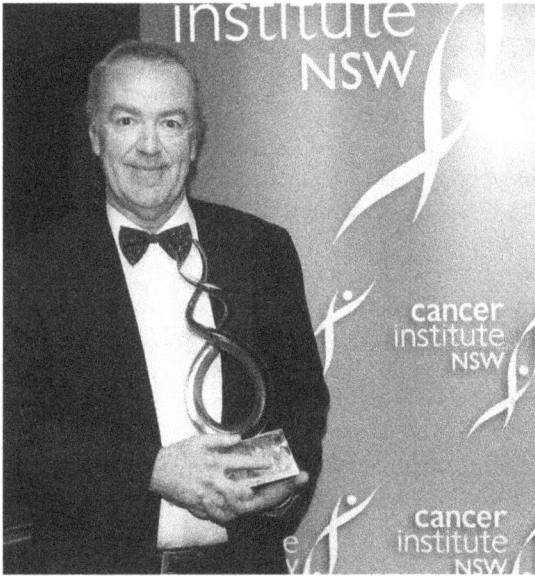

The author in 2008, receiving the NSW Cancer Institute
Award for Outstanding Cancer Researcher of the Year.

I always thought it right to review at least as many papers as I was
writing myself. Most papers you get sent are answering questions that
will make no difference to anything important, some need euthanising,
and a few are destined to be critical bricks in important knowledge
walls. So I still review, but only those that emit that early fragrance from
their abstracts.

I also get oceans of requests from school and university students
to help them with their assignments. Here are 15 questions I'd like
you to answer, says a year 11 student from Adelaide. Can I come and
interview you for a project that's due next week? Sometimes dozens of
these would pour in in a week when a thoughtless teacher or academic
presumably listed my contact details in a handout, as if I was a 24-hour
information service. I also get lengthy, breathless theses from people
wanting me to support their cause, magic potion or paradigm shifting
thoughts that are so far strangely unappreciated.

I have to admit to becoming less accommodating to these sort of requests, as I do try to pursue some pleasures I've never had time for: writing a memoir of growing up in the 1950s and '60s, reading all of Charles Dickens and re-reading Orwell, finding out what the TV series I hear others talk about are all about, and cooking.

But most days, life is not hugely different. Public health challenges are endlessly fascinating; dangerous idiocy and mendacity needs the antiseptic of strong sunlight; and younger colleagues need support and encouragement. I'm writing lots of references!

Academics traditionally have no mandatory retirement age, and some hang on for years in this era of austere academic funding, limiting promotional chances for younger staff. I had no desire to stand in the way of succession and am happy to have a continuing role at my university while releasing my salary.

I took a single sabbatical in 2006, living in Lyon in France, where after breakfast each day, I sat down in a quiet office with no phone at the International Agency for Research in Cancer, where I wrote a daily target of 2,500 words towards a book on public health advocacy.[2] I had the same experience for a month last year in the Rockefeller Centre at Bellagio on Lake Como.

Writing is my first passion, thanks to a wonderful high school English teacher. A day without any writing is a day wasted. I'm planning few wasted days for the foreseeable future. Au revoir, but not adieu.

---

2   Chapman 2008b.

Works cited

Abrams, David, Tony Axéll, Pierre Bartsch, Linda Bauld, Ron Borland et al. (2014). Statement from specialists in nicotine science and public health policy. 26 May. http://bit.ly/2cgLNsw.

Access Economics (2003). *The dementia epidemic: economic impact and positive solutions for Australia*. Canberra: Access Economics, prepared for Alzheimer's Australia. http://bit.ly/2cAW6L2.

Achey, Ted L. (1978). Product information (memo for Lorillard Research). Archived at *Truth Tobacco Industry Documents*. http://bit.ly/2cgmMMJs.

Action on Smoking and Health (n.d.). *Report on the European Consultants Programme, Covington & Burling*. http://bit.ly/2ecDFyw.

Action on Smoking and Health (1988). *Tobacco explained*, 25 June. http://bit.ly/2dwl673.

Agaku, Israel T. and Filippos T. Filippidis (2014). Prevalence, determinants and impact of unawareness about the health consequences of tobacco use among 17,929 school personnel in 29 African countries. *British Medical Journal Open* 8: e005837. http://bit.ly/2ciWNdK.

All About Science (n.d.). What is social Darwinism? http://bit.ly/2cAO4oS.

American Academy of Anti-Aging Medicine (n.d.). Accomplishments. http://bit.ly/2cwYOzg.

American Academy of Anti-Aging Medicine (2002). Official position statement on the truth about human aging. June. http://bit.ly/2cx0MiU.

Anderson, Warwick (2013). *CEO health research translation newsletter*. National Health and Medical Research Council, 20 December. http://bit.ly/2cwZOn4.

Anon (1996). Ethics of using non-traditional sources of income to fund medical and health research. *South African Medical Journal*, 86: 287.

Anon (1992). EPA: butt out of the gutters. *Herald Sun*, 4 March: 1.

Archer, Jeffery, Nicola Fotheringham, Mark Symmons and Bruce Corben (2008). The impact of lowered speed limits in urban and metropolitan areas. Monash University Accident Research Centre, January. http://bit.ly/2d0zxxV.

Arendt, Hannah (1963). *Eichmann in Jerusalem: the banality of evil.* New York: Viking.

Associated Press (2006). Mexican health minister defends tobacco record in bid for top WHO job. *International Herald Tribune*, 17 October.

Australian Competition and Consumer Commission (2005). ACCC resolves "light" and "mild" cigarette issue with BAT. and Philip Morris. 12 May. http://bit.ly/2cIOO7u.

Australian Institute of Health and Welfare (2016). Life expectancy. http://bit.ly/1Hpdhtl.

Australian Institute of Health and Welfare (2014a). *National Drugs Strategy Household Surveys (NDSHS): highlights from the 2013 survey.* Canberra: Australian Institute of Health and Wefare. 17 July. http://bit.ly/YTyEyH.

Australian Institute of Health and Welfare (2014b). *NDSHS 2013 data and references: supplementary tables.* http://bit.ly/1ma2omw.

Australian Institute of Health and Welfare (2011). *Lung cancer in Australia: an overview.* November. http://bit.ly/2cAWgCb.

Australian Institute of Health and Welfare (2008). *2007 National Drug Strategy Household Survey: first results.* April. http://bit.ly/2cgMsuf.

Australian Institute of Health and Welfare (2006). *Cancer in Australia: an overview.* Australian Institute of Health and Welfare. http://bit.ly/2d0zRwM.

Australian Institute of Health and Welfare (2005). *2004 National Drug Strategy Household Survey: detailed findings.* http://bit.ly/2d9hXrW.

Australian Institute of Health and Welfare (2004). *Australian hospital statistics 2003–2004.* Heath Service Series No. 23, AIHW Catalogue No HSE 37. http://bit.ly/2cAVQf4.

Australian Institute of Health and Welfare (2001). *The quantification of drug-caused mortality and morbidity in Australia, 1998.* http://bit.ly/2d4HCGu.

Australian Radiation Protecton and Nuclear Safety Agency (2005). *Code of practice and safety guide: radiation protection in dentistry.* Radiation Protection Series Publication No. 10. December. http://bit.ly/2cUU5cq.

Australian Radiation Protecton and Nuclear Safety Agency (2001). *Code of practice: safe transport of radioactive material.* Radiation Protection Series Publication No. 2. September. http://bit.ly/2cAXqxG.

Back, Chris (2012). Wind turbines: the untold story. Blog post. 9 July. http://bit.ly/
2dK8p6y.

Bandara, Pri (2015). Yes, smart phone and wifi radiation can be deadly! *Ayubowan Health & Lifestyle Education*. 16 June. http://bit.ly/2d0Bp9W.

Barber, K. and S. Sharrock (1994). Morgan consumer review, April–June 1994. Archived at *Truth Tobacco Industry Documents*. http://legacy.library.ucsf.edu/tid/jio32e00.

Barnard, Mike (2012). Bad day in court for anti-wind campaigner Sarah Laurie. *Renew Economy*. 27 November. http://bit.ly/2cIy55O.

Bauld, Linda, Ken Judge and Stephen Platt (2007). Assessing the impact of smoking cessation services on reducing health inequalities in England: observational study. *Tobacco Control* 16: 400–4. http://bit.ly/2cIx8ua.

Bayer, Ronald, Lawrence O. Gostin, Gail H. Javitt and Allan Brandt (2002). Tobacco advertising in the United States: a proposal for a constitutionally acceptable form of regulation. *Journal of the American Medical Association* 287(22): 2990–5.

Bell, Kirsten (2011). Legislating abjection? Secondhand smoke, tobacco control policy and the public's health. *Critical Public Health* 21: 49–62. http://bit.ly/2cUTZl5.

Bhattacharya, Ananyo (2012). Nine ways scientists demonstrate they don't understand journalism. *Guardian*. 17 January. http://bit.ly/2cwZHrv.

Biener, Lois, Rebecca L. Reimer, Melanie Wakefield, Glen Szczypka, Nancy A. Rigotti and Gregory Connolly (2006). Impact of smoking cessation aids and mass media among recent quitters. *American Journal of Preventive Medicine* 30: 217–24. http://bit.ly/2cWjRQx.

Bjartveit, Kjell and Aage Tverdal (2005). Health consequences of smoking 1–4 cigarettes per day. *Tobacco Control* 14: 315–20. http://bit.ly/2d0Bomv.

Blum, Alan (1985). If smoking killed baby seals . . . *New York State journal of medicine* 85: 282–5.

Borland, Ron, Simon Chapman, Neville Owen and David Hill (1990). Effects of a workplace smoking ban on the consumption of cigarettes. *American Journal of Public Health* 80(2): 178–80.

Borland, Ron and David Hill (1991). Public attitudes to smoke-free zones in restaurants: an update. *Medical Journal of Australia* 154: 292–3.

Borland, Ron, Hua-Hie Yong, Bill King, K. Michael Cummings, Geoffrey T. Fong, Tara Elton-Marshall, David Hammond and Ann McNeill (2004). Use of and beliefs about light cigarettes in four countries: findings from the International Tobacco Control Policy Evaluation Survey. *Nicotine and Tobacco Research* 6, supplement 3 (December): s311–21.

Borland, Ron, Hua-Hie Yong, Mohammad Siahpush, Andrew Hyland, Sharon Campbell, Gerard Hastings, K. Michael Cummings and Geoffrey T. Fong (2006). Support for and reported compliance with smoke-free restaurants and bars by smokers in four countries: findings from the International Tobacco Control (ITC) Four Country Survey. *Tobacco Control* 15, supplement 3: iii34–iii41. 10.1136/tc.2004.008748.

Bourke, Latika and Lisa Cox (2014). Philip Morris donated to Liberal Democrat senator David Leyonhjelm. *Sydney Morning Herald*. 1 October. http://bit.ly/1v5f3Gh.

Bowen, Shelley, Anthony Zwi, Peter Sainsbury and Margaret Whitehead (2009). Killer facts, policies and other influences: what evidence triggered early childhood intervention policies in Australia? *Evidence and Policy* 5(1): 5–32. http://bit.ly/2dbVfT2.

Boyse, Sharon (1988). Notes on a special meeting of the UK industry on environmental tobacco smoke. Archived at tobacco.org. http://bit.ly/2eiNXdz.

Brackenridge, Robert D.C. (1985). *Medical selection of life risks: a comprehensive guide to life expectancy for underwriters and clinicians*. London: The Nature Press.

Bradley, M. (2004). Hospitals: now doctors to blame. *Sydney Morning Herald*. 1 April.

Bray, Andrew (2013). Why Waubra residents want their town name back. *The Drum*. 7 November. http://ab.co/2cIxEbx.

Breman, Joel G., Andréa Egan and Gerald T. Keusch (2001). The intolerable burden of malaria: a new look at the numbers. *The American Journal of Tropical Medicine and Hygiene* 64(1): supplement iv–vii.

Brewer, John and Albert Hunter (1989). *Multimethod research: a synthesis of style*. London: Sage.

British American Tobacco (2015). *BAT Annual Report*. http://bit.ly/2d0BRoI.

British American Tobacco. Topline facts and figures. http://bit.ly/2cWlhKT.

Brooke-Taylor, Simon, Janis Baines, Julie Goodchap, Jim Gruber and Tracy Hambridge (2003). Reforms to food additive regulation in Australia and New Zealand. *Food Control* 14(6): 375–82. http://bit.ly/2d0B8DV.

Brose, Leonie S., Sara C. Hitchman, Jamie Brown, Robert West and Ann McNeill (2015). Is the use of electronic cigarettes while smoking associated with smoking cessation attempts, cessation and reduced cigarette consumption? A survey with a one-year follow-up. *Addiction* 110(7): 1160–8. http://bit.ly/1jQTwCb.

Brown and Williamson (1984). Health hazards. Archived at *Truth Tobacco Industry Documents*. http://bit.ly/2cRHokd.

Brown, Jamie, Emma Beard, Daniel Kotz, Susan Michie and Robert West (2014). Real-world effectiveness of e-cigarettes when used to aid smoking cessation: a cross-sectional population study. *Addiction* 109: 1531–40. http://bit.ly/2d9gYrY.

Brownson, Ross, Jian Chang and James Davis (1991). Cigarette smoking and risk of adult leukemia. *American Journal of Epidemiology*, 134: 938–41. http://bit.ly/2d9gnq4.

Callahan, Daniel (1998). False hopes: why America's quest for perfect health is a recipe for failure. New York: Simon & Schuster.

Cancer Council Australia (2015). Clinical practice guidelines PSA testing and early management of test-detected prostate cancer. http://bit.ly/2gdPi5m.

Cancer Council NSW (2014). Mobile phones do not cause brain cancer. http://bit.ly/2cB1rC5.

Cardinale, Alessio, Candida Nastrucci, Alfredo Cesario and Patrizia Russo (2012). Nicotine: specific role in angiogenesis, proliferation and apoptosis. *Critical Reviews in Toxicology* 42: 68–89. http://bit.ly/2cUSZ0r.

Carter, Stacy M. and Simon Chapman (2006). Smokers and nonsmokers talk about regulatory options in tobacco control. *Tobacco Control* 15: 399–404. http://bit.ly/2d0ASoq.

Champion, David and Simon Chapman (2005). Framing pub smoking bans: an analysis of Australian print news media coverage, March 1996–March 2003. *Journal of Epidemiology and Community Health* 59: 679–84.

Channel 4 News (2000). Special reports: dealing with killer industries, studio discussion. 5 December. http://bit.ly/2ciVEDf.

Chapman, Simon (2016a). Symptoms, diseases and aberrant behaviours attributed to wind turbine exposure. Sydney eScholarship Repository: Research Papers and Publications, Public Health. First published 8 June 2015; updated 20 March 2016. http://bit.ly/2cRHWGZ.

Chapman, Simon (2016b). Ten myths about smoking that will not die. *The Conversation*, 10 March. http://bit.ly/1RgEeph.

Chapman, Simon (2015a). Are today's smokers really more "hardened"? *The Conversation*, 14 October. http://bit.ly/2cAXDAP.

Chapman, Simon (2015b). Big Tobacco: "Of all the concerns, there is one – taxation – which alarms us the most". *The Conversation*, 12 November. http://bit.ly/2cAY1zq.

Chapman, Simon (2015c). Smoking: new Australian data to die (or live) for. *The Conversation*, 24 February. http://bit.ly/2cIyCEX.

Chapman, Simon (2015d). With a little help from his friends . . . Joe Cocker's early death. *The Conversation*, 5 January. http://bit.ly/2dbV1v5.

Chapman, Simon (2014a). Beyond statistics: the hidden face of smoking-related cancer. *The Conversation*, 20 January. http://bit.ly/2cUUCet.

Chapman, Simon (2014b). Factoid forensics: have more than 40 Australian families abandoned their homes because of wind farm noise? *Noise and Health* 16(71): 208–12. http://bit.ly/2cAXSMm.

Chapman, Simon (2013a). How Santa and the Tooth Fairy collaborated to allow smoking at Barangaroo. *Sydney Morning Herald*, 29 November. http://bit.ly/2cIy1CQ.

Chapman, Simon (2013b). One hundred and fifty ways the nanny state is good for us. *The Conversation*, 2 July. http://bit.ly/2cLcpCX.

Chapman, Simon (2013c [1998]). *Over our dead bodies: Port Arthur and Australia's fight for gun control*. Sydney: Sydney University Press.

Chapman, Simon (2011). Should the spectacle of surgery be sold to the highest bidder? *British Medical Journal* 342:d237. http://bit.ly/2d9ieLB.

Chapman, Simon (2010). Is the health conference industry exploiting the public sector? *Crikey*, 30 April. http://bit.ly/2cIyKnV.

Chapman, Simon (2009). The inverse impact law of smoking cessation. *The Lancet* 373: 701–3. http://bit.ly/2d4H4jZ.

Chapman, Simon (2008a). Going too far? Exploring the limits of smoking regulations. *William Mitchell Law Review* 34(4): 1605–20.

Chapman, Simon (2008b). *Public health advocacy and tobacco control: making smoking history*. Blackwell Publishing.

Chapman, Simon (2008c). Should smoking in outside public spaces be banned? No. *British Medical Jounral* 337: a2804.

Chapman, Simon (2008d). What should be done about smoking in movies? *Tobacco Control* 17: 363–7. http://bit.ly/2cAQnYS.

Chapman, Simon (2000). Banning smoking outdoors is seldom ethically justified. *Tobacco Control* 9: 95–7.

Chapman, Simon (1995). *The last right? Australians take sides on the right to die*. Port Melbourne, Vic.: Mandarin Books. http://bit.ly/2dbWf9D.

Chapman, Simon (1993). Unravelling gossamer with boxing gloves: problems in explaining the decline in smoking. *British Medical Journal* 307: 429–32. http://bit.ly/2d4H2Za.

Chapman, Simon (1992a). Anatomy of a campaign: the attempt to defeat the NSW Tobacco Advertising Prohibition Bill 1991. *Tobacco Control* 1: 50–6. http://bit.ly/2ciVCet.

Chapman, Simon (1992b). Dogma disputed: potential endemic heterosexual transmission of human immunodeficiency virus in Australia. *Australian Journal of Public Health* 16: 128–41.

Chapman, Simon (1992c). Share accommodation – non-smokers wanted! *Tobacco Control* 4: 248.

Chapman, Simon (1992d). Smoking in the workplace. *The Lancet* 339: 1614.

Chapman, Simon (1989a). On the limitations of econometric analysis in cigarette advertising studies. *British Journal of Addiction* 84: 1267–77. http://bit.ly/2cARlEw.

Chapman, Simon (1989b). The news on smoking: editorial coverage of tobacco and health issues in Australian newspapers, 1987/88. *American Journal of Public Health* 79: 1419–20.

Chapman, Simon (1983). The smokescreen on tobacco advertising. *Sydney Morning Herald*, 7 July.

Chapman, Simon (1985). Stop-smoking clinics: a case for their abandonment. *The Lancet* 325(8434): 918–20.

Chapman, Simon (1980). A David and Goliath story: tobacco advertising and self-regulation in Australia. *British Medical Journal* 281(6249): 1187–90.

Chapman, Simon (1976). Psychotropic drug use in the elderly. *Medical Journal of Australia* 2: 62–4.

Chapman, Simon, Philip Alpers, Kingsley Agho and Mike Jones (2006). Australia's 1996 gun law reforms: faster falls in firearm deaths, firearm suicides, and a decade without mass shootings. *Injury prevention* 12(6): 365–72. http://bit.ly/29xuyrz.

Chapman, Simon, Lamiae Azizia, Qingwei Luoa, and Freddy Sitasa (2016). Has the incidence of brain cancer risen in Australia since the introduction of mobile phones 29 years ago? *Cancer Epidemiology*, 5 May. http://bit.ly/2cAQKmj.

Chapman, Simon and Antony Balmain (2004). Time to legislate for fire-safe cigarettes in Australia. *Medical Journal of Australia* 181: 292–3. http://bit.ly/2dbVihN.

Chapman, Simon, Alexandra Barratt and Martin Stockler (2010). *Let sleeping dogs lie? What men should know before getting tested for prostate cancer*. Sydney: Sydney University Press.

Chapman, Simon and M. Bloch (1992). Policy research: strategic directions. *Tobacco Control* 1 (Supplement): s2–3.

Chapman, Simon, Ron Borland, Ross Brownson, Michelle Scollo, Amanda Dominello and Stephen Woodward (1999). The impact of workplace smoking bans on declining cigarette consumption in Australia and the USA. *American Journal of Public Health* 89: 1018–23. http://bit.ly/2cgO3jH.

Chapman, Simon, Ron Borland, David Hill, Neville Owen and Stephen Woodward (1990). Why the tobacco industry fears the passive smoking issue. *International Journal of Health Services* 20(3): 417–27. http://bit.ly/2cIy8hN.

Smoke Signals

Chapman, Simon and Ronald M. Davis (1997). Smoking in movies: is it a problem? *Tobacco Control* 6(4): 269–71. http://bit.ly/2d9jo9O.

Chapman, Simon and Becky Freeman (2014). *Removing the emperor's clothes: Australia's plain tobacco packaging.* Sydney: Sydney University Press.

Chapman, Simon and Becky Freeman (2010). The cancer emperor's new clothes: Australia's historic legislation for plain tobacco packaging. *British Medical Journal* 340: c2436. http://bit.ly/2dbVuNR.

Chapman, Simon and Becky Freeman (2009). Regulating the tobacco retail environment: beyond reducing sales to minors. *Tobacco Control* 18: 496–501. http://bit.ly/2cLhk6T.

Chapman, Simon and Becky Freeman (2008). Markers of the denormalisation of smoking and the tobacco industry. *Tobacco Control* 17: 25–31.

Chapman, Simon, Abby Haynes, Gemma Derrick, Heidi Sturk, Wayne Hall and Alexis St George (2014). Reaching "an audience that you would never dream of speaking to": influential public health researchers' views on the role of news media in influencing policy and public understanding. *Journal of Health Communication* 19(2): 260–73.

Chapman, Simon and Andrew Hayen (2011). Reviewer refusal rates for 300,866 requested reviews in 20 BMJ Group journals. School of Public Health, University of Sydney. http://bit.ly/2cAYeTc.

Chapman, Simon, Simon Holding, Jessica Ellerm, Rachel Heenan, Andrea Fogarty, Michelle Imison, Ross McKenzie and Kevin McGeechan (2009). The content and structure of Australian TV reportage on health and medicine: a guide for health workers. *The Medical Journal of Australia*, 191: 620–4. http://bit.ly/2cwZPHq.

Chapman, Simon, Quentin Jones, Adrian Bauman and Martin Palin (1995). Incidental depiction of cigarettes and smoking in Australian magazines, 1990–1993. *Australian Journal of Public Health*, 19: 313–5. http://bit.ly/2d0CheH.

Chapman, Simon and Julie Leask (2001). Paid celebrity endorsement in health promotion: a case study. *Health Promotion International* 16: 333–38. http://bit.ly/2d4HQxb.

Chapman, Simon and Jonathan Liberman (2005). Ensuring smokers are adequately informed: reflections on consumer rights, manufacturer responsibilities, and policy implications. *Tobacco Control* 14 (Supplement ii): sii8–sii13. http://bit.ly/2cUVD6p.

Chapman, Simon and Deborah Lupton (1994). *The fight for public health: principles and practice of media advocacy.* London: British Medical Journal Books.

Chapman, Simon and Bernie Mackay (1984). Good for the goose, good for the gander: complaints and judgements about smoking and anti-smoking advertisements under advertising self regulation. *Media Information Australia* 31: 47–55.

Chapman, Simon and Ross MacKenzie (2010). The global research neglect of unassisted smoking cessation: causes and consequences. *PLoS Medicine* 7(2): e1000216. http://bit.ly/2cIRrpz.

Chapman, Simon, Sophie McCarthy and Deborah Lupton (1995). Very good punter-speak. How journalists frame the news on public health. Research Monograph No. 1, Centre for Health Advocacy and Media Research. August. http://bit.ly/2cAQT9w.

Chapman, Simon, Kim McLeod, Melanie Wakefield and Simon Holding (2005). Impact of news of celebrity illness on breast cancer screening: Kylie Minogue's breast cancer diagnosis. *The Medical Journal of Australia* 83: 247–50. http://bit.ly/2cIywgq.

Chapman, Simon, Mark Ragg and Kevin McGeechan (2009). Citation bias in reported smoking prevalence in people with schizophrenia. *Australian and New Zealand Journal of Psychiatry* 43(3): 277–82. http://bit.ly/2cnOgoh.

Chapman, Simon and Juliet Richters (1994). A shattering of glass in Tasmania. *Sydney Morning Herald*, 31 August.

Chapman, Simon and W.N. Schofield (1998). Lifesavers and Samaritans: emergency use of cellular (mobile) phones in Australia. *Accident Analysis and Prevention* 30(6): 815–9. http://bit.ly/2cLhET6.

Chapman, Simon and Stan Shatenstein (2001). The ethics of the cash register: taking tobacco industry research dollars. *Tobacco Control* 10: 1–2. http://bit.ly/2cnPFLH.

Chapman, Simon and Teresa Simonetti (2015). Summary of main conclusions reached in 25 reviews of the research literature on wind farms and health. *Research Papers and Publications. Public Health.* Last updated 10 April 2015. http://bit.ly/2cnPqjT.

Chapman, Simon, Alexis St George, Karen Waller and Vince Cakic (2013). The pattern of complaints about Australian wind farms does not match the establishment and distribution of turbines: support for the psychogenic, "communicated disease" hypothesis. *PLoS one*, 8(10): e76584. http://bit.ly/2dbVzBt.

Chapman, Simon and Stephen Woodward (1993). Australian court decision on passive smoking upheld at appeal. *British Medical Journal* 306: 120–2. http://bit.ly/2cWl1LM.

Chapman, Simon and Sonia Wutzke (1997). Not in our back yard: media coverage of community opposition to mobile phone towers – an application of

Sandman's outrage model of risk perception. *Australian and New Zealand Journal of Public Health* 21(6): 614–20. http://bit.ly/2cWlqxG.

Chen, Xinguang, Jennifer B Unger, Paula Palmer, Michelle D. Weiner, Carl Anderson Johnson, Mamie M. Wong and Greg Austin (2002). Prior cigarette smoking initiation predicting current alcohol use: evidence for a gateway drug effect among California adolescents from eleven ethnic groups. *Addictive Behaviors* 27: 799–817. http://bit.ly/2cIR8eI.

Chesterfield-Evans, Arthur (1992). Test case for passive smoking. *British Medical Journal* 304: 1529.

Chiena, Hung-Yu, Jinn-Ke Jana and Yuh-Min Tseng (2002). An efficient and practical solution to remote authentication: smart card. *Computers and Security* 21: 372–5. http://bit.ly/2d9iwlT.

Clarke, Sarah (2011). Wind sickness doctor fronts Senate inquiry. *ABC News*, 25 March. http://ab.co/2cIQwFY.

Clennell, Andrew (2012). A ban on sunbeds in NSW from 2014. *Daily Telegraph*, 4 February. http://bit.ly/2cLhAmc.

Colebatch, Tim (2013). How mistaken identity and luck won on the day. *Sydney Morning Herald*, 5 October. http://bit.ly/2cUVQ9A.

Colley J.R., Holland Walter, Corkhill RT (1974). Influence of passive smoking and parental phlegm on pneumonia and bronchitis in early childhood. *Lancet*, 2(7888): 1031–4.

Connolly, Gregory and Hillel R. Alpert (2013). Has the tobacco industry evaded the FDA's ban on "Light" cigarette descriptors? *Tobacco Control* 2013. http://bit.ly/2cIA3D9.

Coory, D Michael (2004). Ageing and healthcare costs in Australia: a case of policy based evidence? *The Medicine Journal of Australia* 180: 581–3. http://bit.ly/2cRIs7V.

County of Los Angeles v. R.J. Reynolds Tobacco Company et al. [1996]. http://bit.ly/2cAZcPa.

Crichton, Fiona, Simon Chapman, Tim Cundy and Keith J Petrie (2014). The link between health complaints and wind turbines: support for the nocebo expectations hypothesis. *Frontiers in Public Health*, 11 November. http://bit.ly/2d9hiHh.

Dalton, Madeline A., James D. Sargent, Michael L. Beach, Linda Titus-Ernstoff, Jennifer J. Gibson, M. Bridget Ahrens, Jennifer J. Tickle and Todd F. Heatherton (2003). Effect of viewing smoking in movies on adolescent smoking initiation: a cohort study. *The Lancet* 362: 281–5. http://bit.ly/2d9jgrf.

Daube, Mike, Julia Stafford and Bond Laura (2008). No need for nanny. *Tobacco Control* 17(6): 426–7. http://bit.ly/2cLhDhY.

Davison, Mark (2011). Plain packaging bill to extinguish some tobacco trade marks. *The Drum*, 15 April. http://ab.co/2d0DHGg.

Day, Bob (2015). Wind turbines' inconvenient truth. Blog post. 30 April. http://bit.ly/2ciXO5B.

Department of Community Services and Health (1990). *Tobacco in Australia: a summary of related statistics.* Canberra: Australian Government Publishing Service.

Department of Finance and Deregulation (2013). *Campaign advertising by Australian government departments and agencies: half-year report.* http://bit.ly/2dX73XK.

Department of Health (2016). Introduction of tobacco plain packaging in Australia. 27 May. http://bit.ly/1nWpFFg.

Department of Infrastructure and Transport (2010). *Final regulation impact statement for review of Euro 5/6 light vehicle emissions standards.* http://bit.ly/2cWmQZ3.

Department of Trade and Industry (UK) (2000). Buyers announces investigation into British American Tobacco PLC. 30 October. http://bit.ly/2d0DT8n/

DiClemente, Carlo C. and James O. Prochaska (1982). Self-change and therapy change of smoking behaviour: a comparison of processes of change in smoking and maintainance, *Addictive Behaviours* 7: 133–142.

Doll, Richard, Richard Peto, Jillian Boreham and Isabelle Sutherland (2004). Mortality in relation to smoking: 50 years' observations on male British doctors. *British Medical Journal* 328: 1519. http://bit.ly/2cLiyPq.

Doran, Christopher M., Lisa Valenti, Maxine Robinson,Helena Britt and Richard P. Mattick (2006). Smoking status of Australian general practice patients and their attempts to quit. *Addictive Behaviors* 31: 758–66. http://bit.ly/2d4KaEv.

DuRant, Robert H., Ellen Rome, Michael Rich, Elizabeth Allred, Jean Emans and Elizabeth R. Woods (1997). Tobacco and alcohol use behaviors portrayed in music videos: a content analysis. *American Journal of Public Health* 87: 1131–5. http://bit.ly/2cAZl5q.

Egger, Garry, W. Fitzgerald, G. Frape, A. Monaem, P. Rubinstein, C. Tyler and B. McKay (1983). Results of a large scale media antismoking campaign in Australia: North Coast 'Quit for Life' programme. *British Medical Journal* 287: 1125–8. http://bit.ly/2d4I4Ew.

Elvik, Rune (1999). Can injury prevention efforts go too far? Reflections on some possible implications of Vision Zero for road accident fatalities. *Accident Analysis and Prevention* 31: 265–86.

Environmental Health Branch of the Public and Environmental Health Service, South Australian Health Commission (1995). *Waste control systems: standard for the construction, installation and operation of septic tank systems in South Australia*. March. http://bit.ly/2d0D2Vn.

EPR Expert Reference Group (2015). *Report on the implementation of the New South Wales Extended Producer Responsibility Priority Statement 2004*. Department of Environment and Conservation, New South Wales. http://bit.ly/2cWmYrN.

Etter, Jean-François and Chris Bullen (2014). A longitudinal study of electronic cigarette users. *Addictive Behaviors* 39: 491–4. http://bit.ly/2cAZNjT.

Etter, Jean-François and Chris Bullen (2011). Electronic cigarette: users profile, utilization, satisfaction and perceived efficacy. *Addiction* 106(11): 2017–28. http://bit.ly/2d4JoaG.

Environment Protection Authority (2005). EPA guidelines for responsible pesticide use. http://bit.ly/2cx1NaS.

Fairclough, Gordon (2001a). Philip Morris apologizes for report touting benefits of smokers' deaths. *Wall Street Journal*, 26 July. http://on.wsj.com/2d4JRd0.

Fairclough, Gordon (2001b). Smoking can help Czech economy, Philip Morris-Little report says. *Wall Street Jounral*, 16 July. http://on.wsj.com/2cISCp2.

Farrelly, Matthew C., Kian Kamyab, James Nonnemaker, Erik Crankshaw and Jane A. Allen (2011). Movie smoking and youth initiation: parsing smoking imagery and other adult content. *PloS One* 7(12): e51935. http://bit.ly/2cRJH6S.

Farsalinos, Konstantinos E., Giorgio Romagna, Dimitris Tsiapras, Stamatis Kyrzopoulos and Vassilis Voudris (2014). Characteristics, perceived side effects and benefits of electronic cigarette use: a worldwide survey of more than 19,000 consumers. *International Journal of Environmental Research and Public Health* 11: 4356–73. http://bit.ly/2ciWv6I.

Fernándeza, Esteve, Alessandra Lugod, Luke Clancye, Keitaro Matsuof, Carlo La Vecchiad and Silvano Gallusg (2015). Smoking dependence in 18 European countries: hard to maintain the hardening hypothesis. *Preventive Medicine* 81: 314–9. http://bit.ly/2dbWyBo.

Fiore, Michael C., Thomas E. Novotny, John P. Pierce, Gary A. Giovino, Evridiki J. Hatziandreu, Polly A. Newcomb, Tanya S. Surawicz and Ronald M. Davis (1990). Methods used to quit smoking in the United States. *Journal of the American Medical Association* 263: 2760–5. http://bit.ly/2cAScFd.

Flavor and Extract Manufacturers Association of the United States (2012). *Respiratory health and safety in the flavor manufacturing workplace – 2012 update*. http://bit.ly/2cAZ02D.

Follman, Mark, Gavin Aronsen and Deanna Pan (2016). A guide to mass shootings in America. *Mother Jones*, 18 April. http://bit.ly/U4gk4x.

Fogarty, Andrea and Simon Chapman (2013). What should be done about policy on alcohol pricing and promotions? Australian experts' views of policy priorities: a qualitative interview study. *Biomed Central Public Health* 13: 610.

Fong, Geoffrey T., David Hammond, Fritz L. Laux, Mark P. Zanna, K. Michael Cummings, Ron Borland and Hana Ross (2004). The near-universal experience of regret among smokers in four countries: findings from the International Tobacco Control Policy Evaluation Survey. *Nicotine and Tobacco Research* 6 (supplement 3): s341–51. http://bit.ly/2cgOjip.

Freeman, Becky and Simon Chapman (2007a). Is "YouTube" telling or selling you something? Tobacco content on the YouTube video-sharing website. *Tobacco Control* 16: 207–10. http://bit.ly/2cnPC2z.

Freeman, Becky and Simon Chapman (2007b). Tobacco promotion invades new media. *Lancet Oncology* 8: 973–4. http://bit.ly/2ciWEHB.

Friedman, Lissy (2007). Philip Morris's website and television commercials use new language to mislead the public into believing it has changed its stance on smoking and disease. *Tobacco Control* 16: e9.

Frost, David (2014). Tackling alcohol misuse effectively. Scotch Whisky Association. 12 August. http://bit.ly/2cIAkWL.

Fuoco, Fernanda Carmen, Giorgio Buonanno, Luca Stabile and Paolo Vigo (2014). Influential parameters on particle concentration and size distribution in the mainstream of e-cigarettes. *Environmental Pollution* 184: 523–9. http://bit.ly/2ciXiEJ.

Garfinkel, Harold (1967). *Studies in ethnomethodology.* Englewood Cliffs, NJ: Prentice Hall.

Geertz, Clifford (1973). *The interpretation of culture.* New York: Basic Books.

Gilpin, Elizabeth, John Pierce, Jerry Goodman, David Burns and Donald Shopland (1992). Reasons smokers give for stopping smoking: do they relate to success in stopping? *Tobacco Control* 1: 256–63. http://bit.ly/2cnQSmq.

Giovino G.A., F.J. Chaloupka, A.M. Hartman et al. (2009). *Cigarette smoking prevalence and policies in the 50 states: an era of change—the Robert Wood Johnson Foundation ImpacTeen Tobacco Chartbook.* Buffalo: University at Buffalo, State University of New York.

Glantz, Stanton (2014). 122 public health and medical authorities from 31 countries write WHO DG Chan urging evidence-based approach to ecigs. Centre for Tobacco Control Research and Education, 16 June. http://bit.ly/2cgPwq3.

Greenhalgh, E.M., M. Bayly, and M.H. Winstanley (2015). *Tobacco in Australia, facts and issues: a comprehensive online resource.* Melbourne: Cancer Council Victoria. http://bit.ly/2d0Exmj.

Gostin, Lawrence O. (2002). Corporate speech and the Constitution: the deregulation of tobacco advertising. *American Journal of Public Health*, 92(3): 352–5. http://bit.ly/2cUX8Bo.

Grando, Sergei A (2014). Connections of nicotine to cancer. *Nature Reviews Cancer* 14: 419–29.

Gray, Nigel and Michael Daube (1980). *Guidelines for smoking control.* 2nd Edition. Geneva: International Union Against Cancer.

Haines, Ian (2014). Four reasons I won't have a prostate cancer blood test. *The Conversation*, 5 December. http://bit.ly/1vwfzeM.

Hall, Nina, Peta Ashworth and Hylton Shaw (2012). *Exploring community acceptance of rural wind farms in Australia: a snapshot.* Canberra: CSIRO. http://bit.ly/2ehWH80.

Hart, Carole, Laurence Gruer and Linda Bauld (2013). Does smoking reduction in midlife reduce mortality risk? Results of 2 long-term prospective cohort studies of men and women in Scotland. *American Journal of Epidemiology* 178: 770–9. http://bit.ly/2cRKJjr.

Hart, Julian T. (1971). The inverse care law. *The Lancet* 1: 405–12. http://bit.ly/2cAZl5j.

Hatsukami, Dorothy K., Lindsay F. Stead and Prakash C. Gupta (2008). Tobacco addiction. *The Lancet*, 371: 2027–38. http://bit.ly/2cgPhvb.

Haynes, Abby, Gemma Derrick, Redman Sally, Wayne Hall, James Gillespie, Simon Chapman and Heidi Sturk (2012). Identifying trustworthy experts: how do policymakers find and assess public health researchers worth consulting or collaborating with? *PloS One*, 7(3):e32665. http://bit.ly/2d9j9vv.

Haynes, Abby, Gemma Derrick, Simon Chapman, James Gillespie, Sally Redman, Wayne Hall and Heidi Sturk (2011a). Galvanisers, guides, champions and shields: the many ways that policymakers use public health researchers. *Milbank Quarterly* 89: 564–98. http://bit.ly/2dbY3Q1.

Haynes, Abby, Gemma Derrick, Simon Chapman, Sally Redman, Wayne Hall, James Gillespie and Heidi Sturk (2011b). From "our world" to the "real world": exploring the behavior of policy influential Australian public health researchers. *Social Science and Medicine* 72: 1047–55. http://bit.ly/2cUYKuM.

Health Care Complaints Commission NSW (2003). Investigation report: Campbelltown and Camden Hospitals, Macarthur Health Service. December.

Hill, David, Simon Chapman and Robert Donovan (1998). The return of scare tactics. *Tobacco Control* 7: 5–8. http://bit.ly/2cnQIvn.

Hill, David, Victoria White and Nigel Gray (1991). Australian patterns of tobacco smoking in 1989. *Medical Journal of Australia* 154: 788–9.

Hill, David, Victoria White, R.M. Williams and G.J. Gardner (1993). Tobacco and alcohol use among Australian secondary schoolchildren in 1990. *Medical Journal of Australia* 158(4): 228–33.

Hiscock J (2008). O for obesity at the snack bar. *National Post* (Canada). 16 August.

History.com (2009). Federal legislation makes airbags mandatory. http://bit.ly/1dENnzu.

Hitchman, Sara C., Leonie S. Brose, Jamie Brown, Debbie Robson and Ann McNeill (2015). Associations between e-cigarette type, frequency of use, and quitting smoking: findings from a longitudinal online panel survey in Great Britain. *Nicotine and Tobacco Research* 17(10): 1187–94. http://bit.ly/2dbXsOp.

Hoek, Janet, Ninya Maubach, Rachel Stevenson, Philip Gendall and Richard Edwards (2011). Social smokers' management of conflicted identities. *Tobacco Control* 10. 1136/tobaccocontrol-2011-050176.

Horn, D. (1978). Who is quitting – and why. In J.L. Schwartz (ed.), *Progress in smoking cessation: proceedings of International Conference on Smoking Cessation*. New York: American Cancer Society.

Horovitz, Bruce (2005). NFL strives to ensure superclean Super Bowl. *USA Today*, 4 February. http://usat.ly/2cgPgHw.

Hudson, Phillip (2016). Federal election 2016: voters put their faith in Shorten to handle health. *Australian*, 24 May. http://bit.ly/2dZIx8e.

Hughes, John R (1999). Comorbidity and smoking. *Nicotine and Tobacco Research* 1 (Supplement 2): s149–S152. http://bit.ly/2cAUh3U.

Hughes, John R. and Matthew J. Carpenter (2006). Does smoking reduction increase future cessation and decrease disease risk? A qualitative review. *Nicotine and Tobacco Research* 8: 739–49. http://bit.ly/2cIREZU.

Hughes, John R., Josue Keely and Shelley Naud (2004). Shape of the relapse curve and long-term abstinence among untreated smokers. *Addiction* 99: 29–38.

Hyland, Andrew, Ron Borland, Li Qiang, Hua-Hie Yong, McNeill Ann, Geoffrey T. Fong, Richard J. O'Connor and K. Michael Cummings (2006). Individual-level predictors of cessation behaviours among participants in the International Tobacco Control (ITC) Four Country Survey. Tobacco Control 15: iii83–iii94. http://bit.ly/2cx2ssO.

Hyland, Andrew, Qiang Li, Joseph E. Bauer, Gary A. Giovino, Craig Steger and K. Michael Cummings (2004). Predictors of cessation in a cohort of current and former smokers followed over 13 years. *Nicotine and Tobacco Research* 6 (Supplement 3): s363–69. http://bit.ly/2cx2pNI.

Iacobucci, Gareth (2014). WHO calls for ban on e-cigarette use indoors. *British Medical Journal* 349: g5335. http://bit.ly/2d9kEKb.

Illich, Ivan (1977). *Disabling professions*. London: Marion Boyars.

International Consortium of Investigative Journalists (2000a). Major tobacco multinational implicated in cigarette smuggling, tax evasion, documents show. 31 January. http://bit.ly/2d4K1ky.

International Consortium of Investigative Journalists (2000b). Global reach of tobacco company's involvement in cigarette smuggling exposed in company papers. 2 February. http://bit.ly/2cIAZqX.

Interview with Carl Seltzer (1979). Smoking does not cause heart disease and drinking in moderation actually reduces it (transcript). Channel 0 News (Australia), 4 May. Bates no. LOR03753962/3964.

Jackson, Christine, Jane D. Brown and Kelly L. L'Engle (2007). R-rated movies, bedroom televisions, and initiation of smoking by white and black adolescents. *Archives of Pediatrics and Adolescent Medicine* 161(3): 260–8. http://bit.ly/2d9k6nD.

Jamieson, Patrick E. and Dan Romer (2010). Trends in US movie tobacco portrayal since 1950: a historical analysis. *Tobacco Control* 19: 179–84. http://bit.ly/2cICrcS.

Jankowski, Nicholas W. and Fred Wester (1991). The qualitative tradition in social science inquiry: contributions of mass communications research. In Nicholas W. Jankowski and Klaus Bruhn Jensen (eds), *A handbook of qualitative methodologies for mass communication research*. London: Routledge.

Jick, Todd D. (1979). Mixing qualitative and quantitative methods: triangulation in action. *Administrative Science Quarterly* 24: 602–11. http://bit.ly/2cUXFDz.

Jong, Kathy et al. (2002). *Remoteness and cancer incidence, mortality and survival in New South Wales 1992 to 1996*. NSW Cancer Council. http://bit.ly/2cATqAq.

Joossens, Luk and Martin Raw (2008). Progress in combatting cigarette smuggling: controlling the supply chain. *Tobacco Control* 17: 399–404. http://bit.ly/2d9k0MS.

Keane, Sandi (2012). The Landscape Guardians and the Waubra Foundation. *Independent Australia*, 6 March. http://bit.ly/2dbXu98.

Keferl, Michael (2009). Taspo fail – Japanese reject scarlet letter of smoking. *Japan Trends*, 19 May. http://bit.ly/2cUWuE0.

Kelaher, Margaret, Jennifer Cawson, Julie Miller, Anne Kavanagh, David Dunt and David M. Studdert (2008). Use of breast cancer screening and treatment services by Australian women aged 25–44 years following Kylie Minogue's breast cancer diagnosis. *International Journal of Epidemiology* 37: 1326–32. http://bit.ly/2cAU6FW.

Kendell, Chris (2014). The battle for the electronic cigarette market. *Vaping 360*, 12 September. http://bit.ly/2cnQzYQ.

Khamsi R (2005). Cervical cancer vaccine proves effective. *Nature*, 10 October. http://go.nature.com/2cAUGTY.

Khoo, Deborah, Yvonne Chiam, Priscilla Ng, A. Jon Berrick and H.N. Koong (2010). Phasing out tobacco: proposal to deny access to tobacco for those born from 2000. *Tobacco Control* 19: 355–60. http://bit.ly/2cgT9fy.

King, Hobart (n.d.). REE – rare earth elements and their uses. *Geology*. http://bit.ly/1mJ36Gj.

Kloeden, C.N., A.J. McLean, V.M. Moore, and G. Ponte (1997). Travelling speed and the risk of crash involvement. NHMRC Road Accident Research Unit, University of Adelaide. http://bit.ly/2dpoWeR.

Klein, Richard (1993). *Cigarettes are sublime*. Durham: Duke University Press.

Knight, Jennifer and Simon Chapman (2004). A phony way to show sincerity, as we all well know: tobacco industry lobbying against tobacco control in Hong Kong. *Tobacco Control* 13 (Supplement 2): s13–21. http://bit.ly/2d4KQJZ.

Knopik, W. (1980). Memorandum to W. Kloepfer (Tobacco Institute, USA). 9 September. Bates no. TIMN 0107822/7823.

Koop, Everett C. (2001). Press conference remarks at the launch of NCI Monograph 13, *Risks associated with smoking cigarettes with low machine-measured yields of tar and nicotine*. Washington DC, 23 November. http://bit.ly/2d4KNy5.

Kotz, Daniel, Jamie Brown and Robert West (2014). Prospective cohort study of the effectiveness of smoking cessation treatments used in the "real world". *Mayo Clinic Proceedings* 89(10): 1360–7. http://mayocl.in/2d9jwpP.

Krasnegor, Norman A. (1979). *Cigarette smoking as a dependence process*. National Institute on Drug Abuse. Research Monograph Series 23. http://bit.ly/2cWnG8p.

Kremer, William (2013). E-cigarettes: is a smoking alternative being choked by regulation? *BBC News*, 6 July. http://bbc.in/2cWnsOk.

Kroezen, Marieke, Anneke L. Francke, Peter P. Groenewegen and Liset van Dijk (2012). Nurse prescribing of medicines in Western European and Anglo-Saxon countries: a survey on forces, conditions and jurisdictional control. *International Journal of Nursing Studies* 49(8): 1002–12. http://bit.ly/2cRL2uF.

Lakoff, George (2004). *Don't think of an elephant: know your values and frame the debate*. Vermont: Chelsea Green Publishing.

Laurance, Jeremy (2007). Unveiled: radical prescription for our health crisis. *Independent*, 23 October. http://ind.pn/2d0GgYM.

Laurie, Sarah (2012). Letter to Brad Hazzard. Republished at Wind-watch.org. 24 September. http://docs.wind-watch.org/Laurie-Collector.pdf.

LeGrande, Julian and Divya Srivastva (2009). *Incentives for prevention. Health England report no. 3.* Oxford: Health England. http://bit.ly/2ciXwMf.

Lehrer, T. (1978). Cessation of smoking in clinics the problem of relapse and the "quasi-sick role". In Schwartz JL, (ed.) *Progress in Smoking Cessation: International Conference on Smoking Cessation.* New York: American Cancer Society.

Le Strat, Yann, Jürgen Rehm and Bernard Le Foll (2011). How generalisable to community samples are clinical trial results for treatment of nicotine dependence: a comparison of common eligibility criteria with respondents of a large representative general population survey. *Tobacco Control* 20: 338–43. http://bit.ly/2cx3wgn.

Levin, Myron (2013). Remember when Big Tobacco sold asbestos as the "greatest health protection"? *Mother Jones*, 22 October. http://bit.ly/2cRLx7T.

Levitt, E.E. (1983). Smoking withdrawal: an evaluation of its role in the total effort to eliminate smoking. Paper presented to the 5th World Conference on Smoking and Health, Winnipeg, July 10–15.

Licht, Andrea S, Andrew Hyland, Mark J. Travers and Simon Chapman (2013). Secondhand smoke exposure levels in outdoor hospitality venues: a qualitative and quantitative review of the research literature. *Tobacco Control* 22(3): 172–9. http://bit.ly/2d9lkiD.

Lichtenstein, Edward and Russell E. Glasgow (1992). Smoking cessation: what have we learned over the past decade? *Journal of Consulting and Clinical Psychology* 60: 518¬27.

Ling, Pamela M., Anne Landman and Stanton Aa Glantz (2002). It is time to abandon youth access tobacco programmes. *Tobacco Control* 11: 3–6. http://bit.ly/2cAT2lz.

Livingston, Trish P., Cohen P., Frydenberg M., Ron Borland, Reading D., Val Clarke and David Hill (2002). Knowledge, attitudes and experience associated with testing for prostate cancer: a comparison between male doctors and men in the community. *Internal Medicine Journal* 32(5–6): 215–23. http://bit.ly/2d0FoDs.

Lott, John (1998). *More guns, less crime: understanding crime and gun control laws.* Chicago: University of Chicago Press.

Lum, Kristen L., Jonathan R. Polansky, Robert K. Jackler and Stanton A. Glantz (2008). Signed, sealed and delivered: Big Tobacco in Hollywood, 1927–1951. *Tobacco Control* 17: 313–23. http://bit.ly/2cj0ujC.

MacArthur, Georgina, Melissa Wright, Helen Beer and Shantini Paranjothy Shantini (2011). Impact of media reporting of cervical cancer in a UK celebrity on a population-based cervical screening programme. *Journal of Medical Screening* 18: 204–9. http://bit.ly/2cATvnJ.

Mackenzie R., S. Chapman, A. Barratt and S. Holding (2007). "The news is (not) all good": misrepresentations and inaccuracies in Australian news media discourse on prostate cancer screening. *Medical Journal of Australia* 187: 507–10.

Maguire, Kevin (2000a). Dons furious over tobacco cash. *Guardian*, 6 December. http://bit.ly/2d0FLxK.

Maguire, Kevin (2000b). University accepts tobacco "blood money". *Guardian*, 5 December. http://bit.ly/2cUXXKm.

Mahood, Garfield (1999). Warnings that tell the truth: breaking new ground in Canada. *Tobacco Control* 8:356–61. http://bit.ly/2cAZLZg.

Manley, Cynthia Floyd (2004). National Cancer Institute director envisions end of suffering, death from cancer by 2015. *Reporter*, 13 February. http://bit.ly/2cLjqn1.

Marris, Emma and Daemon Fairless (2007). Wind farms' deadly reputation hard to shift. *Nature*, 24 May. http://go.nature.com/2cgTqiA.

Marsh, A. (1983). Smoking and illness: what smokers really believe. *Health Trends*, February.

Marsh, A. and J. Matheson (1983). Smoking behaviour and attitudes. London: Office of Population Censuses and Surveys.

Marlatt, Alan, Susan Curry and Gordon Judith (1990). A longitudinal analysis of unaided smoking cessation. *Journal of Consulting and Clinical Psychology* 58: 310–6.

Martínez-Sánchez, Jose M., Montse Ballbè, Marcela Fu, Juan Carlos Martín-Sánchez, Esteve Saltó, Mark Gottlieb, Richard Daynard, Gregory N. Connolly and Esteve Fernández (2014). Electronic cigarette use among adult population: a cross-sectional study in Barcelona, Spain (2013–2014). *British Medical Journal Open* 4: e005894. http://bit.ly/2cx2L6R.

Mathews, Rebecca, Wayne D. Hall and Coral E. Gartner (2010). Is there evidence of "hardening" among Australian smokers between 1997 and 2007? Analyses of the Australian National Surveys of Mental Health and Wellbeing. *Australian and New Zealand Journal of Psychiatry* 44:1132–6. http://bit.ly/2cgPUoF.

McKenzie, Nick and Richard Baker (2015). Tobacco company wants schools survey for insights into children and teens. *Sydney Morning Herald*, 19 August. http://bit.ly/1NGpBoM.

Mckie, John and Jeffrey Richardson (2003). The rule of rescue. *Social Science and Medicine* 56: 2407–19. http://cnnmon.ie/2cx2p0g.

McMichael, Anthony (1999). Prisoners of the proximate: loosening the constraints on epidemiology in an age of change. *American Journal of Epidemiology* 149(10): 887–97. http://bit.ly/2d0Iyaa.

McMillen, Robert, Susanne Tanski, Johnathan Winickoff and Nell Valentine (2007). *Attitudes about smoking in the movies.* Social Sciences Research Center, Mississippi State University. http://bit.ly/2cLjuTT.

McNeill, Ann, Brose Leonie S, Robert Calder and Sara C Hitchman (2015). *E-cigarettes: an evidence update. A report commissioned by Public Health England.* Public Health England. August. http://bit.ly/2cnRokd.

Mehta, Stephanie (2007). Carlos Slim, the world's richest man. *CNN Money*, 20 August.

Mekemson, Curtis and Stanton A. Glantz (2002). How the tobacco industry built its relationship with Hollywood. *Tobacco Control* 11 (Supplement 1): i81–i91. http://bit.ly/2cnS2ON.

Mill, John Stuart (1998 [1859]). *On liberty and other essays.* Edited with an introduction and notes by John Gray. Oxford: Oxford University Press.

Miller, Caroline, Melanie Wakefield and Lyn Roberts (2008). Uptake and effectiveness of the Australian telephone Quitline service in the context of a mass media campaign. *Tobacco Control* 12 (Supplement 2): ii53–8. http://bit.ly/2cnROXL.

Milne, Eugene (2005). NHS smoking cessation services and smoking prevalence: observational study. *British Medical Journal* 330: 760. http://bit.ly/2cAUxzV.

Mooney, Marc, Thom White and Dorothy Hatsukami (2004). The blind spot in the nicotine replacement therapy literature: assessment of the double-blind in clinical trials. *Addictive Behaviors* 29(4): 673–84.

Mor, Vincent (2005). The compression of morbidity hypothesis: a review of research and prospects for the future. *Journal of the American Geriatrics Society* 53 (Supplement 9): s308–9.

Motion Picture Association of America (2007). Classification and rating rules.

Mullins, Robyn (1992). *Smoking restrictions in some of Australia's main companies based in Victoria: an update.* Melbourne: Centre for Behavioural Research in Cancer.

Murray, Christopher J.L. and Alan D. Lopez (1996). *The global burden of disease.* A comprehensive assessment of mortality and disability from diseases, injuries and risk factors in 1990 and projected to 2020. Harvard: Harvard University Press.

Nakahara, Shinji, Masao Ichikawa and Susumu Wakai (2005). Smoking scenes in Japanese comics: a preliminary study. *Tobacco Control* 14(1): 71. http://bit.ly/2cgR2bF.

Nakahara, Shinji, Susumu Wakai and Masao Ichikawa (2003). Smoking in children's picture books. *Tobacco Control* 12(1): 110. http://bit.ly/2d0FVVY.

National Association of Attorneys General (1998). *Master Settlement Agreement.* http://bit.ly/2d9mwT6.

National Cancer Institute (2016). Cell phones and cancer risk. 27 May. http://bit.ly/2cx04Cp.

National Cancer Institute (2008). *The role of the media in promoting and reducing tobacco use.* Bethesda, MD: US Department of Health and Human Services, National Institutes of Health, National Cancer Institute, NIH Pub. No. 07-6242, June. http://bit.ly/1NozfQh.

National Health and Medical Research Council (2010). *Wind turbines and health: a rapid review of the evidence.* http://bit.ly/2cnSg8n.

Neff, Linda J., René A. Arrazola, Ralph S. Caraballo, Catherine G. Corey, Shanna Cox, Brian A. King, Conrad J. Choiniere and Corinne G. Husten (2015). Frequency of tobacco use among middle and high school students. *Centers for Disease Control and Prevention* 64(38): 1061–5. http://bit.ly/1j1000Q.

New Zealand Government (2012). *Government response to the report of the Māori Affairs Committee on its* Inquiry into the tobacco industry in Aotearoa and the consequences of tobacco use for Māori *(final response)*. http://bit.ly/2cx3kO3.

Newport, Frank (2013). Most US smokers want to quit, have tried multiple times. *Gallup Wellbeing.* http://bit.ly/1gVxtTy.

Nichols, Michelle (2001). Anti-smoking ad featuring attacks on US condemned. *Scotsman*, 3 November. http://bit.ly/2cLjXFA.

Norberry, Jennifer (1995). Australian pollution laws: offences, penalties and regulatory agencies. In Neil Gunningham, Jennifer Norberry and Sandra McKillop (eds), *Environmental crime.* Canberra: Australian Institute of Criminology. http://bit.ly/2d0GtLx.

Northern Territory Government. Department of Justice (2008). Licensing, regulation and alcohol strategy. http://bit.ly/2cWogCQ.

Nottingham University (2000). Nottingham University Business School to establish International Centre for Corporate Social Responsibility. 4 December. http://bit.ly/2d0GnU3.

Nutt, David J., Lawrence D. Phillips, David Balfour, H. Valerie Curran, Martin Dockrell et al. (2014). Estimating the harms of nicotine-containing products using the MCDA approach. *European Addiction Research* 20(5): 218–25. http://bit.ly/2c40nJK.

Oakes, Wendy, Simon Chapman, James Balmford, Ron Borland and Lisa Trotter (2004). "Bulletproof skeptics in life's jungle": which self-exempting beliefs about smoking most predict lack of intention to quit? *Preventive Medicine* 39: 776–82. http://bit.ly/2cAUvYT.

O'Brien, Jane and Matt Danzico (2011). "Wi-fi refugees" shelter in West Virginia mountains. *BBC News*, 13 September. http://bbc.in/2cB1vC0.

Office of Population Censuses and Surveys (1982). *General Household Survey 1982*. London: HM Stationery Office.

Ontario (2012). Environmental Review Tribunal. *Environmental and Land Tribunal Ontario*, 29 February. http://bit.ly/2cUYwnD.

Osler, William (1905). *Aequanimitas with other addresses: internal medicine as a vocation*. Philadelphia: P. Blakiston's Son & Co.

Osler, William (1904). *Aequanimitas with other addresses to medical students, nurses and practitioners of medicine*. Philadelphia: P. Blakiston's Son & Co.

Papadopoulos, George (2012). Wind turbines and low frequency noise: implications for human health. *National Wind Watch*, 24 September. http://bit.ly/2ciZ7lk.

Parkinson, Giles (2014). Anti-wind, climate denying crusader behind Leyonhjelm RET campaign. *Renew Economy*, 27 November. http://bit.ly/2d9mNp6.

Peachment, Allan (1984). Learning from legislative disasters: the defeat of the Western Australian Government's Tobacco (Promotion and Sales) Bill. *Medical Journal of Australia* 140: 482–85.

Pedersen, Eja, Frits van den Berg, Roel Bakker and Jelte Bouma (2009). Response to noise from modern wind farms in the Netherlands. *Journal of the Acoustical Society of America* 126(2): 634–43. http://bit.ly/2cLlb3D.

Pederson, Linda L. and Neville M. Lefcoe, A psychological and behavioural comparison of ex-smokers and smokers. *Journal of Chronic Disease* 29 (1976): 431–34.

Peto, Richard and Alan D. Lopez (2000). The future worldwide health effects of current smoking patterns. In C.E. Koop, C.E. Pearson and M.R. Schwarz (eds), *Critical issues in global health*. San Fransisco: Jossey-Bass, 2000.

Peto, Richard, Alan D. Lopez, Jillian Boreham, Michael Thun and Heath J.R. Clark (1992). Mortality from tobacco in developed countries: indirect estimation from national vital statistics. *The Lancet* 339: 1268–78. http://bit.ly/2cAUDrl.

Petrie, Keith J., Kate Faasse, Fiona Crichton and Andrew Grey (2014). How common are symptoms? Evidence from a New Zealand national telephone survey. *British Medical Journal Open* 4: e005374. http://bit.ly/2cRMXPx.

Philip Morris International (2007). Philip Morris International announces agreement in principle to acquire additional 30% stake in Mexican tobacco business from Grupo Carso. Press release, 18 July. http://bit.ly/2cgQHpH.

Physicians for a Smoke-Free Canada (2012). Picture based cigarette warnings. http://bit.ly/2cWpVZb.

Pierce, J., T. Dwyer, G. Frape, S. Chapman, A. Chamberlain and N. Burke (1986). Evaluation of the Sydney "Quit. For Life" anti-smoking campaign, part 1: achievement of intermediate goals. *Medical Journal of Australia* 144: 341–4.

Pierce, John P., Sharon E. Cummins, Martha M. White, Aimee Humphrey and
Karen Messer (2012). Quitlines and nicotine replacement for smoking
cessation: do we need to change policy? *Annual Review of Public Health* 33:
341–56. http://bit.ly/2d4KAe4.
Pisinger, Charlotta and Martin Døssing (2014). A systematic review of health
effects of electronic cigarettes. *Preventive Medicine* 69: 248–60. http://bit.ly/
1rUrkkL.
Pisinger, Charlotta and Nina S. Godtfredsen (2007). Is there a health benefit of
reduced tobacco consumption? A systematic review. *Nicotine and Tobacco
Research* 9: 631–46. http://bit.ly/2cnR84I.
Powell, Ronald M. (2015). Symptoms after exposure to smart meter radiation.
EMF Safety Network, 6 March. http://bit.ly/1D1UilG.
Prochaska, James O., Carlo C. DiClemente and John C. Norcross (1992). In search
of how people change: applications to addictive behaviors. *American
Psychologist* 47: 1102–14. http://bit.ly/2cnS9cW.
Proctor, Robert N. (2001). Tobacco and the global lung cancer epidemic. *Nature
Reviews Cancer* 1: 82–6. http://go.nature.com/2d4L0kQ.
Productivity Commission (2005). Economic implications of an ageing
Australia. http://www.pc.gov.au/inquiries/completed/ageing.
Queenan, Joe (2008). Hollywood stogies. *Wall Street Journal*, 21 June.
http://on.wsj.com/2cUYWdw.
Raw, Martin and Julia Heller (1984). *Helping people to stop smoking. The
development, role, and potential of support services in the UK*. London: Health
Education Council.
Rayner, Geof, (2012). Does celebrity involvement in public health campaigns
deliver long-term benefit? No. *British Medical Journal* 345: e6362. 10.1136/
bmj.e6362.
Research and Analysis section (2014). Strong signals: growing use of public wi-fi
hotspots. *Industryacma*, 26 November. http://bit.ly/2cIThXH.
Revkin, Andrew (2005). A new measure of well-being from a happy little
kingdom. *New York Times*, 4 October. http://nyti.ms/2d0HyCZ.
Rice, Tom (2003). Believe it or not: religious and other paranormal beliefs in the
United States. *Journal for the Scientific Study of Religion* 42: 95–106.
http://bit.ly/2cIEMEJ.
Roberts, C., C. Algert, T. Chey, A. Capon and E. Gray (1992). Community
attitudes to smoking in restaurants. *Medical Journal of Australia* 157: 210.
Rosen, Mans and Bengt Haglund (2005). From healthy survivors to sick survivors:
implications for the twenty-first century. *Scandinavian Journal of Public
Health* 33: 151–5.

Roskam, John, James Paterson and Chris Berg (2012). Be like Gough: 75 radical ideas to transform Australia. *IPA Review*, August. http://bit.ly/IC8eKj.

Rosner, David and Gerald Markowitz (2013). Why it took decades of blaming parents before we banned lead paint. *Atlantic*, 22 April. http://theatln.tc/2d4KF1u.

Roxon, Nicola (2008). National Health Security (National Notifiable Disease List) Instrument 2008. Australian Government Federal Register of Legislation, 17 March. http://bit.ly/2ciYfNB.

Ruddick, Graham (2015). Imperial Tobacco plans to drop tobacco . . . from its name. *Guardian*, 16 December. http://bit.ly/2cx3nK5.

Rushe, D. (2000). Tobacco firm backs corporate ethics professorship. *Sunday Times*, 3 December. http://bit.ly/2cx3020.

Ruter, Terri (1996). US journals veto tobacco funded research. *British Medical Journal* 312: 11. http://bit.ly/2dc0vpW.

Sargent, James D., Michael L. Beach, Anna M. Adachi-Mejia, Jennifer J. Gibson, Linda T. Titus-Ernstoff, Charles P. Carusi, Susan D. Swain, Todd F. Heatherton and Madeline A. Dalton (2005). Exposure to movie smoking: its relation to smoking initiation among US adolescents. *Pediatrics* 116: 1183–91. http://bit.ly/2cWotpE.

Schobera, Wolfgang, Katalin Szendreia, Wolfgang Matzena, Helga Osiander-Fuchsb, Dieter Heitmannc, Thomas Schettgend, Rudolf A. Jörrese and Hermann Fromme (2014). Use of electronic cigarettes (e-cigarettes) impairs indoor air quality and increases FeNO levels of e-cigarette consumers. *International Journal of Hygiene and Environmental Health* 217: 628–37.

Schwartz, John (2001). Philip Morris to change name to Altria. *New York Times*, 16 November. http://nyti.ms/2cnSpZA.

Schwartz, Susan (2001). Shock anti-smoking poster rejected. *South China Morning Post*, 2 November. http://bit.ly/2cAVk4f.

Scott, Sophie (2003). The prostate debate. *7:30 Report*, ABC TV, 27 February. http://ab.co/2d0H5kp.

Second Sight (2010). Ill winds. *The Second Sight*, 18 November. http://bit.ly/2cRMpcs.

Shahab, Lion and Robert West (2010). Public support in England for a total ban on the sale of tobacco products. *Tobacco Control* 19: 143–7. http://bit.ly/2cnRTdX.

Shopland, Donald R. (1981). *Bibliography on smoking and health*. Rockville, MD: Office on Smoking and Health.

Siahpush, Mohammad, Melanie A. Wakefield, Matt J. Spittal, Sarah J. Durkin and Michelle M. Scollo (2009). Taxation reduces social disparities in adult

smoking prevalence. *American Journal of Preventive Medicine* 36: 285–91.
http://bit.ly/2dbZn5p.

Sibbald, Barbara (2000). University refuses tobacco-sponsored scholarship.
Canadian Medical Association Journal, 24 November. http://bit.ly/2d4KOlB.

Siegel, J. (2000). Tobacco companies funding research at Israeli universities.
Jerusalem Post, 8 June.

Silagy, C., Tim Lancaster, Lindsay F. Stead, David Mant, G. Fowler (2006).
Nicotine replacement therapy for smoking cessation. *Cochrane Database of
Systematic Reviews* 1: CD000146. http://bit.ly/2cAVTuL.

Slaughter, Elli, Richard M. Gersberg, Kayo Watanabe, John Rudolph, Chris
Stransky and Thomas E. Novotny (2011). Toxicity of cigarette butts, and their
chemical components, to marine and freshwater fish. *Tobacco Control* 20:
i25–i29. http://bit.ly/2cLlcVk.

Slovic, Paul (2000). *The perception of risk*. London: Earthscan.

Smith, Andrea L. and Simon Chapman (2014). Quitting unassisted: the 50-year
research neglect of a major public health phenomenon. *Journal of the
American Medical Association* 311: 137–8. http://bit.ly/2dbZTk4.

Smith, Andrea L., Simon Chapman and Sally M. Dunlop (2015). What do we
know about unassisted smoking cessation in Australia? A systematic review,
2005–2012. *Tobacco Control* 24: 18–27. http://bit.ly/2cAViZR.

Smoke Free Movies (2010a). The problem. http://bit.ly/2cnS6Ou.

Smoke Free Movies (2010b). The solution. http://bit.ly/2cnSuwj.

Smoke Free Movies (2008) Homepage. http://smokefreemovies.ucsf.edu/

Smoke Free Movies (2006). 120,000 lives a year. http://bit.ly/2cB2tOt.

Song, Yun-Mi, Joohon Sung, and Hong-Jun Cho (2008). Reduction and cessation
of cigarette smoking and risk of cancer: a cohort study of Korean men.
Journal of Clinical Oncology 26: 5101–6. http://bit.ly/2cLm5Nr.

South Australian Consolidated Regulations (2011). Controlled Substances
(Poisons) Regulations, Reg. 14. http://bit.ly/2cLlbk6.

Stokes, Patrick (2015). On "nanny states" and race, Leyonhjelm exposes the moral
thinness of libertarianism. *The Conversation*, 30 June. http://bit.ly/1efRbgP.

Stopthesethings (2013a). I am a wind turbine host. *Stop These Things*, 17 February.
http://bit.ly/2d4Mlb5.

Stopthesethings (2013b) Merry Christmas to you and happy birthday to STT. *Stop
These Things*, 25 December. http://bit.ly/2cWq2nJ.

Stopthesethings (2013c). Rally – David Mortimer. *Stop These Things*, 7 July.
http://bit.ly/2cgQoLj.

Straif, Kurt, Dana Loomis, Kathryn Guyton, Yann Grosse, Béatrice
Lauby-Secretan, Fatiha El Ghissassi et al. (2014). Future priorities for the
IARC Monographs. *The Lancet Oncology* 15: 683–4. http://bit.ly/2cnSsEN.

Sweanor, David, Scott Ballin, Ruth D. Corcoran, Alan Davis, Karen Deasy, Roberta G. Ferrence, Rhona Lahey, Sal Lucido, W. James Nethery and Jeffrey Wasserman (1992). Report of the Tobacco Policy Research Study Group on tobacco pricing and taxation in the United States. *Tobacco Control* 1 (Supplement): s31–36. http://bit.ly/2cIUezc.

Taubes, Gary (2013). The science of obesity: what do we really know about what makes us fat? *British Medical Journal* 346: f1050. http://bit.ly/2cIG42x.

Teague, Claude (1973). Some thoughts about new brands of cigarettes for the youth market. Archived at *Truth Tobacco Industry Documents*. http://bit.ly/2cRN91u.

Thomson, A (2000). Special reports: dealing with killer industries. *Channel 4 News* (UK), 5 December. http://bit.ly/2cIUNZG.

Thomson, George, Richard Edwards, Nick Wilson and Tony Blakely (2012). What are the elements of the tobacco endgame? *Tobacco Control* 21: 293–5. http://bit.ly/2ciYzM8.

Thomson, George, Nick Wilson, Richard Edwards and Alistair Woodward (2008). Should smoking in outside public spaces be banned? Yes. *British Medical Journal* 337: a2806.

Thompson, Geoff (2009). 80 million a day. *Foreign Correspondent*, ABC TV, 1 September.

Thorburn, A.W (2005). The prevalence of obesity in Australia. *Obesity Reviews* 6: 187–9.

Tiffany, Stephen (2009). The functional significance of craving in nicotine dependence. *Nebraska Symposium on Motivation*, February 2009. http://bit.ly/2d4LXJI.

Tobacco Control (1994). News analysis. *Tobacco Control*, 3: 200. http://bit.ly/2cAWrko.

Tobacco Institute of Australia (1994). Submission to Senate Community Affairs Reference Committee Inquiry into tobacco industry and the costs of tobacco-related illness. Sydney, Australia. 7 November: 5.

Tocque, Karen, Aaron Barker and Brenda Fullard (2005). Are stop smoking services helping to reduce smoking prevalence? New analysis based on estimated number of smokers. *Tobacco Control Research Bulletin* (SmokeFree North West), March: 1–13. http://bit.ly/2cB2eDa.

Tru Energy Renewable Developments PTY LTD v Regional Council of Coyder & Ords [2014] SAERDC 48 (2014). Environment Resources and Development Court of South Australia. 7 November. http://bit.ly/2cIUqyu.

Tyrrell, Ian (1999). *Deadly enemies: tobacco and its opponents in Australia*. Sydney: UNSW Press.

Tverdal, Aage and Kjell Bjartveit (2006). Health consequences of reduced daily cigarette consumption. *Tobacco Control* 15: 472–80.

United Nations Development Program (2005). *Human development report 2005.* New York: UNDP. http://bit.ly/1GbEyfc.

United Nations Programme on HIV/AIDS (2004). *Report on the global AIDS epidemic.* New York: UNAIDS. http://bit.ly/2cx3PaV.

United Nations Programme on HIV/AIDS (2000). *Report on the global HIV/AIDS epidemic.* New York: UNAIDS. http://bit.ly/2cLlxXY.

Utah Department of Health (2013). *Electronic cigarette use among Utah students (grades 8, 10, and 12) and adults.* http://bit.ly/2cgQRgu.

Vallejo, Justin (2006). No smoking idea no-go for council. *Daily Telegraph*, May, 5: 15.

Van Dijk, Teun (1985). *Discourse and communication.* Berlin: Walter de Gruyter.

Van Weel, Chris and Joop Michels (1997). Dying, not old age, to blame for costs of health care. *The Lancet*, 350: 1159–60.

Vehicle Safety Standards, Department of Infrastructure, Transport, Regional Development and Local Government (2010). Vehicle Standard (Australian Design Rule 10/02 – Steering Column) 2008. Australian Government Federal Register of Legislation. http://bit.ly/2cRNtxj.

Vorrath, Sophie (2015). Anti-wind senators compare turbines to tobacco, pink bats. *Renew economy*, 14 April. http://bit.ly/2cAVsk5.

Wakefield, Melanie A., Kerri Coomber, Sarah J. Durkin, Michelle Scollo, Megan Bayly, Matthew J. Spittal, Julie A. Simpson and David Hill (2014). Time series analysis of the impact of tobacco control policies on smoking prevalence among Australian adults, 2001–2011. *Bulletin World Health Organization*, 92(6): 413–22.

Wakefield, Melanie A., Sarah Durkin, Matthew J. Spittal, Mohammad Siahpush, Michelle Scollo, Julie A. Simpson, Simon Chapman, Victoria White and David Hill (2008). Impact of tobacco control policies and mass media campaigns on monthly adult smoking prevalence. *American Journal of Public Health* 98: 1443–50. http://bit.ly/2d0IqHZ.

Wakefield, Melanie A., Yvonne Terry-McElrath, Sherry Emery, Henry Saffer, Frank J. Chaloupka, Glen Szczypka, Brian Flay, Patrick M. O'Malley and Lloyd D. Johnston (2006). Effect of televised, tobacco company-funded smoking prevention advertising on youth smoking-related beliefs, intentions, and behavior. *Americal Journal of Public Health* 96(12): 2154–60.

Wallmyr, Gudrun and Catharina Welin (2006). Young people, pornography, and sexuality: sources and attitudes. *Journal of School Nursing* 22: 290–5. http://bit.ly/2d4MkE2.

Walsh, Raoul (2011). Australia's experience with varenicline: usage, costs and adverse reactions. *Addiction* 106: 451–2. http://bit.ly/2cIVgeL.

Walsh, Raoul (2008). Over-the-counter nicotine replacement therapy: a methodological review of the evidence supporting its effectiveness. *Drug and Alcohol Review* 27: 529–47. http://bit.ly/2cWq3YH.

Walsh, Raoul and Rob W. Sanson-Fisher (1994). What universities do about tobacco industry research funding. *Tobacco Control* 3: 308–15. http://bit.ly/2d0IgjN.

Wartella, Ellen and Byron Reeves (1985). Historical trends in research on children and the media 1900–1960. *Journal of Communication* 35: 118–33. http://bit.ly/2cWpRsA.

Webb, B (1984). Status of Marlboro development program. Memo to Dick Snyder, PM New York. 7 December. Bates no. PM2023265662/5664.

Wells, James (2012). Lion vs CUB: the state of the beer market. *The Shout*, 7 September. http://bit.ly/2cgQToP.

West, Robert, Emma Beard and Jamie Brown (2016). Trends in electronic cigarette us in England. *Smoking in England*, 10 October. http://t.co/vEpycc28wY.

White, Victoria, David Hill and Williams R (1990). *Cigarette and alcohol consumption among Victorian secondary school children in 1990*. Melbourne: Centre for Behavioural Research in Cancer, Anti Cancer Council of Victoria.

White, Vicki and Tahlia Williams (2015). *Australian secondary school students' use of tobacco in 2014*. Centre for Behavioural Research in Cancer Cancer Council Victoria. http://bit.ly/2cx499N.

Wilson, Cameron (2013). Blowing in the wind. *Bush Telegraph*, ABC Radio National, 7 October. http://ab.co/2cB1rCl.

Wilson, Nick, Deepa Weerasekera, Richard Edwards, George Thomson, Miranda Devlin and Heather Gifford (2010). Characteristics of smoker support for increasing a dedicated tobacco tax: national survey data from New Zealand. *Nicotine and Tobacco Research* 12: 168–73. http://bit.ly/2d4KW4g.

Wilson, Tim (2013a). Advocates of a nanny state assume we are all children. *Courier Mail*, 13 May.

Wilson, Tim (2013b). Removing all doubt. *Freedom Watch*, Institute of Public Affairs, 26 June. http://bit.ly/2cnTujZ.

Wingood, Gina M., Ralph J. DiClemente, Kathy Harrington, Suzy Davies, Edward W. Hook III and M. Kim Oh (2001). Exposure to X-rated movies and adolescents' sexual and contraceptive-related attitudes and behaviors. *Pediatrics* 107(5): 1116–9. http://bit.ly/2dc0Ybv.

Witthöft, Michael and G. James Rubin (2013). Are media warnings about the adverse health effects of modern life self-fulfilling? An experimental study on idiopathic environmental intolerance attributed to electromagnetic fields

(IEI-EMF). *Journal of Psychosomatic Research* 74(3): 206–12. http://bit.ly/2cx4hWC.

Wood, A.A. (1983). The aims of cigarette advertising (letter), *Sydney Morning Herald*.

Worstall, Tim (2014). Astonishing number: Ericsson predicts 5.9 billion smartphone users within 5 years. *Forbes*, 18 May. http://bit.ly/1lBV6C8.

World Health Organization (2014). World Health Organization Conference of the Parties to the WHO Framework Convention on Tobacco Control. Electronic nicotine delivery systems. Sixth Session, 13–18 October, Moscow. Provisional agenda item 4.4.2. http://bit.ly/1AQnpW3.

World Health Organization (2009). *WHO calls for enforceable policies to restrict smoking in movies*. Geneva: World Health Organisation. http://bit.ly/2cIVu5y.

World Health Organization (2008). *Guidelines for drinking-water quality*, 3rd edition. http://bit.ly/2d4LHug.

World Health Organization (1979). *Controlling the smoking epidemic*. Technical Report Series 636. Geneva: World Health Organization.

World Health Organization (n.d.a). *The global burden of disease*. http://bit.ly/16bhvow.

World Health Organization (n.d.b). *Violence and injury prevention*. http://bit.ly/1nNwBF1.

World Health Organisation International Agency for Research on Cancer (2014). *IARC Monographs on the Evaluation of Carcinogenic Risks to Humans. Report of the advisory group to recommend priorities for IARC monographs during 2015–2019*. 18–19 April. http://bit.ly/1IkdfP9.

Worth, Keilah A., Jennifer Gibson Chambers, Daniel H. Nassau, Balvinder K. Rakhra and James D. Sargent (2008). Exposure of US adolescents to extremely violent movies. *Pediatrics* 122(2): 306–12. http://bit.ly/2cIVouD.

Wynder, Ernest L. and Evarts A. Graham (1950). Tobacco smoking as a possible etiologic factor in bronchiogenic carcinoma. A study of six hundred and eighty-four proved cases. *Journal of the American Medical Association* 143: 329–36. http://bit.ly/1ve0TCu.

Zhu, Shu-Hong, Ted Melcer, Jichao Sun, Bradley Rosbrook and John P. Pierce (2000). Smoking cessation with and without assistance: a population-based analysis. *American Journal of Preventive Medicine* 18: 305–11. http://bit.ly/2d0J9ZN.

www.ingramcontent.com/pod-product-compliance
Lightning Source LLC
Chambersburg PA
CBHW071728270326
41928CB00013B/2601